Handbook of Over-the-Counter Herbal Medicines

Penelope Ody studied herbal medicine at the School of Phytotherapy in Sussex, and traditional Chinese medicine at the College of Traditional Chinese Medicine in Guangzhou, and is a member of the National Institute of Medical Herbalists.

Before qualifying as a medical herbalist, more than ten years ago, she worked in business journalism eventually specializing in retail topics and information technology. She edited The Herb Society's magazines *The Herbal Review*, *Herbarium* and *Herbs* from 1988 to 1994 and has written a number of books on both business and scientific topics. Her other herb books include *The Herb Society's Complete Medicinal Herbal* and *Home Herbal*.

She continues to contribute to numerous journals and other publications worldwide, as well as lecturing regularly on herbal topics both in the UK and overseas.

Handbook of Over-the-Counter Herbal Medicines

including licensed remedies, simples and supplements

Penelope Ody

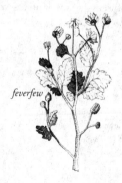

feverfew

KYLE CATHIE LIMITED

To my mother
Mary H Ody

First published in Great Britain in 1996 by
Kyle Cathie Limited
20 Vauxhall Bridge Road
London SW1V 2SA

ISBN 1 85626 235 9

A Cataloguing in Publication record for this title is available from the British
Library.

Designed by Roger Walker Associates
Edited by Gail Dixon-Smith
Illustrations by Juliet Dallas-Conte
Typeset by SX Composing DTP, Essex.
Printed by WBC Book Manufacturers Ltd

Contents

Acknowledgement

Thanks are due to the many suppliers of herbal products who sent details of their remedies and supplements and so patiently answered my numerous queries.

Important Note

The information and advice contained in this book is intended as a general guide to herbs and is not specific to individuals or their particular circumstances. Many plant substances, whether sold as foods or medicines, and used externally or internally, can cause an allergic reaction in some people. Neither the author nor the publishers can be held responsible for claims arising from the inappropriate use of any remedy or healing regime. Do not attempt self-diagnosis or self-treatment for serious or long-term problems before consulting a medical professional or qualified practitioner. Do not undertake any self-treatment while taking other prescribed drugs or receiving therapy without first seeking professional guidance. Always seek medical advice if any symptoms persist.

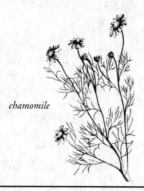

chamomile

Foreword – How to Use this Book

This book is divided into three main sections covering common complaints, herbs and herbal products. Introductory chapters detail the different traditions which have influenced the development of these various remedies and supplements and how the law relates to over-the-counter herbal products.

Of the main sections, the first gives details of ailments that can be effectively treated by herbal remedies. In each case there are suggestions of suitable herbs to use for the particular problem, as well as information about supportive treatments including dietary advice and vitamin or mineral supplements. A list of over-the-counter products which may be relevant is also included.

Because of the legalities of licensing and labelling, suppliers have to be extremely careful about any claims they make for herbal products. Similarly, licences are usually only granted for products designed to tackle simple, self-limiting ailments. Thus, while herbal remedies may be suitable for arthritis or high blood pressure, very few of them will actually say so. The products suggested in this section may be licensed for that particular ailment or indeed for another, or they may be defined simply as food supplements. It should not be assumed that suppliers have made any recommendations for using the product in this way (unless they are so licensed) – the suggestions are purely based on a herbalist's interpretation of the ingredients and their possible efficacy.

The second section of the book is an A–Z of herbs. This lists more than 300 herbs which are included in the over-the-counter products detailed in the following final section. Information is given about the actions and indications of each herb, as well as any cautions as to their use. Several herbs widely used by medical herbalists, such as ephedra, figwort, fumitory and wood betony, are missing from this list. This is quite simply because they are not included in any of the remedies or supplements studied so, although it is possible to buy the crude dried herbs or gather them from hedgerows and use them for a number of ailments, information about them will not be found here. Readers should consult any standard herbal for information about these plants and some suitable sources are given on page 438.

Each herb is followed by a list of the remedies and supplements in which it is used. Herbs are listed by common name and, for consistency, these names are also used throughout the final section, although they will not always be the names that suppliers choose to use on their packaging. Details of preparations, such as capsules and tinctures which contain a single herb (known as simples), are listed separately.

Readers may also find a few unexpected ailments in this listing – "fluid retention" and "cellulite" are not well-defined medical conditions. They are, however, the sort of rather vague ailments for which products have been licensed and therefore it is worth examining just what sort of problems these definitions may cover.

The last section of the book looks at the various remedies and supplements on offer. In all there are more than 800 of these. They range from single powdered herbs in capsules to complex preparations with ten or more ingredients. In most cases information is given about the herbs each product contains, along with details of any recommended dosages, and any ailments for which they could be relevant. Licensed products are indicated here, and throughout the book, by a preceding asterisk.

For the single herbal products containing, for example, garlic, ginkgo, or evening primrose, rather than repeat basic details of individual herbs, the reader should refer in each case to the information given about the plant in the A–Z of herbs.

Over the past few years numerous herbal products have disappeared from the shelves as changes in regulations and the need for product licences take their toll. No doubt many of the remedies listed in this final section will similarly be withdrawn in coming years but others will just as surely appear (indeed already are emerging) to take their place. Likewise a number of suppliers are currently applying for product licences for items now sold as food supplements, so these classifications will certainly change in future as well.

This *Handbook of Over-the-Counter Herbal Medicines* is designed both to help readers match suitable remedies to their particular health problems and to clarify just what ailments individual remedies may be useful for. Under current rules, suppliers of herbal products which are sold as supplements under licence exemptions, cannot specify on the packaging what the plants may be used for. Some suppliers publish leaflets giving information about herbal actions but these are not always readily available so it can be difficult for consumers to select a relevant product. Any suggestions of possible uses for unlicensed products given in this book should not be taken as suppliers' recommendations.

ginger

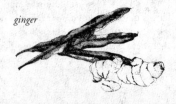

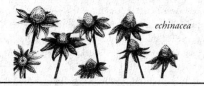

echinacea

All Sorts of Herbal Medicine

Modern herbal medicine represents a complex interweaving of different cultures – a combination of European folk tradition and Eastern influences overlaid by the introduction of New World plants and healing practices and by more recent scientific discoveries. Over-the-counter herbal products draw on this rich mixture with preparations clearly influenced by successive schools of thought. Some – many of them formulated in the 1930s – concentrate on herbs traditionally used by Native Americans, others focus on the more recently discovered healing properties of particular plants, such as circulatory remedies using ginkgo or tonics containing cat's claw.

Because of current licensing and labelling regulations it is not always obvious why a particular product contains the herbs that it does and thus an understanding of the theories which influenced its developers can help clarify the likely therapeutic properties.

While conventional allopathic medicine concentrates on removing symptoms, the usual herbal approach is to "restore balance" and strengthen the system so that the vital energy of the body can combat disease and restore health. Certainly, herbal remedies can be designed simply to relieve symptoms, but most also focus on long-term cures so that – unlike some orthodox drugs – when the sufferer stops taking the tablets the symptoms do not return. A herb like St John's wort, for example, is used as an anti-depressant, but it also acts as a tonic for the nervous system so rather than just providing a short-term uplift in mood it addresses longer term needs. Similarly, while echinacea is an effective anti-bacterial, anti-viral and anti-fungal, it will also help to stimulate the immune system to counter infections more effectively in the future.

European traditions

Herbal medicine has, of course, been practised in Europe for thousands of years and the actions of many of the plants commonly used today were described by such early writers as Pliny and Dioscorides in the first century AD.

Greek and Roman medicine was based on the theory of "humours" which taught that the four vital fluids in the body had to be kept in balance and all illness could thus be defined in terms of humoral imbalance. This model (see Figure 1) was related to the belief that the world was composed of four elements: earth, air, fire and water which each had its corresponding humour. These humours – blood, phlegm, black bile and yellow bile – not only dictated health but also temperament. A person in whom black bile dominated was thus termed "melancholic" and tended to depression while someone with a surfeit of blood was "sanguine" and likely to be cheerful and amusing but probably prone to over indulgence. Although early Greeks like Hippocrates had described the basic humoral theory in the fifth century BC, it was more precisely codified by Galen (AD 131–199) so is often termed "Galenical medicine".

The humours were regulated by various drastic treatments: bleeding the patient to remove a surfeit of blood or giving strong purgatives to clear excess black bile. The humours were also defined in terms of cold or heat, dry or dampness, and herbs were similarly characterized. Phlegm, for example, was associated with cold and dampness so surfeit would be countered by a hot and dry herb to restore balance. Thyme and hyssop both fall into this category and were prescribed for the sort of phlegmatic excess one encounters in the common cold.

Figure 1: The Galenical model relating humours and elements

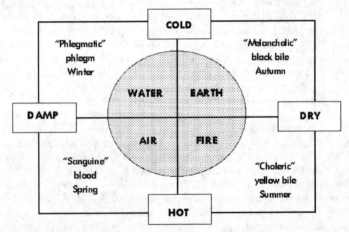

Old herbals often describe the temperature of plants in great detail. John Gerard, writing in 1597, for example, tells us that motherwort is "hot and dry in the second degree" while chickweed is "cold and moist and of a waterish substance".

The appearance of herbs was also important under the Doctrine of

Signatures. This argued that plants contained clues to their medicinal properties in their appearance: yellow flowered herbs, for example, were believed to be helpful for jaundice while pilewort with its nodular roots was clearly ideal for treating haemorrhoids. Some of these interpretations were in fact quite valid (pilewort *is* good for haemorrhoids and yellow-flowered dandelion makes a good liver herb) although others, now largely forgotten, were less accurate.

While most of European herbalism continued to draw on this common Greek and Roman tradition until well into the eighteenth century, there were important regional differences. In Germany, for instance, the visionary nun Hildegard of Bingen had been inspired to produce a herbal in the eleventh century which contained some quite original uses of herbs. She recommended, for example, vervain for skin infections, mint juice for arthritis, and galangal for heart disorders. Some of these ideas derived from local folk traditions; others, Hildegard believed, were instructions from God that came in her visions.

Although Hildegard's writings were largely forgotten until comparatively recently, the sort of cures she advocated remained an underlying influence on herbal use in some parts of Europe. Today, her work has been revived and the practice of "Hildegard medicine" is thriving in many parts of Germany and Austria. Both the Jura pharmaceuticals company in Konstanz and St Hildegard-Posch in Austria make and market over-the-counter herbal remedies based on her theories. Some of these products are now available in the UK.

Since the nineteenth century, use of herbs in mainstream medicine in mainland Europe has remained more widespread than in the UK; indeed "materia medica" – the medicinal herbal repertoire – has continued to be taught in many Central European medical schools until the present day. Herbal products from French, Swiss and German suppliers thus tend to draw more heavily on European traditions than those produced in the UK. Herbs like sanicle, paracress and hemp nettle, which have long-since vanished from the British herbalist's medicine chest, are still used elsewhere in Europe. Some of these remedies and supplements are also marketed in the UK and, as cross-border trade in medicinal products within the EU increases, more will surely follow. Many of these herbs are not listed in commonly available English language herbals so it can be difficult for the average lay person (or indeed their GP) to discover what the actions of a particular remedy may be.

Homoeopathic tradition is also important in mainland Europe. This theory argues that very dilute herbal extracts will cause particular symptoms, while the same brew can then be used to cancel out such symptoms when they occur in illness. Homoeopathy was developed by Samuel Hahnemann in Leipzig between 1811 and 1820 and many of the plants he used were common medicinal herbs. Their use in homoeopathy is, however, generally quite different from mainstream herbalism. Bryony, for example, is a potent herb used for treating bronchial congestion and rheumatic complaints; it is also strongly purgative. In homoeopathy a tincture of this same herb is diluted to such an extent that it is almost impossible to detect its presence, and the remedy is then used for treating certain types of common colds.

Herbs which are extremely toxic and restricted by law to professional practitioners in normal dosages are widely used in homoeopathy; which means that toxic substances like autumn crocus, deadly nightshade or poison ivy may appear in remedies quite safely. Some European suppliers, such as the Swiss company Bioforce, combine both standard herbal extracts and homoeopathic dilutions in their products so, although the contents may seem poisonous, they are actually quite safe. The more dilute a homoeopathic remedy is, the more potent it is believed to be. The number of times the mother tincture has been diluted is indicated after the name of the remedy: "Chamomilla 3×" means that chamomile has been diluted only three times which is a fairly concentrated remedy and therefore less potent; "Arnica 30×" indicates that there have been 30 dilutions and the medicine is considerably stronger.

Not all homoeopathic medicines are herbal: various minerals such as sulphur and graphite are used along with animal products like snake venom (Lachesis) and the poison from honey bees (Apis mellifica).

Also important in European tradition is the anthroposophical medicine developed by Rudolf Steiner in the 1920s. Like Hildegard, Steiner was a visionary and his theories drew on a combination of Galenical theories and homoeopathy combined with his holistic view of health and insights about the healing properties of particular plants. The main aim of anthroposophical medicine is to stimulate the body's natural healing powers and Steiner believed that spiritual well being and the role of the soul were of equal significance in good health.

Anthroposophical medicines are produced worldwide by Weleda, a company which still follows Steiner's precepts. Most of the herbs used are familiar in either herbal or homoeopathic tradition although some of the combinations are more strongly derived from Steiner's unique inspirations.

Physiomedicalists and American influence

While homoeopathy and anthroposophy prospered in mainland Europe, herbal medicine in nineteenth century Britain reached a nadir. The Industrial Revolution drew vast numbers of people into towns, away from their rural roots; herbal folk medicines, which had been maintained in families for generations, were lost and the emphasis was increasingly on patent remedies.

The revival started in the 1840s and 1850s when the unlikely named Albert Coffin and Wooster Beech arrived from the United States with their messages of "Physiomedicalism" and "Eclecticism". The Physiomedical movement had been founded in the 1790s by Samuel Thomson, a New Hampshire herbal practitioner who combined pioneer medical traditions with Native American theories. He believed that all disease was caused by cold (hardly surprising in the bitter New England winters) and he used sweating remedies (popular with many East Coast tribes) to warm his patients. In general, Thomson favoured a combination of emetics and purgatives to clear the system of cold and damp phlegm.

As in Galenical medicine, health to the physiomedicalists meant maintaining internal balance to ensure a healthy "vital force". Herbs were classified as stimulating or sedating, relaxing or astringing and combinations were used to restore balance to both tissues and mental states.

Irritable bowel syndrome, for example, might be treated in a Physiomedical approach with chamomile to sedate the nervous system and relax the digestive tissues, followed by an astringent like agrimony to counter any over-relaxation so caused, and a stimulant such as ginger to encourage the vital force.

The Eclectic school combined herbal remedies and Native American healing traditions with more orthodox medical techniques and at one time the movement boasted 20,000 qualified practitioners in the United States. Wooster Beech's message proved extremely popular in the industrial towns of Northern England and Eclectic systems thrived there until well into the 1930s.

This North American influence can still be seen in many of the herbal remedies produced by traditional UK suppliers such as Potter's and Frank Roberts. American herbs, like bayberry, helonias, Indian tobacco and pleurisy root, are included in their remedies, yet these plants are virtually unknown in mainland Europe. They are often poorly researched, partly because a great deal of herbal study is undertaken in Germany where such traditional New World remedies are little known. These herb do, however, make extremely potent and effective medicines.

The physiomedicalist emphasis on mixtures to counter cold can also be seen in many traditional British products – notably in brews like Potter's Composition Essence.

Modern plant hunters

Plant hunters have been gathering exotic specimens and adding them to the herbal repertoire since the Portuguese set out to navigate the world in the 1450s. The Spanish brought back potatoes and cinchona from South America, missionary Jesuits learned of ginseng in Korea, and an observant Boer farmer first noted the use of devil's claw in the 1930s.

The search goes on, and today, pharmaceutical companies around the world are investigating plants that are used in many ethnic traditions with a view to extracting, and subsequently patenting, active constituents. While some of these plants form the basis of new orthodox drugs (such as taxol extracted from the Pacific yew tree which is being used successfully to treat ovarian cancer), others prove too complex to ever yield a patentable single ingredient and thus join the mainstream herbal repertoire.

Researchers today focus not only on exotic plants from the Amazon rain forests or Kalahari Desert, but also on more mundane European species which thus take on a new lease of life. Butterbur, for example, was regarded as a not particularly important cough cure until the 1950s when Italian researchers discovered that it also had considerable antispasmodic and pain relieving properties and the herb suddenly joined the ranks of digestive remedies. St John's wort has similarly been more recently identified as an immune stimulant, garlic is now well-established as an anti-cholesterol and prophylactic for arteriosclerosis, and feverfew has proven to be a far better migraine remedy than traditional herbals imply.

Over the past few years newcomers such as echinacea, ginkgo and guarana – as well as devil's claw – have started to appear in over-the-counter products. Like commercial companies everywhere, makers of herbal products aim regularly to launch something new and novel to tempt the buying public; sometimes the marketing hype can suggest that these herbs are considerably more potent than they in fact are and occasionally rather inappropriate applications are implied. Ginkgo, for instance, certainly boosts cerebral circulation and can speed recovery after brain surgery, but suggesting that it may be of cosmetic benefit for varicose veins is a little odd.

Suppliers' enthusiasm for a newly discovered plant can also outstrip the popular herbal literature. Peruvian cat's claw, for example, was only identified in the 1970s and reports of its actions in the scientific press largely date from 1989–92. It is now available in capsule form as an over-the-counter tonic – yet the plant is not yet listed in mainstream herbals so potential customers will find information about the product hard to come by. The same applies to other such Amazonian exotics as paratudo and catuaba.

The herbal repertoire is constantly expanding and while it once took decades for a plant to become established and readily available as an over-the-counter product, we are now seeing newcomers appearing on the shelves in health food stores within a year or two of the first significant literature reports. It may give the producers plenty of new lines to promote, but it can be confusing – both for the public who are expected to buy them and for health care professionals who need to advise on suitability and contra-indications.

Ayurvedic medicine

While European and North American traditions are behind the majority of over-the-counter herbal products, both Ayurvedic and Chinese influence are increasingly fashionable and important. Ayurvedic products are largely sold by specialist Indian suppliers, although a few popular herbs – such as gotu kola – are used in Western-style products.

Like Galenical medicine, Ayurveda is based on a model of bodily humours (*doshas*) and a need to maintain the inner life force (*prana*) which is believed to give rise to the fire of digestion and mental energy. *Prana* is linked to breath or oxygen which feeds the fire and if the fire is weak, then the body is weak. This inner fire is called *agni* or *tejas*, while the relationship between *prana* and *tejas* gives rise to *ojas* or good digestion and thus health. This good digestion is equated with juice or sap which in turn produces the six experiences or tastes (*rasas*) that are so crucial in Ayurvedic herbalism – sweet, sour, salty, pungent, bitter and astringent.

Ayurvedic medicines pay great attention to balancing these tastes and popular tonics often combine herbs representing each taste as a means of ensuring balance.

While Galenical theory has four humours, Ayurveda has three: *pitta* (bile linked to the fire element), *vata* (wind associated with the air and aether elements), and *kapha* (phlegm or dampness ruled by the elements of water and earth). These humours can also be seen as the waste products of the digestion process – the end product of the *prana-tejus-ojas* interaction. The more imperfect the digestion, the more waste products there are and the more imbalances in the system.

For good health balance is also needed between the three essential qualities – *sattwa*, *rajas* and *tamas*. *Sattwa* is regarded as purity and enlightenment while *rajas* and *tamas* are the dark side of nature – respectively distraction and dullness. All three are needed, however, and spiritual health is maintained by learning to control *rajas* and *tamas* while developing the calm clarity of *sattwa*. Healthy balance also requires the seven *dhatus* or tissues to be in equilibrium: plasma (*rasa*), blood (*rakta*), muscle (*mamsa*), fat (*medas*), bone (*asthi*), marrow and nerve tissue (*majja*), and semen (*shukra*). There are also numerous *srotas* or "channels" which must be open allowing breath, food and water to flow freely into and around the body. They include such familiar organs as the oesophagus, trachea, arteries, veins and intestines, but the *srotas* can also be compared with the Chinese acupuncture "meridians" which allow energy to flow around the body. Ayurveda also stresses the importance of the three waste products or *malas* – urine, sweat and faeces – which also need to be in balance. *Agni*, the spirit of light or life energy, more prosaically interpreted as digestive function, also needs to be strong.

To perform this complex balancing act, around 800 herbs are used in the "great tradition" of Ayurvedic medicine although some 2,500 medicinal herbs are used throughout India many of them in the "lesser medicine" of folk tradition. Each household has its *maharastra* or "grandmother's purse" filled with healing herbs for the household. The traditions of how to use these have been passed continuously from mother to daughter – or from *sadhu* to *sadhu* – for generations in the tradition of native healers everywhere.

Traditional Chinese medicine

A few years ago it was virtually impossible to buy Chinese herbs in Britain. The intrepid could venture into Soho's Chinatown and, if the language problems were not insurmountable, emerge with a bag of miscellaneous brown things which may, or may not, have been what they wanted to buy. Today, Chinese herbs are being tested in NHS hospitals, the popular media regularly report on the latest "Eastern wonder cure" and the likes of astragalus and reishi mushrooms, if not exactly household words, are becoming increasingly familiar.

As with Galenical and Ayurvedic models, complex theory guides these herbal combinations. Just as the Greeks had four humours and elements, the Chinese have five: earth, metal, water, wood and fire (see Figure 2). These are related to the five main organs of the body (spleen, lungs, kidneys, liver and heart), and five emotions, fluids and tastes (sweet, pungent, salty, sour and bitter).

Echoing Ayurvedic tradition, the taste of herbs is thus extremely significant as it can affect the relevant organs. Sweet herbs, are nutritious and tonifying for the stomach, while salty herbs are associated with fluid balance and kidney function.

As well as the five-element model the Chinese also believe in the duality of vital energy or *Qi* (sometimes spelt as *ch'i*), which has both *yang* and *yin* aspects. *Yang* is associated with male, light and heat, whereas *yin* is seen as female, dark and cold. Herbs are similarly divided: cordyceps, for example, is a *yang* tonic, while American ginseng is considered as benefiting *yin* energy.

Figure 2: The Chinese five element model relates body organs and various other functions to the elements.

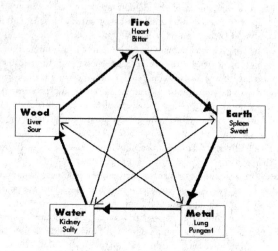

The Chinese almost always use their herbs in combinations rather than singly and these formulae have become strictly codified over the centuries. Herbs are defined in the prescription as the "Emperor" or principle herb, "minister" and "assistant" with the important "harmoniser" (often liquorice or Chinese dates) which blends it all together. There may also be a directional herb which has an affinity for a particular part of the body or acupuncture meridian so directs the mix to that organ. There are several thousands formulae in common use and the mixtures are often sold as ready-prepared pills in Chinese herbal shops. Their names can be quite exotic – Great Protector, Wise Sage or Women's Precious Pills – but as they are currently not widely available they are outside the scope of this book.

A number of Chinese herbs are now being included in mainstream herbal products, ginseng has been available for years, but a newcomer is *Dang Gui* (Chinese angelica) which is defined in Chinese theory as a blood tonic, and there is also considerable interest in the medicinal fungi used in China. These are generally immune-stimulating herbs which have traditionally been used as tonics and to encourage longevity: the group includes the shiitake and reishi mushrooms as well as the rather less savoury cordyceps (a parasitic fungus which feeds on certain sorts of caterpillar).

Currently both Ayurvedic and Chinese herbal products are sold as food supplements rather than licensed medicines, with suppliers usually limiting distribution of ready-made products found in Chinese supermarkets to the professional practitioner sector. As interest in these products grow more of them are likely to be found in the general health foods market.

Consulting a herbalist

While over-the-counter herbal remedies can be helpful for a range of ailments, more serious problems need professional help. Approaches to herbal medicine vary considerably around the world. In the UK, primary health care is dominated by conventionally-trained general practitioners whose attitudes to alternative or complementary therapies range from the sympathetic to the openly hostile: a few GPs may be trained in herbal or homoeopathic medicine or, if not, may be willing to refer patients to suitable practitioners but many more dismiss herbal medicine as "quackery". In France herbal practitioners or "*phytotherapists*" are almost always trained doctors who have studied plant medicine at post-graduate level while in Germany, alternative practitioners qualify as "*heilpraktiker*" and have comparable status to orthodox GPs.

In China, traditional herbal medicine is available in special hospitals as an alternative to Western medicine, while in Japan herbal remedies are available on the equivalent of the National Health Service. In other countries – including some states of the USA – it is illegal for anyone to prescribe herbal remedies or set themselves up as a herbal practitioner, although self-medication with herbs is permitted. In others just about anyone – well trained or not – can set up in business as a medical herbalist and dispense all manner of inappropriate "cures".

Britain is probably unique within Europe in having a well-established and reputable system for training herbal practitioners who have not necessarily obtained any other medical qualifications. The National Institute of Medical Herbalists was founded in 1864 and members qualify by examination after four or five years of specialist study. Many overseas students also attend courses in the UK run by the School of Phytotherapy in Sussex, and there are now two UK universities offering degree courses in herbal medicine. Members of the National Institute use the initials MNIMH or FNIMH after their names which gives the patient some guarantee that they are consulting a suitably trained practitioner.

The UK's other main professional herbal body is The General Council and Register of Herbalists whose members use the initials MH. It has a rather different philosophical approach from that usually adopted by the NIMH practitioners with its members tending more towards homoeopathy: herbal tinctures are likely to be prescribed in drop doses rather than the teaspoonfuls generally favoured by NIMH members. A third, more recently formed organisation, is the Register of Chinese Herbal Medicine whose members largely use a combination of acupuncture and Chinese herbs.

Consulting a professional herbalist is not all that different from visiting a GP, or rather, visiting a GP as one would have done 40 or 50 years ago. Indeed, many herbalists liken their approach to that of the old-fashioned family physician using a lot of patient listening and probing questions to uncover all the relevant symptoms along with time-honoured diagnostic techniques: feeling pulses, looking at tongues, testing urine and with clinical examinations dependent on palpation, auscultation and percussion rather than laboratory tests. A first consultation will generally take at least an hour and subsequent ones 20 minutes or so. A wide range of ailments is commonly treated: both the sort of problems one may normally take to a GP – infections, aches and pains, menstrual disorders, high blood pressure, urinary dysfunction, digestive problems etc – and those chronic conditions for which herbalism is often seen as a "last resort", such as rheumatoid arthritis, ME, emphysema and so on.

As well as reviewing the current illness, the herbalist will ask about medical history – previous health problems that may be contributing to the current imbalance, family tendencies and allergies, diet, lifestyle, stresses and worries.

Examinations may include taking blood pressure and pulses, palpating the abdomen to identify the cause of pain or discomfort, listening to chest wheezes (auscultation) or checking the degree of movement in an arthritic knee or shoulder. Simple clinical tests undertaken on site could include urine analysis or measuring haemoglobin levels using a tiny drop of blood. Existing orthodox medication also needs to be checked.

Herbalists would certainly not recommend dropping vital drugs, but any incompatibility of these with herbal remedies obviously needs to be considered when prescribing plant medicines. Similarly, many patients turn to herbs because they are anxious to phase-out their drugs, for whatever reason, and a safe programme of replacing them with gentler herbal remedies needs to be devised – preferably with the support and co-operation of the patient's GP. Herbal remedies, for example, can be very helpful for sufferers trying to break an addiction to tranquillizers or sleeping pills, or as alternatives for those suffering the side-effects of non-steroidal anti-inflammatory drugs used for arthritis.

At the end of the consultation, the patient does not simply leave with a prescription for the local pharmacist to dispense. In Britain, few pharmacies are willing to stock the hundreds of tinctures, creams, oils, powders, capsules or dried herbs that the medical herbalist needs to keep in stock, so all medical herbalists are permitted under the 1968 Medicines Act and The Medicines (Retail Sale and Supply of Herbal Remedies) Order 1977, to make and dispense their own remedies. As well as a combination of herbs, specially selected to help the unique health problems of each unique individual, the patient may leave the consultation room with a list of dietary suggestions, foods to avoid or details of those to eat more of. There may be recommended relaxation routines to follow or Bach Flower Remedies to help emotional factors affecting physical well-being. Or perhaps the patient will be sent away with a small growing plant to bring a little love and beauty into their life. Whatever the remedy, healing is a two-way process and the patient must take responsibility for their own health and actively participate in any cure. Those who expect a "magic pill" to solve their problems with little of their own effort, may be happier with orthodox therapies.

Generally herbalists like to see patients fairly soon after the first consultation to check on progress – perhaps after two or three weeks – with regular meetings every four to six weeks for six months or more in chronic cases. Herbal medication is likely to be altered slightly after each consultation to reflect changes in the condition.

Just as all patients are different so too are all herbalists. Finding a practitioner with whom you feel empathy and can trust, can be just as important in treatment as taking the right herbs. Some herbalists follow a semi-orthodox path prescribing remedies to ease symptoms just as modern drugs do, others will focus on holistic treatments urging major lifestyle changes. Some will use only Western herbs, others a combination of Chinese or Ayurvedic remedies. Some will talk mainly of pathological conditions, others will suggest *Qi* stagnation, allergies or define just about anything in terms of emotional stress. Some will depend on the consulting couch and the results of clinical tests for diagnosis, others will swing a pendulum or try kinesiology. If possible, choose your practitioner by personal recommendation from like-minded friends to ensure a good relationship with someone who understands your problem and whom you can also understand.

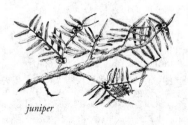

juniper

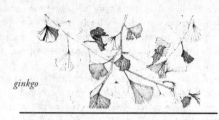

ginkgo

Herbs and the Law

Production and distribution of herbal medicines is, quite rightly, strictly regulated. Despite the popular view that herbs are natural aand therefore "safe", many plants are extremely potent and misuse can have considerable side effects. As the great fifteenth century herbalist Paracelsus argued, "the poison is the dose", meaning that in order to be powerful enough to have some sort of therapeutic impact on the body, the medicine had, in effect, to act as a "poison". Fortunately very few herbs would come under the conventional definition of "poisonous" but they can be powerful medicines and are, quite, rightly, regulated.

It was not always so: prior to the 1968 Thalidomide tragedy, control of both pharmaceutical drugs and herbal medicines was more liberal. Suppliers could make and package what they wanted often providing helpful names like "Blood Pressure Pills" or "Gall Bladder Remedy" to guide the lay public.

After the Thalidomide scandal, the government of the day rushed through a protective piece of legislation aimed at preventing the use of such untested medicines on an unsuspecting public ever again. Those herbal products then on offer were licensed to continue – subject to a thorough review of their contents and efficacy at some later date (a so-called "grandfather clause") – but new products would need to prove safety and efficacy before they hit the shelves. Those granted licences as a right were given a code starting "PLR" and these numbers can still be seen on some anthroposophical products which have yet to undergo a full review.

Under the 1968 Medicines Act medicines are defined as prescription only, pharmacy only and over-the-counter, and all preparations used as medicines and bearing a medicinal claim must be licensed. Herbal remedies are strictly defined under the Act as "medicinal products consisting of a substance produced by subjecting a plant or plants to drying, crushing or any other process", or a combination of such substances and water. An exemption under Section 12 of the Act allows herbalists to make and supply herbal products to their patients without a licence and a second exemption in the same section also means that dried and crushed herbal products also have no need for a licence, provided the manufacturer gives no written recommendation on the package or in any accompanying leaflets about what the product might be used for. This exemption does not apply to imported products.

It means, however, that "echinacea capsules" or "marshmallow and peppermint tablets" do not need a licence and, strictly speaking, are not medicines at all.

Licences are issued by the Medicines Control Agency and companies need to provide clear evidence of efficacy, which is allowed to take the form of research studies or information from official and herbal pharmacopoeias. Information must also be provided about the safety of the product. Licences are generally granted for five years.

The long-awaited review of herbal medicines had, under European Union rules, to be completed by May 1990. For many suppliers, providing the necessary evidence was an expensive business: estimates vary, but most sources suggest that it can cost from around £35,000 to £90,000 to gain a full product licence for a herbal medicine. During the review period a large number of products, presumably deemed unprofitable or unlikely to be granted a licence, disappeared from the shelves.

Product licence details (a code number starting PL) are printed on the packages of licensed herbal remedies and they can make carefully worded claims which generally start: "A herbal remedy traditionally used for the symptomatic relief of . . .". Such products usually also need to include an instruction to "consult your doctor if symptoms persist" on the label.

Often this permitted claim is only a part of the picture. A number of products containing echinacea and little else, for example, are allowed to claim that they can relieve skin problems. However, the same herbal mixture would often be just as adequate for tackling a wide range of infectious conditions, but the suppliers are not allowed to say so. This is partly because product licences are only granted to herbal remedies for self-limiting illnesses such as colds or sore throats. Products are not allowed to make claims for treating chronic problems, like arthritis or high blood pressure, so remedies that can tackle these ailments either have to be sold as suitable for something else, or relegated to the unlicensed "food supplement" category.

Licensed herbal medicines can be prescribed by doctors for conditions other than those specified on the licence, and there has recently been agreement from the Department of Health that such prescriptions will also be fully reimbursed under the NHS. This is an important breakthrough as it means that patients can persuade supportive GPs to supply herbal rather than orthodox remedies. As these can be substantially less expensive than pharmaceutical drugs one imagines that fund-holding GPs would welcome the development. A number of pharmacies are starting to stock herbal remedies to satisfy this demand.

The herbal products issue has been complicated in the years since 1968 by Britain's entry into the European Community (or European Union) and the need for UK legislation on medicinal products to conform to European directives. This caused a major furore back in 1994 when it seemed that the Government intended to overturn Section 12 of the 1968 Medicines Act claiming that the move was required under EU rules. This was not, in fact, the case and a major publicity campaign, which well demonstrated the support for herbal products, persuaded the Government to back down.

The Medicines Control Agency has recently reissued a document known as MAL8, which seeks to define just what a medicinal product is. The key issue is what is written on the label: if a therapeutic claim is made then the item becomes a medicine and needs a licence. If not, it can be regarded as a food. This ruling is expected to tighten up on synthetic supplements which are clearly neither herbs nor foods but are marketed as food supplements when they should be more strictly regulated as medicines.

Of the 800 or so over-the-counter remedies reviewed in this book, under a third are licensed – although several are currently the subject of licence applications. A significant proportion of the unlicensed products are single herb remedies (mostly evening primrose oil, garlic, feverfew, ginseng and ginkgo) exempted under Section 12, but many composite "supplements" are virtually identical to licensed offerings. None of the products in these latter two categories can, of course, imply what you use them for.

For the average customer, faced with the current bewildering array of herbal products on the health food shelves, this careful and necessary protective legislation does little to make remedy choice any easier. Licensed products will tell a little of what they can do, and herbs sold under the Section 12 exemption, nothing at all.

Currently there are no licensed Ayurvedic and Chinese herbal preparations and given the guidelines for demonstrating efficacy it could be difficult to satisfy the MCA requirements: few of the herbs involved figure in European pharmacopoeias and both these forms of traditional medicine use animal and mineral products which are well outside the scope of UK legislation. As these remedies grow in popularity, so too do reports of cases involving toxic side-effects of using them. These are not always justified (witness the case of chaparral, p. 121) but they do encourage a more rigorous approach to regulation. In some countries there are already bans on the importation of certain Chinese herbs, although as yet the UK remains reasonably liberal in its approach. Similarly, many herbal products licensed in other European countries have not been subject to the same rigorous review that the UK undertook back in 1990.

Meanwhile, harmonization of legislation throughout the EU continues and by 1 January, 1998 there is expected to be "mutual recognition" of each country's licensed medicines. This will mean that herbal remedies with a full product licence manufactured in Germany or Italy, for example, should be able to achieve same status in the UK, and vice versa. However, this will only apply to those products which have been fully reviewed and not to those many products from other European nations granted licences as of right (PLRs) which have not been properly assessed.

UK suppliers are confident that export sales of their fully licensed products will be considerable, and we can also expect some interesting additions – reflecting herbal traditions from other parts of Europe – to appear on the shelves of British health food retailers in the next few years.

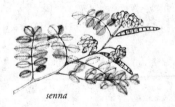

senna

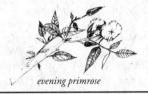

evening primrose

A-Z of Common Complaints

Over-the counter herbal remedies and supplements are available for a wide range of common health problems – but not all. This section covers the range of ailments for which readily available herbal products can be suitable. Herbs can help a great many more disorders than listed here, but in these cases either professional treatment is preferable or there is no suitable product marketed.

Throughout the text remedies marked with an asterisk (*) have been granted a product licence and may also be available on prescription (see page 13).

ACNE AND SPOTS

The characteristic pimples and blackheads of acne are all too familiar to teenagers. Inflamed sebaceous glands are to blame: these glands open into the hair follicles and produce an oily secretion known as sebum. This oil helps to keep the skin soft, moist and supple and it would soon become very dry without this constant lubrication. The sebaceous glands are at their most active during puberty due to the activity of the male hormone androgen. It is a time when the excess oils can block skin pores and lead to bacterial infection with pus-filled pimples, small cysts or blackheads. These also contain dead skin cells which discolour in the air. Typically acne starts in the early teens and usually disappears by mid-20s, although a tendency to spots can be a lifelong problem for some people.

The concentration of sebaceous glands varies over the body and so acne patches tend to be concentrated on the face, back and chest, although the larger sebaceous cysts are more likely to occur on the scalp and genitals. Because the spots are basically caused by infection, sufferers may often be prescribed low-doses of antibiotics on a long-term basis. Most herbalists would argue against such therapy as while antibiotics can effectively clear harmful bacteria, they can also kill the friendly bugs that inhabit our bowels and live on the surface of the skin and this may cause other, long-term problems. Similarly, because overactivity of sebaceous glands can be hormone-related many girls find that spots worsen just before a period when oestrogen levels drop and androgen concentration relatively increases. Indeed, GPs sometimes suggest that teenage girls use the contraceptive pill to try and control their acne. Again, this can have long-term side effects, especially if the menstrual cycle has not yet settled into a regular pattern.

The conventional herbal approach to treating acne is to cut down on the foods which might encourage sebaceous gland activity. This means reducing intake of refined carbohydrates (typically sugar and white flour), fried foods and animal fats. Sweets and chocolates also tend to aggravate the condition – as does excessive intake of alcohol and sweet, sugary drinks. Even excessive amounts of an apparently healthy product like fresh orange juice can cause a flare-up in some sufferers. Herbalists generally also recommend the use of cleansing herbs (known as alteratives) to clear any build-up of toxins from the body: these include burdock, blue flag, clivers, echinacea, red clover, sarsparilla, stinging nettles and yellow dock. All feature in a number of over-the-counter remedies for acne and skin complaints and several are also available as simples.

Deep cleansing with herbal steam baths or limited use of antiseptic herbal lotions can also help: tea tree and eucalyptus oils are included in antiseptic creams while adding camphor, cedar, juniper, lavender or sandalwood oils to a steam bath may also help.

The classic treatment is to rub acne pustules with a cut garlic clove: it's an effective remedy, but not one that teenage sufferers take to with any enthusiasm.

Herbal remedies and supplements which may help

Arkocaps Phytoderma; Arkocaps Phytofluid; Blackmores Echinacea Complex; Blackmores Sarsparilla Complex; Full Potency Herbs Burdock Root Vegicaps; Full Potency Herbs Sarsparilla Root Vegicaps; *Gerard House Blue Flag Root; Heath & Heather Skin; Herbcraft Burdock & Nettle Formula; *HRI Clear Complexion Tablets; *Lanes Kleer; *Potter's Jamaican Sarsparilla; *Potter's Skin Eruptions Mixture .

External: BioCare Dermasorb; Bioforce Echinacea Cream; Gerard House Garlic Ointment; Gerard House Witch Hazel Ointment; *Lanes Kleer Ti-Tree and Witch Hazel Cream; *Lane's Number 44 Skin Ointment; Neal's Yard Echinacea and Propolis Ointment; Nelsons Tea Tree Cream; *Potter's Skin Clear Ointment; Thursday Plantation Antiseptic Cream.

See echinacea simples

AGEING, PROBLEMS OF

Forgetfulness, confusion, incontinence, aches and pains, diabetes, osteoporosis . . . the problems of old age are many and largely inevitable. Herbal remedies cannot turn the clock back, but some can certainly help to relieve the discomforts.

A common problem in the elderly, and one which contributes to an apparent loss of memory and inability to concentrate, is narrowing of the arteries in the brain due to fatty deposits on the blood vessel walls (arteriosclerosis). This sort of damage is not only a contributory cause of strokes (cerebro-vascular accidents) but the reduced blood supply involved can lead to mental dullness as well.

In recent years extracts from the ginkgo tree have been widely promoted as circulatory tonics. The herb can have a beneficial effect on the cerebral circulation and is also regularly prescribed in Germany following strokes and for similar problems. In Ayurvedic medicine gotu kola is used as a traditional restorative for old age and can reputedly help to improve mental clarity while ginseng has long been a favourite with elderly – and affluent – Chinese.

As the body ages metabolism also slows down and thus the quantities of medicines needed can be significantly lower than for adults in their prime. Many OTC products specify reduced amounts for the elderly; if in doubt initially try two-thirds of the recommended adult dose of any product.

Herbal remedies and supplements which may help

Arkocaps Phytoexcel; BioCare Oxydent; Bioforce Arterioforce; Full Potency Herbs Gotu
    Kola Vegicaps; Nature's Plus Ginkgo Combo; Neal's Yard Anti-Oxidant Herbs Elixir;
    Pure-fil Romagen Herbal Antioxidant; Red Kooga Ginseng and Ginkgo Biloba.
See ginseng simples (Table 3)
See ginkgo simples

ANAEMIA

Oxygen is carried to the tissues by haemoglobin which is contained in red blood cells. Any lack of haemoglobin can thus leave the body starved of oxygen with symptoms of fatigue, breathlessness, pallor, insomnia, dizziness, assorted aches and pains, confusion and reduced resistance to infection.

There are many causes of anaemia and professional diagnosis is essential as some – such as leukaemia – can be life-threatening.

A common problem can be dietary deficiency. Production of haemoglobin depends on iron intake and this may either be in short supply or there could be a failure of the transport mechanism used to absorb iron into the body. This can be due to deficiency of vitamin B_{12}, vitamin C or folic acid. Strict vegetarians (vegans) can be especially short of vitamin B_{12} which occurs in most abundance in liver, offal, meat, fish, dairy produce, eggs and brewers' yeast and regular supplements could be necessary. Good sources of folic acid include green vegetables, liver, kidneys, eggs, and whole grains. High alcohol intake can increase the body's requirements for both folic acid and vitamin C, while heavy smokers are often also deficient in vitamin C.

Loss of blood is an obvious cause of anaemia and women who regularly have heavy periods can suffer from undiagnosed anaemia leading to both general fatigue and recurrent infections.

Eating iron-rich foods can help: watercress, apricots, and blackcurrants are all good sources as are those herbs which are said to "rob the soil" – parsley and nettles – and concentrate many important minerals and vitamins in their leaves. Comfrey is also a good source of vitamin B_{12} although internal regular consumption of the plant is no longer recommended as it has been found to contain toxic pyrrolizidine alkaloids.

In traditional Chinese medicine *Dang Gui* is believed to "nourish the blood" and is highly regarded as a woman's tonic. It can be of help in some types of anaemia.

Herbal remedies and supplements which may help

Arkocaps Phytofluid; Bioforce Alfavena; Cantassium Tong Kwai; Full Potency Herbs Dong Quai Vegicaps; Liquid Iron.

ANXIETY, STRESS AND TENSION

The stresses and strains of modern life are all too familiar: jobs are insecure, transport to and from work can be a nightmare, finances are pressurized and demands of children and elderly dependents can strain the most even-tempered.

Herbal remedies should not be seen as an alternative to professional counselling or psychotherapy for those who really cannot cope with their lifestyle, but they can be ideal for occasional use when the stresses mount and tempers become frayed. They also need to be seen as part of a total therapeutic approach: taking herbal sedatives is not going to solve problems caused by over-work and family discord any more than orthodox tranquillizers will. Learning to relax by using techniques like meditation, yoga or *Tai Ch'i* can provide an effective long-term solution. Even the most pressured parent needs to find space for themselves each day in order to cope, and a few minutes of relaxed, deep breathing or listening to a Bach sonata can work wonders.

Remedies fall into a number of categories, including:
• herbal sedatives and relaxants that can ease tensions and feelings of anxiety,
• herbal remedies which can act on the emotions in some way,
• herbal tonics and stimulants which will provide additional short-term energy,
• energy tonics which will help counter stress by strengthening the system and increasing a person's ability to cope.

Many herbs used for insomnia are essentially relaxants and sedatives and there is a considerable overlap in OTC products in this area. The more soporific herbs – such as wild lettuce and hops – are usually reserved for insomnia remedies, while those that have a general relaxing action – valerian, passion flower, skullcap, vervain, chamomile etc – are used both for sleeplessness and relaxing day-time preparations.

The most widely available herbal remedies for the emotions are the Bach

Flower Remedies which have been used since the 1930s and can be very effective for soothing worries, fears and ill-temper. These are very diluted flower extracts preserved in brandy and should be combined as required and further diluted before being taken in drop doses. By this stage the remedies are in homoeopathic dilution and many orthodox herbalists are sceptical of their action. However, a great many people find Bach Flower Remedies extremely helpful and they can be worth trying.

Essential oils, too, can have a direct effect on the emotions. Aromatherapy tends to be regarded in the UK as a massage-based technique but purists in mainland Europe prefer to think of it – as the name implies – as a therapy associated with smells. The powerful aromatic chemicals contained in the oils can have a direct impact on the olfactory nerve and from there are rapidly carried to centres in the brain involved in emotion. Smelling certain oils can be stimulating and uplifting, while others have a more soothing and relaxing effect. Using oils in diffusers to scent rooms can be an easy way to influence the emotions. Alternatively, add a few drops to bath water. Particularly calming are: benzoin, chamomile, camphor, cypress, jasmine, lavender, marjoram, melissa, neroli, rose, and sandalwood.

If a stressful time is looming – such as exams, the school holidays or a heavy work period – then it is worth taking tonic herbs before the event to provide an energy boost rather than depending on short-term stimulants once the stresses mount. Siberian ginseng is particularly useful for helping the body cope more efficiently with stress and improving performance: it was widely used in the 1960s and 1970s by Soviet athletes and long-distance lorry-drivers to increase stamina.

Herbs like gotu kola and reishi can also be valuable: both traditionally act on the spiritual level to bring mental calm and can be helpful for life-stage crises and strengthening resolve to make important changes.

Herbal remedies and supplements which may help

Bioforce Dormeasan; Bioforce Ginsavena; Bioforce Ginsavita; *Bio-Strath Valerian Formula; Blackmores Skullcap & Valerian; Blackmores Valerian Complex; *Cantassium Quiet Days; *Cantassium Quiet Tyme; *Dorwest Scullcap and Gentian Tablets; *Frank Roberts Nerfood Tablets; *Frank Roberts Pulsatilla Compound Tablets; *Frank Roberts Valerian Compound; Full Potency Herbs Chamomile Vegicaps; Full Potency Herbs Scutellariae Vegicaps; *Gerard House Biophylin; *Gerard 99; *Gerard House Motherwort Compound; Gerard House Pulsatilla; Gerard House St John's Wort; Gerard House Sooth-a-Tea; *Gerard House Valerian Compound Tablets; Health Aid Tranquil Capsules with Viburnum; *Heath & Heather Becalm; Herbcraft Passiflora and Valerian Formula; Herbcraft Reishi Shiitake; Herbs of Grace Emotional Balance; *HRI Calm Life Tablets; Jay-Vee Tablets; Kordel's Kalm-Ex; *Lanes Kalms; *Lanes Quiet Life Tablets; *Muir's Head-Ese; *Muir's Pick-Me-Up; *Muir's Stress-Ese; Mycoherb Rei Shi Gen; Mycoherb Rei Gen; Neal's Yard Scullcap Compound Capsules; *Potter's Anased Pain Relief Tablets; *Potter's Newrelax; Super Gre-Caps; *Valerina – Day-Time; *Valerina – Night-Time; *Weleda Fragador Tablets; *Weleda Avena Sativa Comp.

See Bach Flower Remedies; gotu kola, passion flower, Siberian ginseng, and valerian simples

ARTHRITIS

Arthritis simply means inflammation of a joint. There are, however, various types of arthritis requiring rather different treatments, so it is important to be sure of the exact diagnosis.

Osteoarthritis is the sort of "wear and tear" variety that afflicts many of us – some estimates suggest up to 52% – as we grow older. Youthful injuries to joints, that have never fully healed, can often provide the basis for arthritic aches and pains in old age. Obesity can also lead to osteoarthritis with excessive strain on the weight-bearing joints causing damage. Typically in osteoarthritis the protective cartilage between the bones of a joint becomes damaged and wears away causing the bones to rub together and become deformed. Joints often creak, become stiff and painful, and movement may be limited.

Osteoarthritis can be an occupational hazard: coal miners, for example, used to get arthritic knees, while pneumatic drill users may develop the condition in their elbows.

Whereas osteoarthritis tends to affect only a few of the body's joints, rheumatoid arthritis is a more serious and potentially crippling disease. It can affect many joints, usually in a symmetrical pattern so that both hands or feet may suffer, both knees or both sides of the jaw. This sort of arthritis is an inflammatory problem and can be related to a variety of hereditary health problems. The cause is often unknown, although some suggest that viral infection or auto-immune problems can be to blame. Here the membranous capsule covering the joint (the synovium) becomes thickened and inflamed leading to destruction of cartilage and eventually bone. The end result can be severe bone deformity. In the early stage the joint is usually very painful and feels hot to the touch and this later develops into a permanent deformity. Once deformation is complete the condition is usually less painful, although movement can be severely affected.

Women are three times more likely than men to develop rheumatoid arthritis although a related condition affecting the spine – ankylosing spondylitis – most commonly affects younger men.

Arthritis can also occur in children and may be of the inflammatory rheumatoid variety or a more complex syndrome. Juvenile arthritis always needs professional medical treatment. Arthritis – especially in children – may be related to food intolerance and eliminating possible allergens such as dairy products, wheat, gluten, beef or pork can be worth trying in long-standing conditions. Many arthritics also find that refined carbohydrates (e.g. products made from white sugar and white flour), citrus fruits, tomatoes and excessive amounts of red meat increase symptoms, while recent research suggests that generally reducing animal fats in the diet can bring relief.

Localized osteoarthritic problems can respond to topical, long-term treatment, Comfrey, for example, helps to repair the damage from old injuries and rubbing a little comfrey cream into the joint each night, over a period of many months, can help. Herbalists often refer to osteoarthritis as a "cold" condition and regard it as one that can be eased by heat. Oils which help to warm the joint by encouraging increased blood flow to the area – such as those containing cayenne or rosemary – can thus bring symptomatic relief.

Traditional herbalism also sees osteoarthritis in terms of toxins lingering in the body and contributing to the joint damage, so remedies will usually include cleansing herbs, diuretics and digestive stimulants. These can include black cohosh, burdock, celery seed and yellow dock. Anti-inflammatory herbs, such as bogbean and devil's claw, also feature in remedies. Many people use feverfew for arthritis as it is an effective anti-inflammatory although it can have side effects.

Rheumatoid arthritis really needs professional treatment, but the herbal approach will generally put greater emphasis on anti-inflammatory herbs. Some therapists suggest that congenital rheumatic conditions may be due to the body's inability to manufacture *gamma*-linolenic acid and thus supplements of evening primrose or borage oil could be recommended.

Similarly, because certain arthritic conditions might be triggered by a bacterial infection or possibly a virus, herbal arthritic remedies may include anti-bacterials and anti-virals like echinacea or garlic. Calcium supplements may also be helpful, especially among post-menopausal women and kelp can also help to cleanse and stimulate the metabolism.

See also Gout, Osteoporosis, Rheumatism

Herbal remedies and supplements which may help

Arthur's Formula; BioCare Celery Seed; Bioforce IMP (Imperthritica); Blackmores Celery Complex; FSC Ginger and Turmeric; *Gerard House Celery; Health Aid Devil's Claw with Royal Jelly; *Heath & Heather Celery Seed; *Heath & Heather Rheumatic Pain; Kordel's Celery 3000 Plus; Kordel's Feverfew and Willow; Ortis Fresh Devil's Claw Drink.

External: Arthur's Formula Bath and Massage Oil; Arthur's Formula Cream; Bioforce Comfrey Cream; *Culpeper Comfrey Ointment; Dr Shir's Liniment; Frank Roberts Comfrey Ointment; Gerard House Comfrey Ointment; Harpago Gel; Neal's Yard Comfrey Ointment; Phytorhuma; *Potter's Comfrey Ointment.

See bladderwrack, borage oil, devil's claw, evening primrose oil, feverfew, and kelp simples

ASTHMA

Growing pollution in our cities is often blamed for the increase in asthma – especially among children. It can be a life-threatening condition and generally needs professional medical treatment.

In asthma the small bronchial tubes in the lungs tighten making it difficult for the sufferer to breath out and this results in the characteristic wheeze. The tubes also fill with a sticky mucus instead of the usual lubricating fluid phlegm.

Asthma is often an allergic reaction so identifying the allergen is important. Dairy products, wheat or beef can be common culprits while dust and traffic fumes certainly exacerbate the condition. Sulphur dioxide, which is a common air pollutant, can be to blame and this same chemical is often used as a preservative for fruits and wine.

Emotional stress can also play a part: asthmatics often keep their feelings tightly under control and find it difficult to loosen up and relax. Deep breathing, joining a relaxation class or taking up yoga can often help.

Herbal remedies usually include relaxing expectorants and antispasmodics to ease the symptoms. Use of the most potent herbs for asthma (such as Indian tobacco) is restricted to professional practitioners but other suitable plants include gumplant, pill-bearing spurge, sundew and skunk cabbage. Steam inhalations with a few drops of chamomile oil can ease the symptoms of mild attacks.

Herbal remedies and supplements which may help

Blackmores Euphorbia Complex; *Culpeper Cough Relief Mixture; *Frank Roberts Rod-Bron Tablets.

ATHLETE'S FOOT

Athlete's foot (*Tinea pedis*) is a very common fungal infection affecting the space between the toes and toe nails. Depending on the infecting fungus, it can either involve inflammation and itching or may simply cause scaling of the skin and general discomfort. Like all their species, the yeasts causing athlete's foot thrive in warm, damp places so good, sensible foot care – making sure the toes are well dried after bathing and that shoes are comfortable – is important.

Using creams based on anti-fungal herbs, such as marigold, tea tree, and echinacea, can help.

Herbal remedies and supplements which may help

External: BioCare Dermasorb; Bioforce Echinacea Cream; *Lane's Number 44 Skin Ointment; Gerard House Calendula Ointment; Hartwood Aromatics Calendula Ointment; Herbcraft Calendula & Goldenseal Spray; Neal's Yard Calendula Ointment; *Nelsons Calendula Cream; Nelsons Tea Tree Cream; *Potter's Skin Clear Ointment; Thursday Plantation Antiseptic Cream; *Weleda Calendula Lotion.

BABIES AND CHILDREN

Although herbal medicines can often be quite safe for small children, their use does need experience and many over-the-counter remedies specifically exclude children from their recommendations. It is best to err on the side of safety so, unless otherwise directed by a professional practitioner, always follow the guidelines given on the packaging. Some herbal remedies can, however, be helpful for a range of children's ailments.

Bedwetting (enuresis)

Bedwetting only tends to be regarded as a problem when it occurs regularly in children of five years or more. Emotional upsets and insecurity are a common cause, particularly if bedwetting starts in children who have previously been "dry". Nervousness at starting school or changing classes are obvious trigger factors, as are the arrival of new young siblings or parental marital problems. Lots of love and cuddles can help, as can gentle questioning about any school problems – especially bullying or dislike of a particular teacher or type of lesson.

Herbs used for anxiety and tension can help; however, as an additional caution, many licensed herbal remedies often state that they should not be given to children younger than eight or 12. While professional herbalists will generally prescribe low doses of these herbs for children the OTC warning is understandable. Remedies based on chamomile are usually suitable for children as are Californian poppy, lemon balm and passion flower.

Urinary infections can also involve bedwetting so if the child complains of discomfort on passing water this needs professional investigation. Sweet sumach is traditionally used in bedwetting problems and is contained in some OTC products.

Herbal remedies and supplements which may help

Bioforce Cystaforce.

Colic

Small babies can also suffer from colic: this is a severe abdominal pain which tends to come in waves a few seconds or minutes apart. In adults it can be due to an obstruction in the intestine or simply to constipation and can need professional treatment. In babies, colic is usually caused by air becoming trapped in the intestines and is generally associated with feeding difficulties, or a failure to properly "wind" the infant after it has finished sucking.

Babies often remain colicky for the first three months of life which can be extremely wearing on the parents as the child's only reaction to the pain it feels is to cry, loudly. Traditional gripe water is, of course, a herbal remedy usually based on dill extracts. Another suitable option for colic is homoeopathic chamomile (Chamomilla 3×) which is available in drops or pillules.

Herbal remedies and supplements which may help

*Nurse Harvey's Gripe Water; *Weleda Chamomilla 3× Pillules and Drops; *Woodward's Gripe Water

Cradle cap

This affects young babies and is a dandruff-like condition that usually starts with scurf on the head followed by the development of yellow, crusted scaly patches. These can spread over the whole head or simply be confined to particular areas. The condition is quite harmless and some believe that it is related to over-activity of the sebaceous glands in the scalp possibly caused by the mother's hormones. A simple remedy is to gently rub olive or wheatgerm oil into the baby's scalp, allow it to soak well in and then wash the flakes away; infused marigold or heart-sease oils and creams can also be safely used.

Herbal remedies and supplements which may help

External: Bioforce Echinacea Cream; Gerard House Calendula Ointment; Hartwood Aromatics Calendula Ointment; Neal's Yard Calendula Ointment; *Nelsons Calendula Cream; *Weleda Calendula Lotion; *Weleda Calendolon Ointment.

Nappy rash

Nappy rash is an even more common complaint – no matter how frequently babies are changed and dried, most develop a red or sore bottom at some stage. Keeping the affected area as dry as possible (even by blowing with a hair dryer set to the cool setting) is essential.

Ointments are better to use than creams as they form a protective barrier for the skin whereas creams tend to soak in and soften. Marigold, chamomile or comfrey ointment can be helpful and safe to use, as can aloe vera gel. Bacteria in the faeces can react with urine to produce ammonia and this can encourage fungal infections. These are best treated with ointments containing marigold or tea tree.

Herbal remedies and supplements which may help

External: BioCare Dermasorb; Gerard House Calendula Ointment; Gerard House Chamomile Ointment; *Lane's Number 44 Skin Ointment; *Nelsons Calendula Cream; *Nelsons Healing Ointment; Nelsons Tea Tree Cream; *Potter's Comfrey Ointment; *Potter's Skin Clear Ointment; Spring Wind Ointment; Thursday Plantation Antiseptic Cream; *Weleda Balsamicum Ointment; *Weleda Calendolon Ointment.

Sleeplessness

Sleepless babies can be a major problem for the entire family. Check that the room temperature is not too hot or cold and – as the problem can be one of insecurity – give lots of loving cuddles. Chamomile in the bathwater at night can be effective while older children can also be safely given Californian poppy or passion flower products

Herbal remedies and supplements which may help

Arkcaps Phytodream; *Weleda Chamomilla 3× Pillules and Drops.
See also passion flower simples

Teething

Teething generally starts at around six months and can be a gruelling time for all members of the family. Homoeopathic Chamomilla 3× remedies can be very soothing; some babies will take weak chamomile tea from a bottle or it can be added to bath water to encourage more restful nights.

Herbal remedies and supplements which may help

*Weleda Chamomilla 3× Pillules and Drops.

Other ailments

Children also suffer the same complaints as their elders and some over-the-counter products are recommended for children's coughs, constipation and stomach upsets. These are listed below.

For infections, low doses of echinacea are quite safe; however, children's infections can develop into dramatically high fevers with the temperature reaching 39°C/102°F or more. Raising the body temperature is part of the normal defence mechanisms to combat invading organisms and is not generally a problem. However, if the temperature rises above 39°C/102°F for any length of time, professional help is advisable. For milder cases herbal remedies containing elder flower, lime flowers, hyssop, and boneset can be helpful.

See Travel sickness

Herbal remedies and supplements which may help

Bioforce Drosinula Cough Syrup; Bioforce Satasapina Cough Syrup; Bioforce Satasapina Bon Bons; *Cantassium Hay Fever; *CoughEeze; *Culpeper Balm of Gilead Cough Mixture; *Culpeper Cough Relief Mixture; *Culpeper Elder Flower and Peppermint Mixture; *Culpeper Head Cold and Throat Mixture; *Culpeper Influenza Mixture; *Heath & Heather Balm of Gilead Cough Mixture; *Heath & Heather Balm of Gilead Cough Pastilles; *HRI Herbal Catarrh and Rhinitis Tablets; *Lane's Cut-a-Cough; *Lane's Sage and Garlic Catarrh Remedy; *Lanes Biobalm; *Lanes Garlodex; *Lanes Herbelix Specific; *Lanes Honey and Molasses Cough Mixture; *Lanes Kleer; *Lanes Sinotar; *Lusty's Herbalene; *Muir's Catarrh; *Muir's Pick-Me-Up; *Natraleze; Neal's Yard Balm of Gilead; Neal's Yard Echinacea & Mallow Linctus; *Olbas Pastilles; *Potter's Antibron Tablets; *Potter's Antifect; *Potter's Balm of Gilead; *Potter's Catarrh Mixture; *Potter's Elderflowers, Peppermint and Composition Essence; *Potter's Horehound and Aniseed Cough Mixture; *Potter's Life Drops; *Potter's Lightning Cough Remedy; *Potter's Peerless Composition Essence; *Potter's Senna Tablets; *Potter's Skin Eruptions Mixture; *Potter's Vegetable Cough Remover; *Revitonil; *Ricola Swiss Herb Lozenges; *Weleda Carminative Tea; *Weleda Clairo Tea; *Weleda Cough Elixir; *Weleda Herb and Honey Cough Elixir; *Weleda Melissa Comp.

External: *Olbas Oil; *Weleda Catarrh Cream.

BACKACHE, FIBROSITIS, LUMBAGO AND SCIATICA

Backache is reckoned to be one of the most common causes in this country for taking days off work, visiting the GP or seeking alternative medical treatment. Certainly the number of over-the-counter remedies for backache is impressive.

Orthodox treatment usually takes the form of bed rest and pain killers but thorough investigation is also needed to identify the cause of the problem. This can range from pulled muscles and damaged discs (the spongy plugs that separate the vertebra and act as shock absorbers) to poor posture, kidney disease, gynae-cological problems or simply sitting in an awkward position for long periods.

Some sorts of backache are dignified by rather grander names: "lumbago" simply means pain in the lower back (the lumbar region) from whatever cause, whereas "sciatica" is often applied to odd aches and pains in the back but is tech-nically a pain felt along the back and outer side of the thigh, leg and foot, with accompanying back pain and stiffness, generally caused by a damaged disc putting pressure on either the sciatic nerve or one of the other many nerves which start in the lower back area. Both can cause severe pain and leave sufferers unable to straighten up. In acute cases immediate professional medical attention is often needed. "Fibrositis" is an inflammation of fibrous tissue, especially muscle sheaths, which often affects the back muscles. It leads to pain and stiffness and can be treated with anti-inflammatories and the sort of remedies recommended for rheumatic disorders.

Obviously all these different sorts of backache require very different treat-ments so accurate diagnosis is important if therapy is to be relevant. Muscular aches and stiffness can often be associated with recent strenuous exercise – gar-dening or DIY – or perhaps a period of over-work with too long spent bending over computer keyboards or desks. Similarly, if the cause is associated with kidney weakness or a displaced uterus, then these underlying problems need to be tack-led as other backache remedies will only ever provide symptomatic relief.

Several products are available specifically for backache associated with kidney weakness: these remedies generally contain herbs like bearberry, buchu, cornsilk or horsetail.

If the problem really is originating from the back itself then often treatment from an osteopath, chiropractor or acupuncturist can solve the problem. Massage from a remedial masseur or physiotherapist can also give relief, while poor pos-ture can be helped by learning the Alexander Technique through a series of lessons.

The high-tech world of the 1990s is also a major cause of upper back and shoulder pains with "repetitive strain injury" blamed for a variety of problems. By law anyone who has to spend lengthy periods at a computer keyboard must take regular breaks. Ensuring that chair heights are correctly adjusted and that there is space between the keyboard and the desk edge to rest the wrists can also prevent long-term damage. There are similar Health & Safety Executive directives on lift-ing and moving heavy weights at work and it is important to follow these same guidelines in the home as well. Always bend at the knees rather than the waist when stooping to pick something from the ground.

For persistent backache with no obvious cause, changing sleeping arrange-ments can sometimes help. Firm mattresses can be worth trying, while lying on your back with knees bent or curling into a small ball with the spine curved, as in the foetal position, as you fall off to sleep can often bring relief. Putting an extra pillow under the mattress to raise the top of the bed is also worth trying as is experimenting with the various orthopaedic pillows on the market.

Massage oils can be useful – if you have a suitable friend or relative to do the massage – or try a few drops of the same oils added to a hot bath.

Herbal remedies and supplements which may help

*Bio-Strath Willow Formula; *Frank Roberts Buchu Backache Compound Tablets; *Frank Roberts Sciatica Tablets; *Gerard House Ligvites; *Heath & Heather Celery Seed; *Heath & Heather Rheumatic Pain; *Lanes Vegetex; *Muir's Rheumatic Pain; *Muir's Sciatica; *Potter's Backache Tablets; *Potter's Kas-Bah Herb; *Potter's Sciargo; *Potter's Sciargo Herb; *Rheumasol.

External: Amber Massage Salve; Bee Brand Massage Oil; Chirali Old Remedy Strain & Sprain Cream; Dr Shir's Liniment; Neal's Yard Sports Salve; *Potter's Nine Rubbing Oils.

BAD BREATH

Highly spiced foods, garlic, smoking and tooth decay can all contribute to bad breath: it is a problem that is often more embarrassing than health damaging but one which affects many people at some time or another.

Sucking peppermints is a common solution: but these usually contain sugar which can damage the teeth, while too much peppermint oil can be an irritant on the mucous membranes of mouth, upper respiratory tract and stomach.

Traditionally certain herb seeds were chewed to sweeten the breath and it is an old habit worth rediscovering. Try lovage or fennel seeds which have a pleasant flavour; chewing parsley leaves can help to reduce garlic smells (some over-the-counter garlic preparations also contain parsley), although an easier solution is simply to encourage everyone to eat garlic as then no-one notices the smell too much.

Herbal mouthwashes can help combat mouth infections which might contribute to bad breath: use dilute sage or rosemary tinctures or infusions, for example.

Bad breath can often suggest stagnation in the digestive tract with food taking too long to pass through. This is especially likely if there are related symptoms of wind, constipation or abdominal discomfort. Digestive stimulants can often help regulate the system and solve the associated problems.

Herbal remedies and supplements which may help

Herbcraft Fresh Breath Cinnamint Spray.

BLEPHARITIS

See Eye problems

BOILS AND CARBUNCLES

A boil is a tender inflamed area of skin containing pus generally caused by a staphylococcal infection of a hair follicle or a break in the skin. A cluster of boils is known as a carbuncle. Boils are usually a sign of reduced resistance to infection, perhaps because of general debility, chronic illness, exhaustion or over-work. There could also be some deep-seated septic focus – such as a dental abscess adding to the over-all toxicity. Frequent outbreaks of boils can suggest a more serious underlying cause – possibly diabetes or kidney disease. Unskilled lancing of boils can spread infection and is best avoided.

Herbal treatment can include the use of poultices or drawing ointments – often based on slippery elm – to encourage the boil to discharge; anti-bacterial creams containing marigold, echinacea and tea tree are also useful. These can be combined with herbs, such as garlic and echinacea, to boost the immune system and combat bacterial infections.

Herbal remedies and supplements which may help

External: Bioforce Echinacea Cream; Gerard House Calendula Ointment; Golden Yellow Ointment; *Lane's Number 44 Skin Ointment; Neal's Yard Echinacea and Propolis Ointment; *Nelsons Calendula Cream; Nelsons Tea Tree Cream; *Potter's Skin Clear Ointment; *Rickard's Woodsap Ointment; Thursday Plantation Antiseptic Cream; *Weleda Balsamicum Ointment.
See echinacea and garlic simples

BREAST-FEEDING DISORDERS

See Pregnancy and childbirth

BRONCHITIS

Bronchitis is an inflammation of the bronchial tubes, which are the airways bringing air into the lungs. It can be acute, due to an infection, or chronic when it is a serious condition that can lead to lung diseases such as emphysema, and be a major cause of early death.

It is essential for anyone suffering from chronic bronchitis to give up smoking. Alcohol, dairy products, refined carbohydrates and caffeine should also be strictly limited and avoided altogether if possible.

While professional medical treatment is generally needed for bronchitis, herbal remedies can also be supportive. Stimulating expectorants can be used to clear the mucous along with garlic and thyme to combat infections. Lung tonics, such as elecampane and ginseng, can then help to strengthen the system. Warming herbs – like ginger, cayenne and horseradish – can be used for the sort of bronchitis that tends to be worse in damp, cold weather or where there is copious white sputum.

Herbal remedies and supplements which may help

Bioforce Bronchosan; *Frank Roberts Rod-Bron Tablets; St Hildegard Hart's Tongue Fern
    Elixir; Herbcraft Garlic and Horseradish Winter Formula
See Coughs

BRUISES

Everyone suffers bruising at some time or another and the usual colour change from red or pink to purple, bluish and finally a greeny-yellow is very familiar. A bruise is an area of skin discolouration caused by blood escaping from damaged underlying blood vessels following injury and the multi-coloured healing process occurs as the haemoglobin in the escaped blood breaks down into other chemicals before being completely dispersed.

A tendency to bruise easily can be related to problems with the blood's ability to clot or may simply suggest that small blood vessels are comparatively thin and easily damaged. This is often the case in otherwise fit and healthy women who have a tendency to bruise easily. If you do have blood which does not clot readily – or are on blood-thinning drugs – then avoid taking herbs like feverfew which can slow down clotting still further.

An ice pack in the form of a packet of frozen peas provides an ideal emergency treatment to relieve the pain of a new bruise. Alternating that with a hot water bottle can help to encourage reabsorption of blood and bring more rapid relief.

Over-the-counter arnica or comfrey cream applied to unbroken skin will also encourage healing, while if the bruise is the result of some traumatic accident then taking homoeopathic Arnica 6× or Bach Flower Rescue Remedy internally can help calm the sufferer and help to encourage more rapid healing.

Herbal remedies and supplements which may help

Bioforce Comfrey Cream; Bioforce Po Ho Ointment; *Culpeper Comfrey Ointment;
    Frank Roberts Comfrey Ointment; Gerard House Comfrey Ointment; Neal's Yard
    Arnica Ointment; Herbs of Grace Arnica Cream; Neal's Yard Comfrey Ointment;
    *Nelsons Arnica Cream; *Potter's Comfrey Ointment; *Weleda Massage Balm with
    Arnica; *Weleda Arnica Ointment; *Weleda Ruta Ointment.

BUNIONS

These painful swellings of the joint between the big toe and the adjoining bone can be caused by badly fitting shoes although a tendency for them can be hereditary. Ensuring that shoes are the correct size and comfortable is essential – loose slippers or sandals for home use can also help. Comfrey cream applied regularly can be helpful or, if the bunion becomes particularly inflamed and blistered use marigold at night.

Herbal remedies and supplements which may help

External: Amber Massage Salve Bioforce Comfrey Cream; *Culpeper Comfrey Ointment; Frank Roberts Comfrey Ointment; Gerard House Comfrey Ointment; Neal's Yard Comfrey Ointment; *Potter's Comfrey Ointment; Gerard House Calendula Ointment; Hartwood Aromatics Calendula Ointment; Neal's Yard Calendula Ointment; Neal's Yard Hypercal Ointment; *Nelsons Calendula Cream; *Nelsons Hypercal Cream; *Nelsons Hypercal Tincture; *Weleda Calendula Lotion; *Weleda Calendolon Ointment; *Weleda Hypericum/Calendula Ointment.

BURNS (MINOR) AND SCALDS

Burns are potential medical emergencies and only the most minor should be treated at home. Any burn more than about 5 cm/2 in across should be seen by a doctor as soon as possible.

For less severe injuries running cold water over the affected area or using an ice pack (or frozen peas) will cool it down and ease the immediate pain. Keeping the injury cool for two or three hours can often help significantly.

Herbs that can help include aloe vera gel, lavender oil and infused oil of St John's wort.

Herbal remedies and supplements which may help

Herbcraft Aloe Lavender Spray; *Nelsons Burns Ointment; *Potter's Dermacreme Ointment; *Weleda Comburdoron Ointment; *Weleda WCS Dusting Powder.

CATARRH AND SINUS PROBLEMS

From thick mucous making breathing difficult to watery secretions causing a semi-permanent drip – catarrh can take many forms and has many different causes. It is often associated with the common cold and can persist for some time after other symptoms have cleared or it can be a sign of allergic reaction as in hayfever.

Catarrh can be confined to the upper respiratory tract causing nasal congestion, or the mucous can affect the lower airways and be coughed up as phlegm. Lingering catarrh also makes an ideal breeding ground for bacteria and can lead to inflammation of the sinuses. These are cavities in the bones of the face which help prevent the skull becoming too heavy and are found above the nose, around the eyes and across the cheeks. Inflammation here can lead to severe pain made worse by bending forward or blowing the nose.

While orthodox medicine can treat catarrh as a self-contained problem, a more holistic herbal approach regards it in terms of the whole person. Catarrh can indicate that toxic material elsewhere in the body is not being adequately disposed of: the digestive system could be sluggish or the kidneys not working as efficiently as they should. Sinus problems can also be linked to emotional factors.

Suppressed tears can sometimes seem to block the upper respiratory tract and a good cry can often be extremely effective.

Whatever the cause, diet is extremely important and, as in the common cold, foods that encourage mucous formation should be avoided. These include refined carbohydrates, dairy products and alcohol. Eating only fruit for a couple of days helps to clear any lingering toxic wastes, while zinc and vitamin C supplements will help to strengthen the immune system and combat infection.

Steam inhalations can also help clear catarrh. Add five drops of thyme or eucalyptus oil to a basin containing 1litre/1¾ pt of boiling water, cover your head with a towel and inhale the steam for 10 minutes.

Herbal remedies and supplements which may help

Bumbles Propolis, Menthol and Eucalyptus Lozenges; *Cantassium Hay Fever; *CatarrhEeze; *ColdEeze; *Dorwest Garlic and Fenugreek Tablets; *Frank Roberts Catarrh Tablets; *Frank Roberts Sinus and Hay Fever Tablets; Full Potency Herbs Eyebright Vegicaps; *Gerard House Lobelia Compound; *Heath & Heather Balm of Gilead Cough Mixture; *Heath & Heather Balm of Gilead Cough Pastilles; *Heath & Heather Catarrh; Herbcraft Echinacea, Eyebright and Bilberry Formula; Herbs of Grace Expect-Relief; Kordel's Horseradish, Odourless Garlic and Vitamin C; *Lane's Garlodex; *Lane's Herbelix Specific; *Lane's Honey and Molasses Cough Mixture; *Lane's Sinotar; *Lane's Sage and Garlic Catarrh Remedy; *Muir's Catarrh; Neal's Yard Eucalyptus & Menthol Lozenges; *Potter's Antifect; *Olbas Pastilles; *Potter's Catarrh Mixture; *Potter's Chest Mixture; *Ricola Swiss Herb Lozenges
External: *Olbas Oil; *Weleda Catarrh Cream; *Weleda Oleum Rhinale
See also echinacea and garlic simples.

CELLULITE

Cellulite is one of those labels, popular with beauty writers and producers of assorted health aids, that you are unlikely to find in any medical dictionary. It is generally taken to mean the sort of bumpy, "pitted orange peel" skin which can develop on the buttocks, hips, thighs, stomach and arms, and usually indicates stagnant tissues, fat layers and poor lymphatic drainage.

Exercise is important to help tone up the muscles and revitalize the skin while diet should avoid dairy foods, refined carbohydrates, salt, alcohol and junk food. Crash diets, which may damage muscle tissues, followed by rapid weight gain tend to encourage cellulite and should be avoided. Weight needs to be lost gradually with a healthy diet, sensible exercise and no reduction in the vital nutrients the body needs.

Herbal remedies which may be promoted to deal with cellulite are generally similar to the metabolic stimulants, such as kelp, that may be recommended as slimming aids. Others contain pineapple which is rich in an enzyme called bromelain which can stimulate the digestion.

Herbal remedies and supplements which may help

Arkocaps Phytoshape.
External: Neal's Yard Cellulite Oil.

CHILBLAINS

Poor blood flow to the remoter parts of the body, generally in response to cold, is the usual cause of chilblains. In order to maintain a suitably warm temperature for the vital organs and deep tissues of the body, the blood flow to the peripheries is constricted in severe cold, leading to numbness. As the oxygen supply is limited, tissues become more alkaline, so that when the temperature rises and normal blood supply returns, the system starts to restore normal balance and the familiar burning and itching sensation of chilblains is the result.

Wearing adequate clothing on cold days is the easiest way to avoid occasional chilblains while habitual sufferers can improve their circulation with stimulating herbs such as angelica, prickly ash bark or ginger. Rutin is also a good tonic for the small blood vessels and can be taken either pure in tablet form or obtained from herbs like buckwheat. Some research also suggests that ginkgo can improve the peripheral blood circulation, although it is more traditionally regarded as stimulating the blood supply to the brain.

Arnica cream can help relieve the discomfort of chilblains once they've appeared but should not be used on broken skin. Other helpful herbs to relieve symptoms include aloe vera, myrrh or marigold.

Herbal remedies and supplements which may help

External: Bioforce Po Ho Ointment; *Gerard House Dragon Balm Ointment; Neal's Yard Arnica Ointment; *Nelsons Arnica Ointment; *Nelsons Chilblain Ointment; *Weleda Arnica Ointment; *Weleda Frost Cream.
See also Poor circulation

CHILDBIRTH

See Pregnancy and childbirth

COLD SORES

Cold sores are caused by the herpes simplex type 1 virus which is believed to be carried by about 50% of the adult population. The sores are always quite localized and take the form of tiny blisters which usually start with a tingling sensation and develop rapidly to inflamed, red areas generally occurring around the mouth but sometimes found elsewhere on the body. Once a person has been infected, the virus can remain dormant in the body for years usually causing a recurrent outbreak of cold sores if the sufferer is at all run down or over-tired. Women sometimes find that cold sores will coincide with menstruation, and they can often herald a cold or 'flu simply because both can occur when resistance is weakened by exhaustion.

The virus is extremely contagious during the blistering stage and can spread in saliva or by contact, so it is important to avoid touching the cold sore and spreading the infection to other parts of the body.

Cold sores are more of a nuisance than a serious health hazard. They will respond well to herbs and it is best to start treatment as soon as the familiar tingling sensation starts rather than waiting for the full blown sore to develop.

Tea tree cream can be effective as can remedies based on lavender oil, echinacea, or marigold. Garlic and echinacea taken internally will increase resistance to infection and thus reduce the risk of recurrence.

Herbal remedies and supplements which may help

External: Gerard House Calendula Ointment; Hartwood Aromatics Calendula Ointment; Herbcraft Aloe Lavender Spray; Nature's Vyrbrit; Neal's Yard Calendula Ointment; *Nelsons Calendula Cream; Nelsons Tea Tree Cream; *Potter's Skin Clear Ointment; Thursday Plantation Antiseptic Cream; *Weleda Calendula Lotion; *Weleda Calendolon Ointment.

COLD, THE COMMON

Sore throats, blocked noses, coughs and sneezes . . . we are all only too familiar with the symptoms of the common cold. Colds can be caused by any one of hundreds of different viruses. These viruses can only survive in the body's cells and are usually passed from one person to another in droplets of moisture spread by coughs and sneezes. The viruses are constantly changing as they spread, so just because someone has already caught a cold that is "going around" once, immunity to that particular virus will be of little use if there is repeated infection as the virus will have mutated into another form.

Traditionally colds were associated with some sort of external factor such as cold weather or getting soaked in a rainstorm. Modern medicine may dismiss these causes in favour of viruses, but we are certainly more susceptible to colds if we're tired, over-worked, unhappy or, indeed, have been abnormally chilled by the extremes of climate.

Because colds are caused by viruses they cannot be treated by antibiotics which are only good for tackling bacteria. Orthodox medicine tends to rely on remedies to ease the symptoms whereas a herbal approach focuses also on strengthening the body's immune system and thus helping it to fight the virus.

Frequent colds can be a sign of a weakened immunity; they can also indicate a stressful lifestyle or poor diet and no amount of medicines can solve those. Combating a cold at the first sign of symptoms is also important. Rather than trying to ignore the increasing catarrh and sore throat until the cold is in full flood, it is important to start treatment immediately.

Echinacea is one of the best herbs to strengthen the immune system and garlic is especially helpful if the cold develops into a chest infection. Anti-catarrhals such as elder flower and yarrow can ease symptoms. Cut down on refined carbohydrates (sugar and white flour products), as these tend to encourage mucous, and eat plenty of fruit instead. Taking up to 5 g of vitamin C a day can also help.

See also Infections, recurrent

Herbal remedies and supplements which may help

Bioforce Satasapina Cough Syrup; Bioforce Satasapina Bon Bons; *ColdEeze; *Culpeper Elder Flower and Peppermint Mixture; *Culpeper Head Cold and Throat Mixture; *Culpeper Influenza Mixture; *Dorwest Garlic and Fenugreek Tablets; *Frank Roberts Cold Tablets; *Frank Roberts Drops of Life Tablets; *Gerard House Echinacea & Garlic; Gerard House Eez-a-Tea; *Gerard House Garlic Perles; Herbcraft Echinacea Formula; Herbcraft Garlic and Horseradish Winter Formula; *Lane's Cut-a-Cough; *Lanes Garlodex; *Lanes Herbelix Specific; *Lanes Honey and Molasses Cough Mixture; Neal's Yard Elderflower, Peppermint & Composition Essence; *Olbas Pastilles; *Potter's Elderflowers, Peppermint and Composition Essence; *Potter's Life Drops; *Potter's Peerless Composition Essence; *Revitonil; Rio Vitalis Lapacho.

External: Bioforce Po Ho Oil and Ointment; *Olbas Oil; Power Health Head Clear.

See also echinacea and garlic simples

COLIC

See Babies and children

COLITIS

See Irritable bowel syndrome

CONJUNCTIVITIS

See Eye problems

CONSTIPATION

Constipation used to be referred to as "the English disease" as Britons seemed to have an obsessive preoccupation with bowel motions and "keeping regular". Laxative products remain among the country's best selling over-the-counter products worth many millions of pounds every year.

However, prolonged use of laxatives should certainly be avoided: many work by irritating the bowel to encourage movement and over the years such constant irritation leads to weakness and damage, with the risk of diverticulosis.

There is no "standard pattern" of "normal" bowel movements. Some people go every day, others every other day or perhaps twice a day. Diet is, obviously, significant, with vegetarians and those eating a high fibre diet likely to have a more frequent pattern of bowel motions than someone eating mainly meat and refined carbohydrates. The food we eat also influences how long it can take to be excreted: for traditional people in the Third World it normally takes around 12 hours or less for food to pass through whereas for those eating a conventional Western diet it can be as long as 72 hours.

Low fibre diet combined with a lack of exercise – and often coupled with a sluggish lifestyle or personality – leads to what is sometimes called "flaccid" or "atonic" constipation. Constipation can also be associated with nervous tension and a hectic life style with little time to respond to the normal urge to defaecate. The sufferer is often so tense and stressed that the digestive system is unable to relax and allow normal functioning to progress. Stools are sometimes described as resembling rabbit droppings. This type of constipation can alternate with bouts of diarrhoea and may lead to the catch-all label of "irritable bowel syndrome".

Atonic constipation can be helped by exercise, a high fibre diet (or the use of a bulking laxative such as isphaghula) and abdominal massage. The stronger herbal laxatives which contain chemicals called anthraquinones and work by irritating the bowel, are useful for short-term treatments: this group includes senna, cascara sagrada, alder buckthorn, rhubarb root, aloes and yellow dock.

The "tension" variety of constipation often responds to bowel relaxants such as chamomile, valerian or wild yam. Gentle sources of fibre are preferable in this type of constipation so conventional "roughage" – such as bran – should be avoided, as should the anthraquinone herbs. Relaxation classes and a general reduction in stress levels are also important.

Carminatives, such as fennel seed, are often added to OTC constipation remedies to reduce the griping pains which strong laxatives can cause.
See Haemorrhoids, Irritable bowel syndrome

Herbal remedies and supplements which may help

Arkocaps Phytoclense; Arkocaps Phytosenalax; Arkocaps Phytofibre; BioCare Colon Care; Bioforce Linoforce; Blackmores Cape Aloes and Cascara; Discovery Coliclens; *Dorwest Natural Herb Tablets; *Frank Roberts B & L Tablets; Frank Roberts Constipation Tablets; Full Potency Herbs Liquorice RootVegicaps; *Fybogel; *Gerard House Gladlax; *Gerard House Pilewort Compound Tablets; *Heath & Heather Inner Fresh; Herbs of Grace BTA; Herbs of Grace BTB; Herbs of Grace Bulking Agent; *Herbulax; *HRI Golden Seal Digestive; *Lanes Dual-Lax Extra Strong; *Lanes Pileabs; Natural Flow Colonite; *Lusty's Herbalene; Natural Flow Psyllium Husks; Natural Flow Regular Ten Powder; Neal's Yard Cascara Capsules; Ortilax; Ortisan; Ortis Fruit & Fibres; * Potter's Cleansing Herb; *Potter's Out of Sorts

Tablets; *Potter's Senna Tablets; Power Health Pure Isphaghula; Professional Herbs Cascara and Rhubarb; *Regulan; Solgar Psyllium Seed Husks; Trimulina Isphaghula; *Weleda Clairo Tea; *Weleda Laxadoron Tablets; *Weleda Digestodoran Tablets.

CONVALESCENCE AND DEBILITY

Herbs have long been used as "pick-me-ups" and tonics when recovering from illness and exhaustion. Some can be quite specific: elecampane, for example, is an excellent tonic after influenza and is particularly useful for clearing lingering coughs. Others are more general and can be used whenever tiredness becomes a problem. Stimulant herbs in this category include ginseng, gotu kola and guarana.
See Tiredness and fatigue

Herbal remedies and supplements which may help

Arkocaps Phytoenergyze; Bioforce Neuroforce; *Fo Ti Tieng; Full Potency Herbs Astragalus Root Vegicaps; Full Potency Herbs Cat's Claw Tablets; Health Aid Liquid Herbal Booster; *Muir's Pick-Me-Up; Mycoherb Tri Myco Gen; *Potter's Strength Tablets; Power Health Pure Guarana; Reevecrest Bom-Dia; Rio Amazon Guarana Buzz Gum; Rio Amazon Guarana Jungle Elixir; Rio Amazon Guarana; SX Formula; Weleda Blackthorn Elixir.
See ginseng simples (Table 3), Siberian ginseng simples

COUGHS

Coughing is the body's natural response to any blockage of the airway. That can include dust and traffic fumes or mucous resulting from infection. Coughing can also be a symptom of more serious illness so professional medical attention is needed for any cough which persists for more than a few days or where there is no obvious cause.

Coughs can be dry and irritating or "productive" with phlegm which can vary in shade from white to green. Coloured phlegm generally indicates an infection and if it is streaked with blood then, again, professional medical help is needed. Dry coughs can often linger for weeks following a cold and in some cases coughing can be nervous habit.

There is a very wide choice of herbal cough remedies ranging from the strongly expectorant, which will encourage the production of phlegm, to the cough suppressants which can ease a persistent dry, tickling cough. Taking the wrong sort of remedy can do more harm than good. If there is an infection then suppressing the cough and keeping the infected phlegm in the lungs is not a good idea. Equally if there is no phlegm then taking an expectorant will just make a tickling cough more violent. Many herbal expectorants are believed to work by irritating the stomach lining which causes a reflex action in the lungs encouraging coughing. In large doses these herbs are often emetics (they cause vomiting) so taking extra doses in the hope of clearing the cough more rapidly can lead to nausea. Herbal expectorants are sometimes classified as either "stimulating" – which encourage ever more productive coughing – or "relaxing", which have a more soothing effect and loosen phlegm rather than encouraging its violent removal.

As well as expectorants and suppressants, herbal cough remedies usually include demulcents, which soothe irritated mucous membranes, and antibacterials to combat infection.

When buying over-the-counter herbal cough mixtures it is important to match the action of the herbs they contain to the cough symptoms. Relaxing expectorants and demulcents for asthmatic and irritable coughs, stimulating expectorants for congestive conditions or suppressants for lingering irritating or nervous coughs.

- Stimulating expectorants include: asafoetida, balm of gilead, bloodroot, bryony, ipecacuanha, queen's delight, squill, white horehound, cowslip, bittersweet, elecampane
- Relaxing expectorants include: coltsfoot, marshmallow, ribwort plantain, liquorice, aniseed, lungwort, lungmoss, hyssop, gumplant, pleurisy root, sundew, pill-bearing spurge
- Demulcents include many of the relaxing expectorants: marshmallow, ribwort plantain, mullein, lungwort, lungmoss, Iceland moss, Irish moss
- Antibacterial herbs found in cough remedies include: garlic, thyme, hyssop
- Herbal cough suppressants include: wild cherry bark, aniseed and sedatives like wild lettuce

Herbal remedies and supplements which may help

Arkocaps Phytocoff; Bioforce Bronchosan; Bioforce Drosinula Cough Syrup; Bioforce Petasan Syrup; Bioforce Satasapina Cough Syrup; Bioforce Satasapina Bon Bons; Bioforce Usneasan Cough Lozenges; *Bio-Strath Thyme Formula; Blackmores Euphorbia Complex; Blackmores Liquorice Complex; Bumbles Propolis, Aniseed and Liquorice Lozenges; *ColdEeze; *CoughEeze; *Culpeper Balm of Gilead Cough Mixture; *Culpeper Cough Relief Mixture; *Dorwest Garlic and Fenugreek Tablets; *Gerard House Garlic Perles; *Gerard House Lobelia Compound *Hactos Cough Mixture; *Heath & Heather Balm of Gilead Cough Mixture; *Heath & Heather Balm of Gilead Cough Pastilles; *Heath & Heather Catarrh; Herbcraft Echinacea Formula; Herbcraft Echinacea, Eyebright and Bilberry Formula; Herbcraft Mullein Formula; *Höfels Original One-a-Day Garlic Pearles; *Höfels One-a-Day Garlic with Parsley; *Lane's Cut-a-Cough; *Lane's Sage and Garlic Catarrh Remedy; *Lanes Honey and Molasses Cough Mixture; *Lusty's Garlic Perles; Neal's Yard Balm of Gilead; Neal's Yard Echinacea & Mallow Linctus; Neal's Yard Horehound & Honey Lozenges; Neal's Yard Horehound & Aniseed Linctus; *Potter's Antibron Tablets; *Potter's Balm of Gilead; *Potter's Chest Mixture; *Potter's Horehound and Aniseed Cough Mixture; *Potter's Lightning Cough Remedy; *Potter's Vegetable Cough Remover; *Ricola Swiss Herb Lozenges; *Weleda Cough Drops; *Weleda Cough Elixir; *Weleda Herb and Honey Cough Elixir.

CRAMP

The severe pain of cramp is caused by a sudden contraction of the muscles. Commonly this occurs in calf muscles which become hard and tense. Rubbing the muscle vigorously can bring rapid relief. It can be caused by unusual exercise, stress, tiredness or poor posture or there might be an imbalance in body salts. In hot weather cramp is often due to a shortage of salt related to dehydration. In hot climates salt tablets can be useful for those prone to cramps.

Herbal massage oils – such as those containing cypress, marjoram or basil – can be helpful and internal remedies containing wild yam, black haw, black cohosh or cramp bark can help relax muscles.

Herbal remedies and supplements which may help

Gerard House Wild Yam; Gerard House Cramp Bark; *Gerard House Ligvites
External: *Weleda Massage Balm with Calendula

CUTS AND GRAZES

Herbal alternatives to the usual mixture of orthodox antiseptic creams which fill the average domestic first aid box are now readily available. Always bathe cuts and grazes before applying creams. Either rinse the wound under running water or use cotton wool soaked in warm water taking care to wipe from the centre to the edge of the graze to clear any grime. Infusions of antiseptic herbs, such as marigold, also make a good wash. Pressing a clean tissue or gauze pad over the injury for a few minutes will stop bleeding.

Marigold, echinacea or tea tree creams are suitably antiseptic and can be used on open wounds. Aloe vera creams can also be used on grazes and there are also various combinations with St John's wort. In the past, comfrey was also generally recommended to encourage healing. However, since recent concerns over the toxic alkaloids it contains, most over-the-counter remedies based on comfrey advise that it should not be used on open wounds.

Herbal remedies and supplements which may help

Bioforce Echinacea Cream; Gerard House Garlic Ointment; Gerard House Calendula Ointment; Hartwood Aromatics Calendula Ointment; Herbcraft Aloe Lavender Spray; *Lanes Kleer Ti-Tree and Witch Hazel Cream; Herbs of Grace Calendula Cream; Herbs of Grace Witch Hazel Cream; *Lane's Number 44 Skin Ointment; Neal's Yard Echinacea and Propolis Ointment; Neal's Yard Calendula Ointment; Neal's Yard Hypercal Ointment; *Nelsons Calendula Cream; *Nelsons Hypercal Cream; *Nelsons Hypercal Tincture; Nelsons Tea Tree Cream; *Nelsons Healing Ointment; *Potter's Skin Clear Ointment; *Potter's Dermacreme Ointment; Thursday Plantation Antiseptic Cream; *Weleda Balsamicum Ointment; *Weleda Calendula Lotion; *Weleda Calendolon Ointment; *Weleda Hypericum/Calendula Ointment.

CYSTITIS

Cystitis simply means inflammation of the bladder and is generally caused by infections ascending through the urethra – the tube that links the bladder to the outside world – to affect the bladder lining. It tends to be more common in women as their urethras are much shorter: approximately 3.5 cm/1½ in compared with about 20 cm/8 in in men. It is one of the commonest of ailments affecting around half of all women at some point during their lives.

The symptoms will be familiar to many: a burning sensation on passing urine, a frequent need to do so, and a dull ache in the lower abdomen.

Like all opportunist infections the bugs which cause cystitis are common and only tend to get out of control when the sufferer is run down. Cystitis often occurs when the individual is tired, over-worked or under additional emotional stress. The bacterium which usually causes cystitis is *Escherichia coliform* (also referred to as *E. coli*), which normally lives quite happily in our bowels. The bacteria can be spread to the urethra by poor personal hygiene – wiping from back to front rather than front to back after a bowel motion – or they can be accidentally encouraged towards the urethra when inserting tampons or by sexual intercourse.

Indeed, cystitis can follow intercourse with monotonous regularity for some women, leading to a reluctance to make love that can put considerable strains on a relationship.

Washing the area between urethra and anus (the perineum) after each bowel motion can help reduce the risk of counter infection as can emptying the bladder within 10 or 15 minutes of intercourse and again washing the area. Bacteria thrive in warm, damp conditions so wearing loose panties, preferably cotton, and stockings instead of tights can help to keep the area around the urethra cool. Maintaining a more alkaline urine also discourages the bacteria so opt for a more vegetarian diet limiting meat intake, and avoiding acidic foods like rhubarb, oranges and pickles.

Recent research has highlighted that cranberry juice can relieve the discomfort of cystitis and a number of preparations containing cranberry extracts are now appearing. Also useful are the urinary antiseptics such as bearberry, couchgrass and juniper.

Herbal remedies and supplements which may help

Arkocaps Phytosistitus; BioCare CP227; BioCare UR 228; Bioforce Cystaforce; Bioforce Golden Grass Tea; Blackmores Cornsilk Complex; Cantassium Concentrated Cranberry; Frank Roberts Black Willow Compound Tablets; Frank Roberts Uva-Ursi Compound Tablets; FSC Cranberry Concentrate Tablets; Herbs of Grace Uroton; Neal's Yard Buchu Compound Capsules; *Potter's Antitis Tablets; *Potter's Kas-Bah Herb; Power Health Cranberry Juice; Solgar Natural Cranberry Extract with Vitamin C Vegicaps; Solgar Herbal Water Formula Capsules; *Uvacin.

DANDRUFF AND SEBORRHOEIC DERMATITIS

The familiar scurf of dandruff is generally made up of larger than usual flakes of dead skin which, in the normal course of events, would be more discreetly replaced every 28 days or so. Dandruff can also be caused by seborrhoeic eczema where over-production of sebum (the natural oil secretion which lubricates the hair) leads to oily, yellow flakes and often sore red patches on the scalp.

Both sorts of dandruff are believed to be caused, in part, by a fungal infection (due to *Pityrosporum ovale*) although unlike similar infections this is not contagious as it seems to depend on an individual over-response to the fungus.

Wearing hats can make dandruff worse – the hot, damp environment so produced is ideal for encouraging fungal growth – and use of medicated shampoos can sometimes worsen the condition because of the effect the detergents they contain have on scalp secretions and natural bacteria populations.

Cleansing herbs taken internally (as for other skin problems) can help with seborrhoeic eczema, while a diet low in fats and refined carbohydrates and high in fresh fruits and vegetables can also help.

Herbal shampoos containing West Indian bay (or bay rum), rosemary or stinging nettle extracts can be helpful.

Herbal remedies and supplements which may help

*Potter's Adiantine; *Potter's Medicated Extract of Rosemary.

DEPRESSION

While we all tend to feel down from time to time, clinical depression is a debilitating illness that needs professional help – preferably counselling and psychiatric help rather than anti-depressant drugs which can have side effects and will not necessarily provide a long-term cure. In traditional medicine depression was regarded as "melancholia" and was the result of too much "black bile" in the system. Black bile was considered as one of the four body "humours" (along with blood, phlegm and yellow bile) which had to be in balance to ensure good health.

An excess of black bile was treated with strong purgatives and digestive remedies to clean out the system. Interestingly, depression is often accompanied by constipation as intense sadness seems to shut down the digestive system.

A herbal approach generally involves countering any physical exhaustion and debility which may be contributing to the problem, stimulating the digestive system if need be, and using herbs which strengthen the nervous system. Herbs in this category which are found in over-the-counter remedies include wild oats, damiana, vervain, ginseng, lemon balm, skullcap, St John's wort and rosemary. While few herbal medicines will actually claim they can be used for depression, many will suggest they can help "counter everyday stresses" or can soothe anxiety or insomnia.

Bach Flower Remedies can also be particularly helpful, especially gentian, gorse and mustard; essential oils including basil, bergamot, chamomile, camphor, clary sage, jasmine, lavender, lemon balm, neroli, patchouli, rose, rose geranium, sandalwood and ylang ylang can also be included in massage treatments or added to bath water.

Herbal remedies and supplements which may help

Arkocaps Phytophrodisiac; Bioforce Ginsavena; Bioforce Ginsavita; Bioforce Neuroforce; Bioforce Hyperiforce; Blackmores Hypericum; *Frank Roberts Strength Tablets; *Frank Roberts Supa-Tonic Tablets; Gerard House St John's Wort; Gerard House Vig-a-Tea; Herbatone; Kira; Neal's Yard Scullcap Compound Capsules; *Potter's Strength Tablets.

DERMATITIS

See Eczema

DIABETES, LATE-ONSET

Late-onset diabetes is an all-too-common result of a lifetime of the worst Western diets with too many sugars and an irregular pattern of meals. While insulin-dependent diabetics should take great care with using hypoglycaemic herbs, unless under professional guidance, late-onset diabetes can generally be controlled by diet, with careful monitoring of blood or urine sugar levels, and here hypoglycaemic remedies can be beneficial.

Herbs to reduce blood sugar levels include: alfalfa, aloes, bean pods, bilberry, burdock, celery, cornsilk, damiana, elecampane, eucalyptus, fenugreek, garlic, ginger, ginseng, juniper, marshmallow, myrrh, sage and stinging nettle. Of these alfalfa, bean husks, bilberry, fenugreek, garlic and ginseng are probably the most practical to take as regular dietary supplements.

Given UK product licensing laws, no over-the-counter remedies can actually claim to help diabetes, but a number of continental brews are specifically marketed elsewhere in Europe as diabetic aids.

Herbal remedies and supplements which may help

Arkocaps Alfalfa; Arkocaps Phytoslim; Arkocaps Phytovainetone; Bioforce DBT (Diabetisan); Blackmores Alfalfa Tablets; Full Potency Herbs Fenugreek Vegicaps; Lamberts Alfalfa Extract; Solgar Alfalfa Tablets; Power Health Alfalfa
See also garlic simples (Table 2), ginseng simples (Table 3)

DIARRHOEA

Frequent loose or liquid bowel motions can be the all-too-familiar result of infection or irritation in the digestive tract. Excessive bowel motions can lead to cramping pains and general soreness in the anal area, while symptoms may include nausea and vomiting. Causes can range from food poisoning and over-eating to stress and anxiety.

Sudden diarrhoea is most commonly caused by some sort of gastro-intestinal infection – especially if others who shared the same meal are similarly affected. This is a common problem for holidaymakers who may find that local standards of hygiene in exotic locations are not quite the same as back home. When travelling in high risk areas never eat raw salads, always wash and peel fruit, avoid ice cubes in drinks and regard street-side hawkers selling "bottled water" with some suspicion.

Diarrhoea and vomiting are the body's natural reaction to an infecting organism and are often the best way of getting rid of it quickly. Taking the sort of anti-diarrhoeals which simply put a stop to the process can cause more harm than good and it is often best simply to soothe the digestive tract with astringent herbs and let nature take its course. Strong, cold tea is rich in tannins and can ease an excessively over-worked gut if nothing better is available.

"Gastric 'flu" and stomach chills can also lead to diarrhoea. Again symptoms are likely to be short lived and using astringent herbal mixtures (such as those containing agrimony or tormentil) combined with anti-infection mixtures, like echinacea, can help. Diarrhoea is very dehydrating and it is important to increase fluid intake during such bouts. This is especially important for small children Regular diarrhoea is more likely to be stress-related. This can range from that irritating, but largely harmless, increased frequency before exams or job interviews to debilitating disorders like ulcerative colitis which require professional help and can lead to long-term, chronic illness.

This sort of diarrhoea can be helped by the addition of calming and sedative herbs (such as valerian and skullcap) to the mixture.

See also Irritable bowel syndrome

Herbal remedies and supplements which may help

Bioforce Tormentavena; *Gerard House Cranesbill Tablets; *Potter's Spanish Tummy Mix; *Weleda Melissa Comp.

DIVERTICULITIS

Diverticulosis is a problem which usually affects the elderly and often follows a life-long history of constipation and excessive use of laxatives.

The problem is caused by a weakening of the muscular wall of the bowel so that small areas of the mucous membrane form pouches, or diverticulum, in which food remnants (particularly pips and seeds) can be trapped leading to inflammation (diverticulitis). The result is severe cramping pain often accompanied by fever.

Around 25% of adults suffer from some degree of diverticulosis in the large intestine and thus run the risk of diverticulitis. Avoiding foods which are likely to produce small, hard residues can be helpful, although the diet should remain high in roughage to prevent constipation which can similarly exacerbate the condition. Bulking laxatives, such as isphaghula, may be useful, as can soothing, mucilaginous herbs like liquorice, wild yam or marshmallow.

If an infection develops, echinacea, golden seal or myrrh can help and fenugreek will also help to relieve discomfort.

Herbal remedies and supplements which may help

Frank Roberts Golden Seal Compound Tablets; *Frank Roberts Althaea Compound Tablets; Full Potency Herbs Fenugreek Vegicaps; *Gerard House Fenulin; Gerard House Wild Yam; *Lanes Biobalm
See also isphaghula simples

DYSPEPSIA

See Indigestion and heartburn

ECZEMA AND DERMATITIS

Eczema and dermatitis are both terms used to describe non-contagious inflammatory skin conditions. The skin is usually red and itching with a rash or spots which can resemble small blisters which "weep" – ooze clear fluid which forms a crust. "Dry eczema" involves a thickening and drying of the skin. There are very many causes for the problem: commonly an allergen is involved, which can be fairly obvious. In "contact dermatitis", for example, chemicals (especially cleaning materials) spilt on the skin may cause a rash to develop rapidly or rashes could result from metallic clasps such as ear-rings or bra fastenings. Nickel and chromium are often to blame and it is worth remembering that stainless steels generally contain nickel.

Other allergens are less apparent, as happens with eczema in small children where an underlying milk allergy is to blame and can be difficult to identify. Other dietary culprits include wheat, eggs, fruits and vegetables that are rich in salicylates (especially tomatoes, oranges, berry fruits, peppers and aubergines), or shellfish. Washing-up powder is another common culprit, as are house-dust mites and household pets.

Tension and anxiety can be contributory factors and eczema sufferers often find symptoms increase when they are worried or under additional work or family pressures.

In the elderly, poor circulation caused by inadequate venous return of blood can lead to yet another type of eczema – varicose eczema. This may sometimes (but not always) be associated with a tendency to develop varicose ulcers.

Herbal remedies for eczema and dermatitis are generally taken internally: as with other skin problems they tend to focus on cleansing herbs like burdock, yellow dock, red clover and heartsease.

External remedies often include chamomile or marigold which are good anti-inflammatory herbs. Essential oils, including lavender, rosemary or rose, can also be added, while evening primrose oil can be both applied externally or taken in capsule form.

Herbal remedies and supplements which may help

Arkocaps Phytoderma; Blackmores Echinacea Complex; Blackmores Sarsparilla Complex; Full Potency Herbs Burdock Root Vegicaps; *Gerard House Blue Flag Root; Gerard House Seaweed and Sarsparilla Tablets; Heath & Heather Skin; Herbcraft Burdock & Nettle Formula; *Lanes Kleer; *Potter's Jamaican Sarsparilla; *Potter's Skin Eruptions Mixture.

External: Bioforce Echinacea Cream; Gerard House Calendula Ointment; Gerard House Calendula Ointment; Gerard House Chickweed Ointment; Hartwood Aromatics Calendula Ointment; Health Aid Eczem Oil; Herbs of Grace Calendula Cream; Herbs of Grace Chamomile Cream; Herbs of Grace Chickweed Cream; *Lanes Kleer Ti-Tree and Witch Hazel Cream; *Lane's Number 44 Skin Ointment; Neal's Yard Stellaria Ointment; Neal's Yard Calendula Ointment; *Nelsons Calendula Cream; *Potter's Eczema Ointment; *Potter's Herbheal Ointment; *Potter's Skin Clear Ointment; *Rickard's Woodsap Ointment; Spring Wind Ointment; *Weleda Calendula Lotion; *Weleda Calendolon Ointment; *Weleda Dermatodendron Ointment.

See borage oil and evening primrose oil (Table 1) simples

EYE PROBLEMS

Herbal remedies can be helpful for a number of eye problems although if symptoms persist it is always best to seek professional treatment.

Blepharitis

This is an inflammation of the eye-lid. It can be an allergic reaction to cosmetics and is often accompanied by white scales on the lashes. In chronic cases the eyelid can become ulcerated with a yellow crust, the eyelashes are often matted and may fall out. Immune stimulants such as echinacea can help internally, while bathing the eye with diluted tincture or weak infusion of chamomile, elderflower or red clover can also help.

Herbal remedies and supplements which may help

*Gerard House Blue Flag Root; *HRI Clear Complexion Tablets; *Potter's Skin Eruptions Mixture.

External: Gerard House Chickweed Ointment; Neal's Yard Stellaria Ointment; *Potter's Herbheal Ointment.

See echinacea and garlic simples (Table 2)

Conjunctivitis

Also known as red eye, conjunctivitis is an inflammation of the fine membrane (conjunctiva) covering the eye-ball. Sufferers usually complain of severe pain, watering and a "gritty feeling" on blinking. Eye-baths containing well-diluted eyebright, elderflower, chamomile, marshmallow or marigold tincture can be helpful. Immune stimulants internally can also help.
See echinacea and garlic simples (Table 2)

Styes

Styes are an acute inflammation of a gland at the base of an eyelash usually caused by bacterial infection. They can indicate lowered resistance due to stress, over-work or repeated infection. Marigold cream may be helpful.

Herbal remedies and supplements which may help

Gerard House Calendula Ointment; Hartwood Aromatics Calendula Ointment; Herbs of Grace Calendula Cream; Neal's Yard Calendula Ointment; Neal's Yard Hypercal Ointment; *Nelsons Calendula Cream; *Nelsons Hypercal Cream; *Nelsons Healing Ointment; *Nelsons Hypercal Tincture; *Weleda Calendula Lotion; *Weleda Calendolon Ointment; *Weleda Hypericum/Calendula Ointment.

See also Infections, recurrent

Tired Eyes

We've all suffered from sore, tired eyes after too much reading or too much time spent in a highly polluted atmosphere. Eye-baths containing well-diluted eyebright tincture can be helpful or pads soaked in distilled witch hazel and applied for 5-10 minutes. Used chamomile or fennel tea bags also make a soothing compress, as do slices of cucumber.

Herbal remedies and supplements which may help

Kordel's I-Vista; *Weleda Larch Resin Lotion.

FIBROSITIS

See Backache

FLATULENCE

Wind – whether it goes up or down – is usually more of an embarrassment than indicator of serious health problems. Flatulence can be accompanied by stomach pains, bloating and cramps with rumblings in the lower bowel adding to the embarrassment.

Diet is often the problem. Some foods are essentially very "windy": old herbals usually stress this point when discussing beans and brassicas. Traditional recipes usually added carminative herbs in cooking to reduce the problem. Adding fennel, dill, rosemary or sage to our cooking not only improves the flavour but also adds herbs to stimulate and soothe the digestive system and reduce the risk of wind and indigestion.

Orthodox treatments usually concentrate on antacids whereas a herbal approach will be based on carminative herbs which interfere less with stomach acid secretions. Look for remedies containing such herbs as peppermint, fennel, anise, lemon balm and chamomile.

See Indigestion and heartburn

Herbal remedies and supplements which may help

*Culpeper Herbal Mixture for Acidity, Indigestion and Flatulence; Frank Roberts Acidosis Tablets; *Gerard House Golden Seal Compound; *Gerard House Ginger; *Gerard House Papaya Plus Tablets; *Heath & Heather Indigestion & Flatulence; Herbcraft Peppermint Formula; *HRI Golden Seal Digestive; Lamberts Peppermint Oil Capsules; *Lanes Biobalm; *Lanes Digest; *Natraleze; Obbekjaers Peppermint; *Potter's Indian Brandee; *Potter's Indigestion Mixture; *Potter's Slippery Elm Stomach Tablets; *Weleda Carminative Tea; *Weleda Digestodoran Tablets.

See ginger simples

FLUID RETENTION

Numerous over-the-counter herbal remedies will suggest – either in their promotional material or by a suitably watery name – that they can be used for some sort of abnormal "fluid balance" or "water retention". Some of these are aimed at easing symptoms of premenstrual syndrome (PMS) but others are thinly disguised slimming aids that can help reduce weight by acting as potent diuretics. As such they could be potentially damaging leading to an artificial dehydration that may appear to cut the kilograms but does little for general health. Popular diuretic herbs used in such remedies include parsley, celery seed, dandelion leaf, buchu, juniper berries and boldo. Some of these have significant side-effects. Juniper berries, for example, will lead to kidney damage in prolonged use and should never be taken continuously for more than three or four weeks without professional guidance. Such herbal preparations are inappropriate as "slimming aids" and should be avoided.

Where fluid retention is associated with PMS then treatment should be aimed at restoring balance to the cycle rather than simply encouraging urinary action, and "fluid retention" remedies should be seen as only part of the picture. Herbs like chastetree, which acts on the hormonal system, or Chinese angelica root (*Dang Gui*) can be more effective at solving the underlying menstrual disorders leading to the fluid imbalance.

Excess fluid retention can contribute to raised blood pressure and diuretics are often prescribed to reduce the fluid in the system and thus the volume in blood vessels and so reduce blood pressure. Do not take herbal remedies for "fluid retention" if you are suffering from raised blood pressure, without professional advice.

Herbal remedies and supplements which may help

*Aqualette; BioCare Celery Seed; *Cantassium Boldo Aid; *FSC Waterfall; *Gerard House Helonias Compound; *Heath & Heather Water Relief; Health Aid Super Boldo; HRI Water Balance Tablets; Kordel's Celery and Juniper; *Lanes Cascade; *Muir's Water-Ese; Neal's Yard Buchu Compound Capsules; *Potter's Diuretabs; *Potter's Watershed Mixture; Professional Herbs Uva Ursi and Parsley.

See chastetree simples

GASTRITIS

Gastritis means an inflammation of the stomach lining and is often the result of over-indulgence in rich foods and alcohol. Symptoms are similar to food poisoning with nausea, vomiting and diarrhoea. Chronic gastritis increases the risk of developing stomach or duodenal ulcers and is often associated with smoking or alcoholism.

Those prone to gastritis should avoid irritant foods – spices, tea, coffee, alcohol, fried foods and pickles – and eat smaller meals more regularly. Orthodox remedies, as with indigestion and flatulence, usually concentrate on reducing stomach acidity which can lead to other digestive problems. A herbal approach is more likely to include soothing mucilages and anti-inflammatories with herbs that will cover and protect the stomach lining and encourage healing. Slippery elm is one of the most popular remedies and is available in tablets or as powder which simply needs mixing with water.

Other popular herbs include meadowsweet, liquorice, chamomile and marshmallow. Older remedies often included comfrey, which is an effective healer for damaged mucous membranes, however, recent concerns over the potentially toxic alkaloids it contains have discouraged any internal use of the plant.

Herbal remedies and supplements which may help

Bioforce Gastrosan; *Frank Roberts Althaea Compound Tablets; FSC Bromelain Plus; *Gerard House Fenulin; *Gerard House Golden Seal Compound; Lamberts Chewable Bromelain with Papain; *Lanes Biobalm; Neal's Yard Slippery Elm; Solgar Bromelain Tablets; *Weleda Melissa Comp.

GOUT

For non-sufferers, gout tends to be in the musical-hall joke category associated with over-indulgence of port or rich food. The reality is quite different with this acutely painful disease which is often an inherited condition and not always afflicting those who eat or drink too much.

The pain is caused by a build-up of uric acid crystals in the joints – commonly the big toe joint – associated with an inability to break down a group of chemicals called purines that are found in shellfish, red meats and offal. Eliminating these from the diet will often reduce symptoms as will cutting out foods rich in fruit sugars (including sweet wines and port). Some suggest that a vegetarian diet is ideal for gout sufferers.

Oxalic acid, found in rhubarb, sorrel and spinach, is another food residue that can exacerbate the problem, so these foods too should be avoided.

Herbal remedies for gout generally contain celery seed which can help clear excess uric acid from the system.

Herbal remedies and supplements which may help

BioCare Celery Seed; *Gerard House Celery; Kordel's Celery 3000 Plus; *Heath & Heather Celery Seed; *FSC Waterfall.
See devil's claw simples

GUM DISEASE – GINGIVITIS, BLEEDING GUMS

Gum disease is usually the result of poor oral hygiene and if untreated can lead to loosening and eventual loss of teeth. Regular and correct brushing is important as is eating foods which contain roughage that can help clean the teeth as they are chewed. The traditional "apple a day" is an extremely effective herbal remedy! Herbal mouthwashes can help bleeding or inflamed gums. Remedies containing myrrh, sage or marigold can be particularly effective.

Herbal remedies and supplements which may help

*Bio-Strath Chamomile Formula; Reevecrest Gum Thyme
External: *Weleda Medicinal Gargle

HAEMORRHOIDS

See Piles

HALITOSIS

See Bad breath

HANGOVERS

Headaches, nausea and diarrhoea are the usual result of excessive intake of alcohol. The obvious solution is to drink only in moderation, but for the occasional over-indulgence herbs can bring relief. Remedies for gastritis (such as those containing slippery elm and marshmallow) can ease the nausea and heartburn while large doses of evening primrose oil (1-2 g on the morning after) can help to normalize liver funtion.

A useful herb is milk thistle seed which actually helps to repair the liver damage that can result from alcohol abuse. It is also very protective: milk thistle seed taken before the binge will often prevent unpleasant side effects next morning, but the herb should not be regarded as a passport to pain-free drinking! Also important is kudzu vine which is known to reduce the desire for alcohol and has been used successfully in treating alcoholics.

Herbal remedies and supplements which may help

*Bio-Strath Artichoke Formula; BioCare Silymarin Complex; FSC Milk Thistle Tablets; Full Potency Herbs Milk Thistle Vegicaps; Lamberts Silymarin Extract.
See evening primrose simples (Table 1)

HAY FEVER AND ALLERGIC RHINITIS

Although hay fever is associated with pollen allergies in the summer months, the symptoms can be triggered by a range of all-year problems including house dust, animal hairs and car fumes.

Strictly speaking, hay fever refers just to problems caused by grasses, but many sufferers find their symptoms can start in spring when flowering currants and elders start to bloom and they continue through to late autumn when the fungal spores arrive.

Typical symptoms include sneezing, sore and watering eyes, running noses and drowsiness. Around one in six teenagers in the UK tends to be affected and it is a major cause of missed exams and absenteeism. The physical symptoms are largely due to the body's production of histamine as it attempts to rid itself of the allergen and orthodox treatments are generally based on anti-histamines.

The herbal approach involves strengthening the mucous membranes to help reduce the likely allergic response: useful herbs include ribwort plantain, elder flowers, golden seal and ground ivy. Anti-allergenic herbs like chamomile and thyme oil can help reduce symptoms while eyebright, primarily an anti-catarrhal, can be very effective.

Herbal remedies and supplements which may help

*Cantassium Hay Fever; *Frank Roberts Sinus and Hay Fever Tablets; Full Potency Herbs Eyebright Vegicaps; Kordel's Horseradish, Odourless Garlic and Vitamin C; *Lanes Herbelix Specific.
External: *Weleda Gencydo Ointment.

HEAD LICE

Epidemics of head lice are very common in schools and the usual medicated shampoos suggested often contain quite potent chemicals that parents are understandably reluctant to use on children.

Lice are tiny brown insects about the size of a pinhead and they lay six to eight eggs a day at the base of the hair shafts (usually at the nape of the neck or behind the ears). These eggs hatch to produce white nymphs and discarded egg husks (nits). These live for about 20 days in an immature form – happily feeding on blood from the scalp – before pupating to the mature insect. Lice do not fly or jump they simply walk from one head to another which is easily achieved in the close confines of the classroom or playground.

Traditionally, parents would regularly comb their children's hair with a fine-toothed comb and the child would lean forward over a piece of plain paper or a mirror to see if any lice, nits or nymphs fell out. It is still the easiest way to detect their presence if a child seems to be scratching his or her head more than usual.

A useful alternative to chemical treatments is tea tree oil which is one of the very few essential oils that can be used directly on the skin without dilution. Use a fine-toothed comb sprinkled with a little oil and comb the hair well; in addition add 10–20 drops of oil to a pint of warm water and use as a final hair rinse after shampooing. Repeat the combing treatment every day for two weeks and then repeat as required.

A strong immune system is said to help prevent infestation so taking garlic supplements may help.

See tea tree simples

HEADACHES AND MIGRAINES

Herbalists tend to regard a headache as a symptom of some underlying disorder rather than an illness in its own right. Causes are numerous and the location and character of the pain is often an indication of what the problem may be. Headaches that seem centred behind the eyes can often suggest an underlying digestive disturbance, those that seem to start at the back of the neck and creep forward are generally tension headaches, while pain and sensitivity around the eyes or above the nose can be caused by a sinus problem.

For some people, tension headaches are extremely common at stressful times; others may find that stress highlights a different area of weakness with stomach upsets or urinary problems. Relaxing herbs, such as vervain, skullcap, lavender and St John's wort can be helpful to ease symptoms while Siberian ginseng can improve one's stress tolerance and thus reduce the risk of headaches in the first place.

Muscle strain in the shoulders and neck can also contribute to head pain. Sitting or working awkwardly, hunched over a desk or computer keyboard can easily lead to headaches. Massage oils containing herbs such as thyme, lavender, eucalyptus or juniper rubbed into the affected areas can also help prevent headaches developing.

Migraine is an especially common problem and is typically preceded by visual disturbances: jagged lights at the edge of the visual field or a sense that there is a strange out-of-focus area in what one sees. Sometimes the attack may simply comprise these visual upsets and there is no following headache, although sadly for sufferers this is rarely the case. Other symptoms include increased sensitivity to light which can often only be relieved by lying in a darkened room.

Migraines can be associated with gastric disturbance (nausea and vomiting) and frequent bilious attacks in a child may lead to migraine as it grows older. Identifying the cause is again important: this may be food intolerance or be stress related. Red wine, chocolate, pork, citrus fruits, coffee and cheese are all common culprits. Attacks are believed to be caused by a sudden constriction of the blood vessels in the brain followed by over-relaxation and increased blood flow. Generally only one side of the body is affected: the pain is usually one sided and there might be pins and needles in one arm or hand as well.

Many sufferers find that chewing feverfew leaves can help prevent attacks. This herb can cause ulceration of the mucous membranes in sensitive individuals (usually in the form of mouth ulcers) and it should not be taken if this side-effect develops. Lavender oil massaged into the temples can sometimes help prevent an attack developing, while among herbs that can ease the pain once it starts are Jamaica dogwood, valerian, or lavender.

Persistent or sudden unusually severe headaches, lasting for three days or more should be referred to a medical practitioner.

Herbal remedies and supplements which may help

Kordel's Feverfew and Willow; *Potter's Anased Pain Relief Tablets.
See feverfew simples

HEARTBURN

See Indigestion and heartburn

HEAVY PERIODS (MENORRHAGIA)

See Menstrual problems

HIGH BLOOD PRESSURE

High blood pressure generally needs professional treatment rather than over-the-counter remedies. Causes vary but can involve arteriosclerosis with narrowing of the arteries, heart disease, anxiety and tension or kidney disease.

Herbal relaxants help to ease the stresses contributing to the problem, while several plants are also effective at dealing with arteriosclerosis. Garlic is probably the best known remedy for countering the fatty deposits which build-up in the arteries, and has been shown to reduce the levels of cholesterol circulating in the blood after a fatty meal. Remedies containing ginkgo, gugulon, lime flowers and mistletoe are also worth considering. Rutin supplements can help improve the quality of arteriole walls and buckwheat is a good natural source.

As well as treating the underlying cause, herbal remedies for blood pressure often take an orthodox approach combining herbs which dilate the blood vessels with diuretics so that the capacity of the system is increased while the volume of fluid in the circulation is reduced, so leading to an over-all reduction in pressure. Diuretics commonly used in OTC preparations include dandelion leaf, juniper berries, parsley, cornsilk and clivers. Relaxants include cramp bark, yarrow and lime flowers. Hawthorn is a widely used herbal treatment for high blood pressure: it improves the coronary circulation and acts as a heart tonic stabilizing the blood pressure.

A remedy from Hildegard of Bingen that can be useful is galangal which is particularly useful where the high blood pressure is associated with angina pectoris.

Herbal remedies and supplements which may help

Arkocaps Phytochol; Bioforce Arterioforce; Blackmores Cactus & Hawthorn; East West Ju Hua Tea; Frank Roberts BP Tablets; Full Potency Herbs Hawthorn Berry Vegicaps; Gerard House Hawthorn; Herbs of Grace Beat Easy; Potter's Buckwheat Tablets; Power Health Hawthorn; Rutivite.

HIVES

See Urticaria

HYPERTENSION

See High blood pressure

INDIGESTION AND HEARTBURN

Rushed meals, wearing tight belts, eating irregularly or while feeling tense, or perhaps too many rich and potentially irritant foods can all contribute to those feelings of heartburn, pain in the lower chest, flatulence and nausea that go under the label of indigestion.

The vast majority of indigestion sufferers never seek professional help, accepting the disorder as "just one of those things" and trying an assortment of antacid remedies to solve the problem. Unfortunately artificially trying to reduce the normal acid secretions of the stomach often simply stimulates it to produce more in an attempt to restore balance and ensure that the digestion process runs smoothly, so antacids can be counter productive.

Herbal remedies take a rather different approach: relaxing herbs, such as chamomile and lemon balm, will help to reduce the anxiety and tension which can contribute to indigestion while aromatic carminatives will ease flatulence and nausea. Fennel, lemon balm, dill, cinnamon, ginger, chamomile and peppermint are all effective.

Other herbs, such as meadowsweet, Irish moss and slippery elm, will help to protect the stomach from high acid secretions while bitter remedies like yellow gentian, dandelion root or barberry all help to stimulate the digestive process and restore normal function.

Heartburn can be a particular problem in both chronic obesity and pregnancy where the stomach is forced upwards and the muscle, which divides the oesophagus from the stomach and normally prevents food returning to the gullet, is weakened. Acid reflux thus occurs with the highly acidic contents of the stomach returning to the oesophagus which can lead to inflammation and eventually ulceration. A hiatus hernia, where part of the stomach is forced upwards through the diaphragm, causes similar high acidity problems. Raising the head of the bed by 15–20 cm/6–8 in by putting normal house bricks under the legs will prevent acid flowing out of the stomach at night and can prove a very simple way of reducing symptoms.

The pain of indigestion can be confused with heart pain from disorders like angina pectoris. This sort of pain eases with rest, while heartburn is generally worse when the sufferer lies down.

Sudden severe "indigestion" in someone who has previously been symptom free should always be professionally investigated for a possible underlying heart condition. Chronic indigestion can also be a sign of peptic ulcers, gall bladder disorders, liver problems or cancer and expert diagnosis is essential.

Herbal remedies and supplements which may help

BioCare Gastroplex; BioCare Eradicidin Forte; *Bio-Strath Artichoke Formula; Blackmores Slippery Elm; *Box's Far Famed Indigestion Tablets; *Culpeper Herbal Mixture for Acidity, Indigestion and Flatulence; *Dorwest Digestive Tablets; Frank Roberts Acidosis Tablets; *Frank Roberts Nervous Dyspepsia Tablets; Full Potency Herbs Chamomile Vegicaps; *Gerard House Ginger; *Gerard House Golden Seal Compound; Gerard House Marshmallow and Peppermint; *Gerard House Papaya Plus Tablets; *Gerard House Slippery Elm Tablets; *Heath & Heather Indigestion & Flatulence; Herbcraft Peppermint Formula; Lamberts Peppermint Oil Capsules *Lanes Biobalm; *Lanes Digest; *Natraleze; Neal's Yard Slippery Elm; Obbekjaers Peppermint; *Potter's Acidosis; *Potter's Appetiser Mixture; *Potter's Indian Brandee; *Potter's Indigestion Mixture; *Potter's Slippery Elm Stomach Tablets; Power Health Peppermint Oil; *Weleda Digestodoran Tablets.

INFECTIONS, RECURRENT

Persistent colds, crops of boils, chronic fatigue or repeated urinary infections, can often indicate reduced resistance. The body's immunity can be stretched by stress, over-work and food allergies making it harder to combat bacteria, viruses and fungi. Many common organisms are extremely opportunist and while we all harbour numerous potentially lethal bacteria, if the system is weakened in any way these can very rapidly get out of hand.

Many tonic herbs have a reputation for strengthening the immune system and anyone feeling generally run down or suffering constant minor infections may benefit. Garlic, echinacea and the various types of ginseng have long been used in this way and all are generally best taken for short periods of three or four weeks followed by a break.

A number of traditional Chinese tonics can also boost the immune system and some are becoming available in the West: astragalus, reishi, and shiitake mushroom can all be very effective. Other more modern arrivals on the health food shelves include guarana and cat's claw.

Herbal remedies and supplements which may help

Arkocaps Phytoenergyze; BioCare Buccalzyme; BioCare Ginkgo Plus; Full Potency Herbs Astragalus Root Vegicaps; Full Potency Herbs Cat's Claw Tablets; Full Potency Herbs Echinacea/Goldenseal/Cat's Claw Complex Vegicaps; Health Aid Liquid Herbal Booster; Herbcraft Reishi Shiitake; Imuno-Strength; Mycoherb Bai Mu Gen; Mycoherb Cordy Gen; Mycoherb Grifo Gen; Mycoherb Myco Forte; Mycoherb Rei Gen; Mycoherb Rei Shi Gen; Mycoherb Shi Gen; Mycoherb Tri Myco Gen; Power Health Pure Guarana; Reevecrest Bom-Dia; Rio Amazon Guarana Buzz Gum; Rio Amazon Guarana Jungle Elixir; Rio Amazon Guarana; Three G's.
See also echinacea and garlic simples (Table 2)

INFLUENZA

Influenza is caused by a virus and thus will not respond to conventional antibiotic treatments. True influenza can be severe and in cases life-threatening with headaches, painful muscles, weakness and high temperature, as well as all the usual symptoms of a bad cold. An attack will typically last for about a week but will often leave the sufferer feeling depressed and debilitated for some time. 'Flu is a particular problem for the elderly, very young, diabetics and those suffering from chronic chest, heart or kidney disorders.

Herbal remedies will generally be similar to those used for the common cold with particular emphasis on plants like boneset, pleurisy root, garlic, ginger, horseradish and elder. Plenty of echinacea can also help with fever remedies as appropriate.
See Common colds, Convalescece and debility, Coughs

Herbal remedies and supplements which may help

Bioforce Bronchosan; *ColdEeze; *Culpeper Elder Flower and Peppermint Mixture; *Culpeper Influenza Mixture; *Frank Roberts Cold Tablets; *Gerard House Echinacea & Garlic; *Potter's Life Drops; Rio Vitalis Lapacho.

External: Power Health Head Clear

See echinacea and garlic simples (Table 2)

INSECT BITES AND STINGS

For most people insect bites and stings in Britain lead to little more than local irritation which eases in a few days. For an unfortunate minority stings can lead to severe allergic reactions and may be fatal. Typical symptoms include dizziness, sickness, breathing problems and marked swelling of the affected area. Immediate emergency medical treatment is vital in such cases.

Bees will only sting if they or their hive are attacked, as the hooked barb on the sting cannot be withdrawn and the insect dies defending itself. Wasps have a straight sting and can, rather unpleasantly, repeatedly attack their victims. Bee stings are acidic and in traditional first aid were treated with blue-bag (an alkaline starch used in washing) or bicarbonate of soda, while alkaline wasp stings were soothed by vinegar. Both, however, respond well to slices of onion.

Mosquitoes and gnats can be equally troublesome in the summer and in sensitive individuals can lead to weeping sores that will take several days to heal.

Over-the-counter herbal creams based on St John's wort, marigold, sage or lemon balm can bring relief. Aloe vera plants also contain a cooling sap that will reduce irritation and commercially available aloe vera ointment can be used as an alternative. If bites become infected echinacea or tea tree creams can be helpful.

Keeping the insects away is another method of tackling the problem and several herbal oils will help here. Tea tree, lemon balm and lemongrass oils can all help to keep insects at bay: spray some of these oils, well-diluted in water, over clothing and exposed skin.

Herbal remedies and supplements which may help

External: Bioforce Echinacea Cream; Golden Yellow Ointment; *Lane's Number 44 Skin Ointment; *Nelsons Pyrethrum Spray; Nelsons Tea Tree Cream; *Potter's Skin Clear Ointment; Thursday Plantation Antiseptic Cream; Thursday Plantation Walkabout; *Weleda Comburdoron Ointment.

INSOMNIA

See Sleeplessness

IRRITABLE BOWEL SYNDROME

Irritable bowel syndrome is a convenient label for a range of symptoms typical of poor digestive function, anxiety or food intolerance. Sufferers usually complain of bloating, flatulence, abdominal pain and alternating bouts of diarrhoea and constipation. Stools may contain mucus and blood or else resemble rabbit droppings.

Food intolerance is a very common cause: one study suggests that two-thirds of IBS sufferers actually display some sort of food allergy. Main culprits include dairy foods, gluten (found in wheat, oats, barley and rye), caffeine-containing drinks, alcohol, cigarettes, eggs and red meat. If food intolerance is the cause then it is important to identify and avoid the problem categories. Eliminating them from the diet and then gradually reintroducing each one usually pinpoints the culprit but the process really needs professional guidance.

Soothing herbs such as marshmallow, wild yam and meadowsweet can help, as can digestive tonics and stimulants like angelica, hops, peppermint, golden seal and milk thistle. Astringents such as American cranesbill and agrimony are often added to remedies to ease the symptoms of diarrhoea.

Herbal remedies and supplements which may help

BioCare Salicidin; Bioforce Gastrosan; *Culpeper Herbal Tonic for Digestive Disorders; *Frank Roberts Althaea Compound Tablets; Frank Roberts Golden Seal Compound Tablets; FSC Bromelain Plus; Full Potency Herbs Goldenseal Root Vegicaps; *HRI Golden Seal Digestive; Lamberts Chewable Bromelain with Papain; *Muir's Gastric-Ese; Solgar Bromelain Tablets; *Weleda Melissa Comp.

LARYNGITIS

Laryngitis is an inflammation of the voice box or larynx and vocal cords usually due to a viral or bacterial infection. It can cause hoarseness or even a complete loss of voice. If symptoms persist for more than a few days then professional investigation is needed in case there is some major problem such as a growth causing the hoarseness. Minor cases can be relieved by gargles containing sage or rosemary, and steam inhalations.
See Sore throats; Catarrh and sinus problems

Herbal remedies and supplements which may help

Bioforce Satasapina Cough Syrup; Bioforce Satasapina Bon Bons; Bioforce Po Ho Oil; Bioforce Usneasan Cough Lozenges; *Culpeper Head Cold and Throat Mixture; *Lanes Honey and Molasses Cough Mixture; Neal's Yard Lemon & Honey Lozenges; *Olbas Pastilles; *Ricola Swiss Herb Lozenges; Thursday Plantation Throat Lozenges; *Weleda Medicinal Gargle.

External: Bioforce Po Ho Ointment; Herbcraft Calendula & Goldenseal Spray; Herbcraft Liquorice and Propolis Spray.

LIBIDO, LOSS OF

Stress, over-work, alcohol, excess caffeine from too much coffee-drinking – the causes of low libido and problems with sexual intercourse are numerous. In chronic conditions professional help can be needed but more often than not a more relaxed approach to love making will be enough.

For centuries many herbs have been regarded as aphrodisiacs and although several of these traditional remedies are of doubtful efficacy, a few do have a demonstrable effect on the body's hormones and over-the-counter offerings include a variety. Few serious offerings will blatantly advertise their use as sex aids on wrappers and most prefer to emphasis their relevance as "traditional restoratives" or through slightly suggestive brand names.

For women, chastetree is widely used as an aphrodisiac in the Middle East where it grows wild, and although Western herbal medicine emphasizes its use in regulating female hormones, those taking it for PMS are occasionally surprised to discover its other effects. Schisandra has a similar reputation in the East for both men and women.

For men the most popularly used Western herbal aphrodisiac is probably damiana which features in numerous remedies. This is a good herb for countering tension and fatigue. Ginseng is another tonic herb which can also improve sexual performance and invigorates male energies, or for something more exotic, consider catuaba. Among essential oils, jasmine, ylang ylang, rose, patchouli and sandalwood all have an aphrodisiac effect and can be used in body massage or diffusers.

Herbal remedies and supplements which may help

Arkocaps Phytophrodisiac; *Gerard House Curzon; La Gelee Royale; *Potter's Elixir of Damiana and Saw Palmetto; Reevecrest Libidex 5; Rio D'Amor Catuaba.

LIVER AND GALL BLADDER PROBLEMS

The liver is the largest organ in the body and is often described as acting as its chemical factory: processing fatty acids, producing essential enzymes and storing nutrients. It is also important in maintaining the quality of blood, making the clotting agents fibrinogen and prothrombin, and acting as the storeroom for iron which is essential for haemoglobin (responsible for carrying oxygen around the body). The liver also helps to regulate blood sugar levels and produces vitamin A from precursors in the diet. It is important in the production of bile which is needed to digest fatty foods.

The liver is in the front line of the body's defences as it breaks down the various chemicals absorbed in digestion and prevents harmful substances reaching the circulation and brain. In our polluted world, the liver is thus under considerable stress to ensure that only safe and familiar substances are absorbed into the body.

Hardly surprising then, that this over-worked organ can become a little sluggish and lead to digestive problems. Many herbs have a potent effect on the liver to cleanse and stimulate, and while liver disorders in general require expert treatment, several OTC herbal preparations are offered as liver tonics of one sort or another. Some of these are simply marketed as general digestive stimulants, while a few can claim to regulate liver or gall bladder function.

Bile produced in the liver is stored and concentrated in the gall bladder. This can become infected or inflamed and gallstones can be formed if certain substances, such as cholesterol, become particularly concentrated in the bile. Gallstones may be quite symptomless, but if they become large enough to obstruct the gall duct they can lead to jaundice and severe pain. Heartburn after eating fatty meals often suggests that the gall bladder is not working as efficiently as it should.

Herbal cholagogues can often help normalize gall bladder function. These stimulate bile flow to improve the digestion and often have a laxative effect. They include greater celandine, barberry, silver birch, blue flag, golden seal, rosemary, sage, butternut, boldo, turmeric, globe artichoke, black radish, boneset, yellow dock, fringe tree and dandelion.

Bitter herbs generally act as liver stimulants. These include: globe artichoke, yellow gentian, centaury, dandelion root, wormwood, calumba, greater celandine, barberry, chicory, Oregon grape, boldo, bogbean, hops, white horehound, southernwood, white willow, holy thistle and gotu kola.

Others act as liver tonics to repair cells and restore normal function: milk thistle seeds, black root, dandelion root, globe artichoke, centaury, hart's tongue and bittersweet.

Herbal remedies and supplements which may help

Arkocaps Dandelion; Arkocaps Phytodigest; BioCare Liv243; BioCare Silymarin Complex; *Bio-Strath Artichoke Formula; Bioforce Boldocynara; *Blackmores Dandelion Complex; Frank Roberts Black Root Compound Tablets; FSC Milk Thistle Tablets; Full Potency Herbs Dandelion Root Vegicaps; Full Potency Herbs Goldenseal Root Vegicaps; Full Potency Herbs Milk Thistle Vegicaps; Herbcraft Dandelion Formula; Lamberts Silymarin Extract; *Potter's GB Tablets; Schoenenberger Artichoke Juice; Schoenenberger Black Radish Juice.

LUMBAGO

See Backache

MASTITIS

See Pregnancy and childbirth

MENOPAUSE

For most women the menopause passes by with little more inconvenience than occasional hot flushes and night sweats. Periods often stop suddenly without further problem or else gradually fade away in an irregular pattern. For others, the picture is quite different. It can be a time of major emotional upheaval, depression, weight gain and heavy bleeding. Today, many of these symptoms may be treated by hormone replacement therapy which boosts oestrogen levels, although critics still have doubts about the long-term effects of such treatment.

For some women (including those with a high risk of osteoporosis) this is a preferred solution, but for those who want to complete this transition period, then herbal remedies can prove beneficial in both relieving the more troublesome symptoms and helping the body to adjust to new levels of functionality. A normally healthy life style with good diet, regular exercise, a happy and fulfilled outlook and acceptable stress levels is obviously important. Anyone who starts out being depressed, overworked or malnourished is unlikely to pass through the menopause without trauma.

While professional herbalists generally aim to use a hormone-balancing mixture of herbs to help ease the change, OTC remedies usually focus on relieving symptoms, often with generous use of herbal relaxants.

Herbs with a hormonal action include chastetree, wild yam, helonias, sage and life root. Useful nervines for emotional stress include skullcap, lemon balm or valerian.

Among the more specific symptomatic remedies used for menopausal symptoms are golden seal, which can help with excessive hot flushes, and sage which reduces sweating. Hawthorn and motherwort can also be used for palpitations, another frequent menopausal symptom.

Vaginal dryness can often be helped with creams containing vitamin E and marigold.

Herbal remedies and supplements which may help

Arkocaps Phytomenopause; Bioforce Menosan; Efacal; Equillence; *Frank Roberts Motherwort Compound Formula; Full Potency Herbs Goldenseal Root Vegicaps; Glanolin 500; Healthcrafts GEB6 Combination; Herbs of Grace Menotune; Ladies Meno-Life Formula; LadyCare: For Women Going Through the Menopause; *Lanes Athera; Melbrosia PLD; *Potter's Wellwoman Herbs; *Potter's Wellwoman Tablets; Rio Paratudo Pfaffia.

External: Galen Calendula and Vitamin E Cream.

See chastetree, borage oil and evening primrose oil simples (Table 1)

MENSTRUAL PROBLEMS

Herbs have a long history of use for gynaecological problems and in many cases their very names suggest the association – motherwort, mother's hearts, lady's mantle, squaw weed and so on. Several of these plants can have a direct effect on the reproductive organs while others have a more general application. Pasque flower, for example, is often specifically used to relieve pain while raspberry leaf is well known for tonifying the womb, preparing for childbirth, and providing relief from some symptoms of premenstrual syndrome.

Although herbs have been used since long before hormones were ever dreamed of, a number do stimulate production of these essential chemicals. Chastetree berries (agnus castus) are widely used for menstrual problems. They act on the pituitary gland to encourage production of a number of sex hormones; it can help to normalize the cycle, relieve premenstrual tension and be useful at the menopause. Sage, too has a hormonal action.

Several herbs are used for period pain and their choice will depend on the nature of the discomfort. Herbalists tend to divide period pain into two types:

- Congestive pain which builds up shortly before the period starts. It is associated with blood stagnation and blood congestion and can involve bloating and fluid retention. It eases once the period has started.
- Spasmodic pain due to uterine cramps once flow starts and can be linked to a prostaglandin imbalance and emotional tension.

Motherwort and helonias are included in remedies to ease the stagnation sort of pain while pasque flower, black haw and black cohosh are included in remedies to help cramping pain.

Herbs can also ease excessively heavy periods: often these have no apparent cause and some women's periods are always heavier than others. However, it is important to seek medical advice if the pattern of flow changes significantly. Shepherd's purse (also known as mother's hearts) can be helpful as can American cranesbill and marigold.

Premenstrual syndrome also responds well to herbal remedies. Symptoms can include abdominal bloating, emotional disturbances and breast tenderness and the problem tends to be associated, in orthodox terms, with a too rapid fall in progesterone levels in relation to oestrogen. Conventional treatments thus tend to concentrate on hormone levels, and certainly chastetree berries make an ideal herbal alternative. Helonias, too, acts as a stimulant for ovarian hormones and may help as well. Herbalists, however, tend to regard PMS as rather more multi-dimensional than simply a case of hormones out of balance. Chinese medicine regards menstruation as involved with liver function and PMS remedies focus on energizing and tonifying this organ. Chinese angelica (*Dang Gui*), for example, is regularly used in China to "nourish the blood" and is a regular component of menstrual remedies.

Evening primrose oil has become almost a herb of choice for many PMS sufferers in recent years. The *gamma*-linolenic acid it contains is believed to help with production of the prostaglandin PGE_1. GLA is also contained in borage seed oil (often sold as starflower oil) and blackcurrant seed oil. It can be particularly helpful for relieving fluid retention and breast tenderness.

Numerous licensed herbal remedies are marketed for "fluid retention". These vary from simples containing chastetree to complex combinations of diuretics. Some are ideal for PMS symptoms but it is worth checking ingredients carefully rather than hoping that assorted diuretics will solve a complex syndrome.

Herbal remedies and supplements which may help

BioCare PT208; Arkocaps Phytopremenstrual; Cantassium Tong Kwai; Frank Roberts Alchemilla Compound; Full Potency Herbs Dong Quai Vegicaps; Gerard House Fem-a-Tea; *Gerard House Helonias Compound; *Heath & Heather Water Relief; Heath & Heather Raspberry Leaf; Glanolin 500; Health Aid FemmeVit; LadyCare: For Women with Monthly Periods; *Potter's Prementaid; *Potter's Raspberry Leaf.
• *See borage oil, evening primrose oil (Table 1), chastetree, and raspberry leaf simples*

MIGRAINE

See Headaches and migraine

MORNING SICKNESS

See Pregnancy and childbirth

MOUTH ULCERS

Mouth ulcers – or aphtha – are commonly occurring lesions found on the tongue, roof of the mouth and inside the cheeks. They usually start with a red, sore patch of blisters erupting to produce a greyish white ulcer. They can occur singly or in groups and most of us experience them at some time or another. They will usually clear of their own accord after a week or so but can be so painful that eating becomes almost impossible.

No-one really knows why mouth ulcers happen, although they can sometimes have an obvious cause as the result of ill-fitting dentures. They usually erupt when the sufferer is tired, over-stressed or fighting infections and they can sometimes be associated with digestive disorders and stomach upsets. Mouth ulcers are generally more common in those suffering from yeast infections and can be exacerbated by high sugar intake. Regular bouts of mouth ulcers can suggest some underlying weakness and a course of immune stimulant herbs and tonics can help: taking garlic pearles or ginseng for a month can help boost the system although it is better to save echinacea for short sharp bursts of treatment.

Herbal mouth washes using sage, cloves, rosemary, myrrh or echinacea can help relieve symptoms.

Herbal remedies and supplements which may help

*Bio-Strath Chamomile Formula; Bioforce Po Ho Oil; *Weleda Medicinal Gargle.
See echinacea, myrrh and sage simples

MUSCULAR ACHES, PAINS, STRAINS AND SPRAINS

Pulled muscles and twisted joints can be acutely painful and if they are the result of some accidental, traumatic injury then an X-ray can be necessary to identify possible fractures.

Strains involve a slight tearing of a muscle or the tendon attaching it to a bone and are generally caused by over-stretching. Sprains are a tear in the joint capsule or associated ligaments caused by twisting. Muscular aches and pains can also be associated with rheumatic problems and inflammation of the muscle or associated soft tissues.

Comfrey and arnica are ideal for treating any damaged tissue and are used in a number of over-the-counter creams. Arnica can be particularly useful for relieving pain while comfrey actually increases the rate of cell growth and so speeds healing. Avoid using both ointments if the skin is broken: arnica can be irritant while comfrey is under suspicion for containing toxic alkaloids. Homoeopathic preparations based on poison ivy and rue are also helpful.

Twisted or strained muscles can often respond well to herbal rubs. Massage oils containing eucalyptus, lavender, thyme, rosemary or camphor can be effective.

See also Rheumatism, Repetitive strain injury, Backache

Herbal remedies and supplements which may help

*Bio-Strath Willow Formula; *Frank Roberts Prickly Ash Compound Tablets; *Potter's Anased Pain Relief Tablets

External: Amber Massage Salve; Bioforce Comfrey Cream; Chirali Old Remedy Strain & Sprain Cream; *Culpeper Comfrey Ointment; *Culpeper Healing Ointment; Dr Shir's Liniment; Frank Roberts Comfrey Ointment; Gerard House Comfrey Ointment; Golden Yellow Ointment; Herbs of Grace Arnica Cream; Neal's Yard Arnica Ointment; Neal's Yard Comfrey Ointment; Neal's Yard Ginger and Juniper Warming Oil; Neal's Yard Rhus Tox and Ruta Ointment; Neal's Yard Sports Salve; *Nelsons Rhus Tox Cream; *Nelsons Strains Ointment; *Olbas Oil; Phytorhuma; *Potter's Comfrey Ointment; *Potter's Nine Rubbing Oils; *Weleda Arnica Ointment; *Weleda Massage Balm with Arnica; *Weleda Ruta Ointment; *Weleda Massage Balm with Calendula; *Weleda Rhus Tox Ointment.

NAPPY RASH

See Babies and children

NASAL CONGESTION

See Catarrh and sinus problems

NAUSEA AND VOMITING

Nausea and vomiting can be associated with a wide range of illnesses: from life-threatening fevers and stomach problems to motion sickness, migraines and indigestion.

It is important to seek professional help for severe and persistent problems but minor disorders, with a clear cause, can be helped by herbal remedies at home. Many herbs are, however, quite unpleasant to taste and for sufferers who really do dislike the flavour they can increase rather than ease symptoms.

For nausea associated with stomach upsets herbs such as lemon balm, dandelion, angelica or marshmallow can be helpful. Ginger is probably the most effective anti-emetic and is readily available.

See Indigestion, Travel sickness, Pregnancy and childbirth.

Herbal remedies and supplements which may help

Bioforce Gastrosan; *Dorwest Digestive Tablets; *Frank Roberts Nervous Dyspepsia Tablets; *Gerard House Golden Seal Compound; *Weleda Melissa Comp.
See ginger simples

NETTLE RASH

See Urticaria

NEURALGIA

Neuralgia means nerve pain and usually involves an inflammation of the nerve fibres. It can occur anywhere but is perhaps most common as an inflammation of the trigeminal nerve which runs along the side of the face and scalp. The pain is often exacerbated by cold and draughts and in very severe cases surgical treatment is recommended to cut the nerve. Herbalists use nerve tonics, such as vervain or St John's wort, as well as painkillers, circulatory stimulants (for example ginger and cayenne) and sedatives. Local application of lemon oil, lavender oil, St John's wort oil, or wintergreen oil may also help. Suitable internal nerve tonics include St John's wort, wild oats, damiana, skullcap and vervain.

Herbal remedies and supplements which may help

Blackmores Hypericum; Gerard House St John's Wort; Kira; *Potter's Anased Pain Relief Tablets.
External: *Nelsons Hypercal Tincture.

OSTEOPOROSIS

Many post-menopausal women these days are concerned about the risk of osteo-porosis with its loss of bony tissue leading to brittle bones, a tendency to fracture, and the characteristic "dowager's hump" as the spine bends. Small women with light "bird like" bones are believed to be at greater risk.

There are various theories as to the cause of osteoporosis in older women and one school of thought firmly blames hormones, urging hormone replace-ment therapy as a preventative. The value of this therapy is debatable, with HRT bringing its own health risks and the effectiveness of such treatments as a preven-tative for bone loss not fully proven.

Certainly regular exercise can prevent osteoporosis while a diet rich in cal-cium also helps. This could come from the numerous food supplements available or from eating calcium-rich foods, such as sesame seeds and paste (tahini), plenty of green vegetables and a reasonable amount of dairy products.

Sage tea was traditionally taken as a counter to old age and it is now known to have a hormonal effect – rather, perhaps, like weak HRT.

A number of calcium preparations are available combined with other useful supplements like fish oils (known to help counter rheumatic and arthritic disor-ders) and evening primrose oil which contains valuable essential fatty acids.

Herbal remedies and supplements which may help

Bioforce Urticalan; Efacal; Hartwood Aromatics Especially Yours; Herbs of Grace Phyto Calc.

See borage oil simples, evening primrose oil simples (Table 1)

PERIOD PAIN (DYSMENORRHOEA)

See Menstrual problems

PILES

Piles, or haemorrhoids, are a type of varicose veins which can easily be felt, like bunches of grapes, around the rectum. Around 50% of the adult population is likely to suffer from piles at some time or other in their life. When severe they can be extremely uncomfortable and make sitting quite painful, they can also bleed and have discharges of mucous.

Piles are often associated with constipation and over-straining. Although less severe piles can often be cured completely, once formed they do have a ten-dency to recur later in life and they can often be rekindled by over-exertion, such as lifting heavy weights or excessive physical exercise, as well as by recurrent bouts of constipation.

Established piles, which have prolapsed through the anus, can usually be easily felt at the rectum and fresh blood seen in the lavatory pan when passing stools. Internal piles, which remain inside the anus, are usually painless although they can give a blood-stained discharge and may be associated with anal itching. Numerous herbal remedies are available for treating piles: most contain an assortment of laxatives, such as aloes, senna and cascara sagrada, as well as astringent herbs that help to tonify the varicosed vein. Pilewort is an extremely popular remedy usually contained in ointments; other astringents used in pile remedies include agrimony and American cranesbill.

See Varicose veins

Herbal remedies and supplements which may help

Arkocaps Phytovarix; Culpeper Pilewort Tablets; *Frank Roberts Pilewort Compound Tablets – Green Label; *Frank Roberts Pilewort Compound Tablets – Orange Label; *Gerard House Pilewort Compound Tablets; Herbs of Grace Pilease; *Lanes Pileabs; *Potter's Piletabs.

External: *Culpeper Haemorrhoidal Ointment; *Frank Roberts Anti-irritant Ointment; *Frank Roberts Pilewort Ointment; *Lanes Heemex; *Nelsons Haemorrhoid Cream; *Potter's Pilewort Ointment.

POOR CIRCULATION

While poor circulation can be a sign of more serious heart problems it is often simply an inherited tendency bringing with it regular bouts of chilblains and the likelihood of "dead" fingers (Raynaud's phenomenon) in cold weather.

Herbal circulatory stimulants can often help: they include ginger, cayenne, cinnamon, angelica, and prickly ash. Buckwheat – a good source of rutin – can also help strengthen the blood vessels. Ginkgo is widely promoted as a circulatory remedy although its main action is on the cerebral rather than peripheral circulation.

Herbal remedies and supplements which may help

BioCare Ginkgo Plus; Blackmores Cactus & Hawthorn; FSC Ginger and Turmeric; Full Potency Herbs Butcher's Broom Vegicaps; Full Potency Herbs Bilberry with Ginkgo Biloba Vegicaps; Full Potency Herbs Cayenne Capsules; Gerard House Prickly Ash Tablets; Herbcraft Garlic and Horseradish Winter Formula; Herbs of Grace Vari-VN; Herbs of Grace Vital Flow; St. Hildegard-Posch Galangal and Fennel Tablets; Potter's Buckwheat Tablets; Power Health Circulating Compound; Professional Herbs Cayenne & Ginger; Pure-fil Rutin; Reevecrest Nutrimental Plus; Rutivite.

See ginger and ginkgo simples

PREGNANCY AND CHILDBIRTH

Herbs have a long tradition of use for easing the pains of childbirth and the ills of pregnancy: for generations of women they were the only available remedies and much folklore – as well as hard scientific evidence – testifies to their efficacy. Unfortunately, modern medicine and legislation means that few women in the West have the opportunity to use herbs in this way today and the choice of suitable over-the-counter products is extremely limited.

Like most orthodox drugs, many herbs will cross the placental barrier so it is unwise to take remedies unless you really have to. The list of herbs to be avoided in pregnancy (in therapeutic doses at least) is also quite long, and growing as suppliers increasingly err on the side of caution. Most licensed herbal remedies caution against use in pregnancy and lactation. With some remedies this is wise advice, with others it is questionable. Without specific professional guidance it is always better to follow the instructions on the packet to the letter.

Suitable over-the-counter remedies can be found, however, for some of the more common problems of pregnancy.

Morning sickness

This affects many pregnant women in the first three months and is, fortunately for most, confined to a few minutes on rising. For some sufferers, symptoms can last all day and extend through much of the nine months as well. Researchers have found that ginger is extremely effective even in these very severe cases. Up to one gram per dose has been used quite safely in hospital trials. Other herbs that can help include fennel, lemon balm, chamomile and peppermint. These are often best taken in drop doses of tincture.
See ginger simples.

Heartburn and constipation

Heartburn can be safely treated with slippery elm or marshmallow while for constipation (often exacerbated by the use of supplementary iron tablets) stay with the gentler remedies – isphaghula, butternut, yellow dock or dandelion root – rather than the more powerful anthraquinone laxatives (senna, cascara sagrada, alder buckthorn or rhubarb).

Herbal remedies and supplements which may help

Arkocaps Dandelion; Blackmores Slippery Elm; Full Potency Herbs Dandelion Root Vegicaps; *Gerard House Slippery Elm Tablets; Neal's Yard Slippery Elm Tablets
See isphaghula simples

Childbirth

Raspberry leaf has long been used to help women prepare for childbirth and helps to tonify the uterus and aid contractions. It should only be taken in the last six weeks of pregnancy. To help recover from the birth itself, homoeopathic Arnica 6× tablets taken every 15–30 minutes for a few hours will help repair stressed tissues.
See raspberry leaf simples.

Breast-feeding problems

Sore nipples in breast-feeding are commonplace: the cause is often poor positioning of the baby who should suck at the whole areola (the dark area around the nipple) rather than just holding on to the nipple itself. Marigold and chamomile creams can help considerably. Many herbs also encourage milk flow – fennel, dill, fenugreek and milk thistle – and can be taken in teas.

To dry up milk at weaning take sage tea.

Mastitis, an inflammation of the breast generally caused by bacterial infection through damaged nipples is also commonplace in breast-feeding. It can sometimes involve the discharge of pus and is extremely painful. The traditional herbal remedy is to apply a crushed cabbage leaf between breast and bra and, simple though this may seem, it is surprisingly effective. Echinacea taken internally can help combat infection.

Herbal remedies and supplements which may help

External: Bioforce Seven Herb Cream; Gerard House Chamomile Ointment; Gerard House Calendula Ointment; Hartwood Aromatics Calendula Ointment; Herbs of Grace Calendula Cream; Neal's Yard Calendula Ointment; *Nelsons Calendula Cream; *Nelsons Healing Ointment; *Weleda Calendula Lotion; *Weleda Calendolon Ointment.

See echinacea simples
See also Anaemia, Backache, High blood pressure, Insomnia, Piles, Thrush , Varicose veins

Herbs (mentioned in this book) to avoid in therapeutic dose in pregnancy, unless under professional guidance

alder buckthorn, angelica, autumn crocus, barberry, basil oil, black cohosh, blood root, cascara sagrada, cayenne, celery seed, chamomile oil, cinnamon, coltsfoot, cowslip, *Dang Gui,* fennel, fenugreek, feverfew, ginseng, golden seal, greater celandine, juniper, lady's mantle, lavender, male fern, marjoram, mistletoe, motherwort, myrrh, nutmeg, parsley, poke root, rhubarb root, rue, sage, senna, shepherd's purse, southernwood, thyme, vervain, wild yam, wormwood and yarrow.

Small quantities of the culinary herbs mentioned above, used in cooking, are quite safe.

PREMENSTRUAL SYNDROME

See Menstrual problems

PROSTATE DISORDERS

The prostate gland is one of the male sex organs and produces an alkaline fluid that forms part of the semen. It opens into the urethra, below the bladder. In elderly men the gland often becomes enlarged causing problems with passing water: the flow is reduced and residual urine often remains in the bladder leading to infection. Urine can also travel back from the bladder to the kidneys because of pressure differences, and can cause damage and reduced kidney function. Benign prostate enlargement is thought to be caused by accumulation in the prostate of the male sex hormone, testosterone, where it is converted to a potent chemical called dihydrotestosterone (DHT) which causes the spurt in growth. Although enlargement is generally benign, there is always the possibility of prostate cancer so professional diagnosis is important.

Orthodox treatment usually involves removing part of the prostate gland. However, the remnants will still retain the tendency for enlargement so the treatment may need to be repeated in time.

Saw palmetto berries are a proven treatment for benign prostate enlargement and are included in a number of OTC products. These do not always specify their use for prostate problems because of the licensing regulations, and tend to be offered as remedies for assorted urinary disorders or even promoted as aphrodisiacs.

Other useful herbs for prostate problems include horsetail, Siberian ginseng and cornsilk. Zinc supplements can also help and pumpkin seeds, a good source of zinc, make a valuable dietary supplement.

Herbal remedies and supplements which may help

Bioforce Prostasan; Frank Roberts Black Willow Compound Tablets; Full Potency Herbs Saw Palmetto Berries Vegicaps; *Gerard House Waterlex Tablets; Nature's Plus Prost-Actin; *Potter's Antiglan Tablets; *Potter's Protat; Power Health Pumpkin Seed Oil; Prostex; *Sabalin; Serenoa-C.

PSORIASIS

Psoriasis is one of the commonest skin complaints affecting around one in 100 people in the UK. It is characterized by itchy, dry skin covered in silvery scales that flake off to reveal inflamed, red areas. These can vary in size from less than 1 cm/½ in in diameter to covering almost the entire body in especially severe cases. Knees, legs, elbows, forearm and scalp are more commonly affected.

The cause of psoriasis is complex and related to auto-immune disease where the body's immune system seems to turn on itself and, in this case, causes an over-production of the epithelial cells which form the outer layer of the skin. Instead of skin cells dividing and shedding in the normal 25–28 days the entire process can take place once or twice a week.

Psoriasis often runs in families and in some cases it can be associated with arthritis. Anxiety can aggravate the condition and it can be linked to an over-tense personality unwilling to form close relationships and eager to keep people at arm's length. Severe shock can often trigger the start of the disorder or a recurrence.

Psoriasis generally starts in the late teens or 20s and can become a life-long problem. It tends to come and go for no apparent cause and will often disappear completely in the summer in response to plenty of sunshine and sea-bathing.

Herbal treatment usually involves cleansing skin herbs like burdock, nettles, red clover, Oregon grape vine or clivers as well as the use of nervines like skullcap or valerian to relieve any underlying anxiety and reduce tension. Bach Flower Remedies can be especially helpful. Heart and circulatory tonics can also be included in remedies as the constant over-production of skin can, in severe cases, put considerable strains on the system.

Alcohol should be strictly avoided as it dilates the peripheral blood vessels and so encourages skin cell production still further.

Herbal remedies and supplements which may help

Arkocaps Phytoderma; Full Potency Herbs Burdock Root Vegicaps; Heath & Heather Skin Tablets; Herbcraft Burdock & Nettle Formula; *Lanes Kleer; *Potter's Skin Eruptions Mixture.

External: Frank Roberts Phytolacca Cream; Frank Roberts Cade Oil Ointment; Heloderm CT Ointment; Heloderm CT Shampoo; *Potter's Parasolv Ointment; *Rickard's Woodsap Ointment; Spring Wind Ointment.

REPETITIVE STRAIN INJURY

RSI has become a *cause célèbre* in recent years with organizations like the National Union of Journalists vociferously campaigning on behalf of members who, it is claimed, are suffering a lifetime of ill-health as a result of using computer keyboards for many hours each day.

In the past similar ailments tended to be categorized by occupation: "upholsterer's hands" or "fisherwoman's fingers", but any repetitive task, be it typing, scanning bar codes in a supermarket or playing a musical instrument can lead to physical problems.

Repetitive strain injury often manifests as cramp-like pain or a burning sensation in the hands, arms, shoulders or back leading ultimately to fatigue, an inability to work effectively and depression.

Taking regular breaks from work is often easier said than done but it is important to try and vary the routines which have contributed to the problem. Baoding balls – Chinese massage balls slightly larger that golf balls – can help. These need to be rotated in the palm for 5–10 minutes each day, a slightly cumbersome skill that is not difficult to learn. Start with smaller ping-pong balls if you prefer.

Massage oils containing lavender, thyme, rosemary or eucalyptus can also provide some relief while internal muscle relaxing remedies containing wild yam, cramp bark or Indian tobacco can also be worth trying.

Herbal remedies and supplements which may help

Gerard House Cramp Bark; Gerard House Wild Yam.

External: Amber Massage Salve; Bee Brand Massage Oil; *Weleda Massage Balm with Arnica; *Weleda Massage Balm with Calendula.

RHEUMATISM

Rheumatism is a very non-precise term used to describe the various aches and pains suffered in joints or muscles at some time or other by most of us. It can include arthritis, fibrositis and lumbago, or may be referred to as "myalgia" which just means pain in the muscles.

Orthodox medicine generally prescribes painkillers while the herbal approach usually involves the use of cleansing herbs to remove any chemical toxins lingering in the tissues. Diuretics, digestive stimulants, circulatory stimulants and laxatives are all likely to be found in herbal remedies for rheumatism: kelp supplements are also sometimes recommended as additional support. Herbal painkillers – which offer a more gentle action than orthodox drugs – and anti-inflammatories are often included. Typical remedies are white willow, devil's claw, black cohosh, celery, guiaicum, burdock, clivers, bogbean or prickly ash.

Externally, as with osteoarthritis, remedies are likely to focus on warming herbs that will also stimulate the circulation by encouraging blood flow to a particular area. Plasters, soaked in stimulating oils like eucalyptus, camphor or rosemary can sometimes be found over-the-counter – especially from shops specialising shops in oriental medicine.

Herbal remedies and supplements which may help

Arthur's Formula; Bioforce IMP (Imperthritica); *Bio-Strath Willow Formula; *Cantassium Rheumatic Pain; Blackmores Celery Complex; *Culpeper Rheumatic Tablets; *Dorwest Kelp Seaweed; *Dorwest Mixed Vegetable Tablets; *Frank Roberts Rheumatic Pain Tablets; *Frank Roberts Prickly Ash Compound Tablets; *Gerard House Celery; *Gerard House Ligvites; Gerard House Prickly Ash Tablets; Gerard House Seaweed and Sarsparilla Tablets; Health Aid Devil's Claw with Royal Jelly; *Heath & Heather Celery Seed; *Heath & Heather Rheumatic Pain; Kordel's Celery 3000 Plus; *Lanes Vegetex; *Muir's Rheumatic Pain; Ortis Fresh Devil's Claw Drink; *Potter's Malted Kelp Tablets; *Potter's Rheumatic Pain Tablets; *Potter's Tabritis; *Rheumasol; Weleda Birch Elixir.

External: Arthur's Formula Cream; Arthurs Formula Bath and Massage Oil; Bee Brand Massage Oil; Chirali Old Remedy Strain & Sprain Cream; Frank Roberts Cajuput Rub; *Gerard House Dragon Balm Ointment; Harpago Gel; Neal's Yard Rhus Tox and Ruta Ointment; *Nelsons Rhus Tox Cream; Phytorhuma; *Potter's Nine Rubbing Oils; *Weleda Rhus Tox Ointment.

See devil's claw simples

SCIATICA

See Backache

SINUSITIS, SINUS PAIN

See Catarrh and sinus problems

SKIN PROBLEMS

See Acne, Babies and children, Eczema, Psoriasis, Urticaria

SLEEPLESSNESS

There's an old country saying that a woman needs six hours sleep, a man seven and only a fool needs eight. Few would wholeheartedly agree with such beliefs, but it is certainly true that the amount of sleep we each need varies and that at some times we need rather more sleep than at others.

Sleeplessness becomes a problem when sufferers feel tired and unable to concentrate during the day or when it becomes a worry in itself with seemingly endless hours spent tossing and turning in bed at night. In general the body will catch up eventually and a few bad nights are usually followed by a period of restful and restorative sleep.

There are many causes for disturbed sleep patterns: heavy meals late at night can lead to disturbed digestion, painful joints and muscles or irritating coughs will keep most people awake, while catnapping during the day simply fills up the sleep quota and there is no need for further rest.

Commonly, insomnia is associated with tension and worries and a failure to relax before bedtime. The majority of herbal OTC remedies for sleeplessness are based on sedative and relaxing herbs which will help to reduce anxieties, calm an over-active mind and encourage sleep. Unlike orthodox treatments they are non-addictive, although some find that with regular use the potency of herbal insomnia remedies is reduced and it can be worthwhile changing the mix regularly if long-term use is likely.

As always with herbal medicine, it is far better to identify and treat the cause of a problem rather than simply tackle the symptoms. If inability to relax or over-anxiety is the root cause of insomnia, meditation classes or a review of lifestyle might be a better solution than endless use of OTC relaxants. Herbal insomnia remedies are usually very similar in formulation to day-time treatments for anxiety and tension: look for those containing hops, wild lettuce, passion flower or Californian poppy as well as general-purpose relaxants like chamomile, skullcap, valerian, vervain or lemon balm.

Herbal remedies and supplements which may help

Arkocaps Phytodreams; Arkocaps Phytopremenstrual; Bioforce Dormeasan; *Bio-Strath Valerian Formula; *Cantassium Quiet Nite Sleep; Culpeper Valerian Tablets; *Dorwest Scullcap and Gentian Tablets; *Frank Roberts Calmanite Tablets; FSC Valerian

Formula; Full Potency Herbs Chamomile Vegicaps; Full Potency Herbs Valerian Root Vegicaps; *Gerard House Valerian Compound Tablets; Gerard House Sooth-a-Tea; *Healthcrafts Night Time; *Heath & Heather Quiet Night; Herbcraft Passiflora and Valerian Formula; Herbs of Grace Sweet Sleep; HRI Night Tablets; Kordel's Quiet Time; *Lanes Kalms; *Lanes Quiet Life Tablets; *Natrasleep; *Potter's Anased Pain Relief Tablets; *Potter's Nodoff Mixture; Power Health Passion Flower Oil; Professional Herbs Valerian; *Valerina – Night -Time; *Weleda Avena Sativa Comp.
See passion flower simples

SLIMMING

Around 20–25% of the population is reckoned to be seriously overweight and risking an array of obesity-related diseases – from heart problems to arthritis – as a result. At the opposite extreme, the desire to be fashionably thin can encourage an equally unhealthy attitude towards eating with the risk of such disorders as anorexia nervosa and bulima. Both these groups need professional help with their problems.

In between are vast numbers of people, at worst, slightly over-weight who spend much time trying out various diets and slimming products in the hope of shedding a few pounds.

Regular exercise and controlled eating are usually the best ways of losing weight, but they require discipline and usually need to be maintained for many months. It is all too easy to be tempted by the publicity blurb of some over-hyped slimming remedy which seems to promise instant thinness. Many of these products are based on herbs, the majority are unlicensed and several contain totally unsuitable plants.

While some herbs can have an effect on metabolism and could help with weight control, many herbal slimming products are basically a combination of diuretics and laxatives which cause weight loss by tampering with normal digestion. Certainly they can reduce weight in the short term, but it is a purely artificial effect. Over-use of laxatives can lead to disorders like diverticulitis in later life while too many diuretics can cause dehydration and interfere with the body's normal sodium and potassium balance leading to heart irregularities. Slimming products which contain laxative and diuretic herbs, like senna, cascara sagrada, alder buckthorn, rhubarb root, juniper berries, bearberry or boldo, should never be taken for longer than a few days at a time.

Other slimming products are bulking agents which fill up the stomach and discourage further eating. These can help to prevent over-eating but their misuse can also lead to cutting down too drastically on food intake. Some of the products sold as bulking agents for slimming also have a laxative effect, such as isphaghula husks: these do actually help reduce consumption of fats and create a feeling of fullness which discourages over-eating, however, the long-term use purely as a slimming aid should still be discouraged.

Various seaweeds (kelp or bladderwrack) are often included in slimming formulae. These are rich in iodine and other minerals and can help increase thyroid activity and thus metabolism so have gained a reputation as a slimming aid. However, consuming large amounts of kelp for a long period carries the risk of thyrotoxicosis and heart damage from thyroid overactivity.

Several herbal slimming products also contain malabar tamarind (*Garcinia cambogia*) which is believed to affect the metabolism of carbohydrates and thus preventing fat being deposited in tissues and prevent over-eating.

Herbal remedies and supplements which may help

Arkocaps Phytoshape; Arkocaps Phytotrim; Arkocaps Phytofibre; BioCare CitriMax Forte; Citri-Trim; *Dorwest Kelp Seaweed; *Frank Roberts Kelp and Nettle Compound; *Frank Roberts Reducing (Slimming) Tablets; Full Potency Herbs Green Tea Vegi-caps; *Gerard House Kelp; Gerard House Sleek-a-Tea; Health Aid Boldo Plus; Natural Flow CitriMax Fat Control Nutritional Complex; Phoenix Nutrition CitriMax; *Potter's Boldo Aid to Slimming Tablets; *Rickard's Slimwell Herbal Anti-Fat Tablets; Trimulina Isphaghula; Weight Logic.

SMOKING, GIVING UP

Tobacco smoking is reckoned to kill some 100,000 people in the UK every year through an array of smoking-related disorders that can include bronchitis, lung cancer and circulatory disease. Passive smoking can be just as harmful and is increasingly regarded as an anti-social activity adding to the pressures to give up the habit.

Stopping any addiction is extremely difficult and, not surprisingly, there is a wide assortment of products purporting to make it easier. Conventional remedies usually contain nicotine, which is the main addictive alkaloid in tobacco. By taking nicotine in the form of gum or absorbing it through the skin from patches, runs the theory, cigarette smokers can wean themselves off the habit. It is then supposed to be a simple matter to cut out the nicotine gum.

Heavy smokers faced with long-haul flights in non-smoking aircraft also resort to these various remedies. Some do report that excessive sucking of nicotine lozenges on such occasions can cause sores to develop in the mouth and gums.

Herbal treatments sometimes include Indian tobacco, which contains alkaloids that are similar to nicotine but are non-addictive. They thus allow the smoker to break the habit without becoming dependent on a nicotine substitute. Some smokers who have used these products claim that they are extremely effective as they appear to cause severe nausea if you use tobacco while taking them – which proves to be an extremely effective deterrent.

Herbal cigarettes, which are nicotine free but are said to provide the "tactile pleasure of holding and smoking a cigarette" during those first fraught weeks of withdrawal, are also popular and some claim they work well.

Herbal remedies and supplements which may help

Honeyrose Herbal Cigarettes; *Potter's Antismoking Tablets.

SORE THROATS

For many people a sore throat can be the first sign of a developing cold or it can suggest pharyngitis, tonsillitis or German measles. The inflammation may be caused by viral or bacterial infection and recurrence can be associated with stress or reduced resistance to infection.

Mild cases will often clear in two or three days with or without treatment but the discomfort can be eased by many of the over-the-counter throat lozenges and pastilles available.

Gargles are also helpful: use such herbs as sage, raspberry leaf or lady's mantle either in infusion or as 5 ml/1 tsp of tincture to a tumbler of water. Echinacea, golden seal or myrrh tincture are all just as effective although the taste is not so pleasant!

Herbal remedies and supplements which may help

Bioforce Satasapina Cough Syrup; Bioforce Satasapina Bon Bons; Bumbles Propolis Aniseed & Liquorice; Bumbles Propolis, Menthol & Eucalyptus; *Culpeper Head Cold and Throat Mixture; *Lanes Honey and Molasses Cough Mixture; Neal's Yard Lemon & Honey Lozenges; *Olbas Pastilles; *Potter's Elderflowers, Peppermint and Composition Essence; *Potter's Life Drops *Ricola Swiss Herb Lozenges; Thursday Plantation Throat Lozenges.

External: Bioforce Po Ho Oil; Bioforce Po Ho Ointment; Herbcraft Liquorice and Propolis Spray; *Weleda Medicinal Gargle.

STOMACH UPSETS

Minor stomach upsets with abdominal pain, nausea, diarrhoea and vomiting affect us all at some time. They can often be associated with food poisoning, an excess of rich food or too much alcohol when soothing herbs like slippery elm and marshmallow can bring relief. Other stomach upsets are linked to chills when warming herbs such as cayenne and ginger can be useful.

Some people are rather more prone to stomach upsets than others and the problem can be stress-related with an increase in nervous tension or anxiety levels usually accompanied by digestive problems. Relaxing carminatives such as lemon balm and chamomile can be useful in these cases.

Digestive stimulants such as yellow gentian and holy thistle are also included in some remedies.

See Gastritis

Herbal remedies and supplements which may help

Bioforce Gastrosan; *Bio-Strath Liquorice Formula; *Culpeper Herbal Tonic for Digestive
       Disorders; *Frank Roberts Cranesbill Compound Tablets; *Gerard House Fenulin;
       *HRI Golden Seal Digestive; Lamberts Chewable Bromelain with Papain; *Lanes
       Biobalm; *Muir's Gastric-Ese; *Potter's Appetiser Mixture; *Potter's Stomach Mix-
       ture; Solgar Bromelain Tablets; *Weleda Melissa Comp.

STYES

See Eye problems

SUNBURN

Given the publicity in recent years of the risks of skin cancer from sunbathing in
our ozone-depleted environment, one would imagine that we would all remain
well-protected under sunhats and long-sleeved shirts. Perhaps because the sun's
rays are more penetrative in our polluted atmosphere sunburn seems even more
commonplace. St John's wort oil is a useful standby for emergencies while products using aloe vera, lavender and chamomile can be useful for minor problems.
See also Burns (minor) and scalds

Herbal remedies and supplements which may help

External: Herbcraft Aloe Lavender Spray; Spring Wind Ointment.
See St John's wort simples

TENNIS ELBOW

Tennis elbow is a painful inflammation of the tendon at the outer edge of the
elbow usually caused by excessive exercise – hence the name. As this is an inflammatory problem, herbal anti-inflammatories applied topically can be helpful.
Massage oils containing St John's wort, yarrow or chamomile oils are worth looking for.

Herbal remedies and supplements which may help

External: Arthur's Formula Bath and Massage Oil; Bee Brand Massage Oil; Dr Shir's Lini-
       ment; Neal's Yard Ginger and Juniper Warming Oil; Neal's Yard Rhus Tox and Ruta
       Ointment; Neal's Yard Sports Salve; *Nelsons Rhus Tox Cream; *Weleda Massage
       Balm with Arnica; *Weleda Rhus Tox Ointment.

TENSION HEADACHES

See Headaches and migraines

THREADWORMS

See Worms

THRUSH AND YEAST INFECTIONS

Information about yeast infections or candidiasis has become much more widespread in recent years and a wide assortment of products aimed at tackling the problem is now available.

There are some 60–70 yeasts which can affect the body although *Candida albicans* tends to be the commonest. These yeasts, like various familiar bacteria, reside in large numbers in our guts and on the surface of the skin. Like bacteria they usually cause us few problems, but if resistance is weakened by over-work, stress or illness, then – being opportunist creatures – they can proliferate and affect our well-being. This proliferation not only leads to yeasts in the bowel competing with the other more friendly bacteria which normally live there, thus upsetting the digestion, but is also believed to cause the yeasts to take on a fungal form and be absorbed into the bloodstream. In this fungal form they can travel to any part of the body and their normal chemistry can conflict with our own causing a wide variety of health problems.

Although many practitioners remain sceptical about the exact role yeast infection can play in ill health, exponents of the candidiasis theory suggest that these fungal yeasts can interfere with neurotransmitters leading to anxiety and panic attacks. The chemicals they produce are also believed by some to mimic human hormones leading to menstrual problems while others suggest that yeast intolerance can be the root cause of numerous aches and pains, chronic fatigue problems and persistent infections.

A number of over-the-counter remedies, based on combinations of vitamins, minerals or plant extracts, have been launched in recent years and several of these include recognised anti-fungal herbs, like garlic and pau d'arco, others are based on caprylic acid which is a derivative of coconut oil.

A more obvious sign of yeast infection is thrush which affects the mucous membranes especially of the mouth (usually in babies) and vagina. Like candidiasis, thrush usually starts when the body is out of balance and resistance is low. Typical symptoms are irritation, soreness, characteristic white patches on the membrane lining and – in vaginal thrush – a white, cheesy discharge. Yeasts thrive in warm, damp conditions and thus women, prone to repeated vaginal thrush infections should wear cotton pants and stockings instead of tights, to ensure that the perineum remains cool and dry. High blood sugar levels will also encourage yeast proliferation so it can be a problem for diabetics; non-diabetics should reduce sugar intake to a minimum. Use of antibiotics also wipes out many of the bacteria which keep the more opportunist yeasts, like *Candida albicans*, under control, so thrush can often follow another infection and antibiotic treatment. Taking capsules of friendly bacteria, such as *Lactobacillus acidophilus*, or eating live yoghurt while on antibiotics can help.

Orthodox treatment involves potent anti-fungals, but because *Candida albicans* is always resident on the surface of our bodies, reinfection is commonplace. Herbal treatment focuses more on improving resistance and restoring balance as well as providing symptomatic relief with anti-fungal herbs. Tea tree is a useful topical anti-fungal which is available OTC in creams and pessaries.

Herbal remedies and supplements which may help

BioCare Biocidin; BioCare Candistatin; BioCare Candicin; BioCare Eradicidin Forte; Cantassium Didamega; Full Potency Herbs Pau d'Arco Vegicaps; Full Potency Herbs Yucca Vegicaps; Herbs of Grace Anti-Fung; Rio Vitalis Lapacho.

External: Gerard House Calendula Ointment; Hartwood Aromatics Calendula Ointment; Herbs of Grace Calendula Cream; *Lane's Number 44 Skin Ointment; Neal's Yard Calendula Ointment; *Nelsons Calendula Cream; Nelsons Tea Tree Cream; *Potter's Skin Clear Ointment; Thursday Plantation Antiseptic Cream; *Weleda Calendula Lotion; *Weleda Calendolon Ointment.

TIREDNESS AND FATIGUE

One of the commonest presenting symptoms for patients visiting both GPs and alternative practitioners is tiredness: a general lack of energy that falls short of clinical exhaustion but can interfere with enjoyment and performance. Severe tiredness can be characteristic of chronic fatigue syndrome or myalgic encephalomyelitis (also referred to as post-viral syndrome) and professional help is needed in such cases.

At one time low-grade tiredness was regularly treated with artificially stimulating drugs, although this practice has, fortunately, fallen from favour. However, many GPs are too willing to put the problem down to "depression" and prescribe powerful anti-depressants which may do little to solve the underlying cause. A herbal approach will in general encourage a reassessment of lifestyle, using relaxation techniques or meditation to help prevent the sufferer from dissipating energies by over-activity. Sooner or later most people will learn that it really is not a good idea to "burn the candle at both ends" for any length of time.

Herbal stimulants are, of course, familiar to all: coffee, tea and chocolate which are rich in caffeine, theobromine and related alkaloids are regularly used as a short-term restorative. Cola drinks, similarly, are caffeine rich and provide the same artificial boost. Coca Cola takes its name from the original herbal ingredients: coca leaves, the source of cocaine, and cola nuts which are an extremely rich source of caffeine. The drinks producer has long since replaced these plant ingredients with synthetic (and milder) substitutes, but cola nuts are still very widely used in herbal remedies.

Opting for longer-term energy tonics is generally the preferable option: ginseng, a Chinese herb, has become extremely popular in the West in recent years. In traditional Chinese medicine, ginseng tends to be regarded as boosting the *yang* energies and while it can be taken by women other tonics are often preferable. Both American and Siberian ginsengs are regarded as more *yin* in character and so can be more suitable for women. Another favourite Chinese tonic for women (which can sometimes be suitable for men as well) is *Dang Gui* (Chinese angelica): this is very widely used in the East and is starting to appear in Western OTC products as well. Other popular tonic herbs available in over-the-counter preparations are gotu kola, guarana and cat's claw – a more recent addition to the herbal repertoire. Interest is also growing in the various medicinal fungi popular in China – notably reishi and shiitake mushrooms – and these are now becoming more readily available.

See also Anxiety, stress and tension, Convalescence and debility

Herbal remedies and supplements which may help

Arkocaps Phytoexcel; Arkocaps Phytophrodisiac; Arkocaps Phytosuperior; BioCare Oxy-B15; Bioforce Neuroforce; *Bio-Strath Elixir; *Dorwest Damiana and Kola Tablets; East West Amachazuru Tea; East West Shi Hu and Gan Cao Tea; *Fo Ti Tieng; *Frank Roberts Avexan Tablets; *Frank Roberts Strength Tablets; *Frank Roberts Supa-Tonic Tablets; FSC Siberian Ginseng; Full Potency Herbs American Ginseng Root Vegicaps; Full Potency Herbs Cat's Claw Tablets; Full Potency Herbs Gotu Kola Vegicaps; *Gerard House Curzon; Gerard House Vig-a-Tea; Health Aid Herbal Booster; Health Aid Liquid Herbal Booster; Healthcrafts Korean and Siberian Ginseng; La Gelee Royale; Melbrosia Executive; *Muir's Pick-Me-Up; Natural Flow Triple Ginseng; Nature's Plus Ginkgo Combo; *Potter's Chlorophyll Tablets; *Potter's Strength Tablets; Super Gre-Caps; SX Formula; Three G's; Weleda Blackthorn Elixir.

See ginseng simples (Table 3), guarana simples

TONSILLITIS

The tonsils are small packs of lymphatic tissue at the back of the throat which help protect the body from infection. Recurrent tonsillitis can often indicate some underlying stress on the system, such as food allergy, with the immune system having to work overtime to combat the problem. In severe cases the tonsil can become filled with pus causing an abscess or quinsy which can need surgical treatment.

Tonsillitis can be severe and requires professional medical help. As a short-term, self-help measure gargling with echinacea, thyme or pineapple juice can help while poke root or echinacea taken internally can help combat infection.

Herbal remedies and supplements which may help

Bioforce Usneasan Cough Lozenges; *Frank Roberts Catarrh Tablets.

External: Herbcraft Calendula & Goldenseal Spray; Herbcraft Liquorice and Propolis Spray; *Weleda Medicinal Gargle.
See echinacea simples

TOOTHACHE

Toothache caused by tooth decay should almost be a thing of the past thanks to regular dental check-ups. Apart from such obvious damage as a cracked filling or broken tooth, these days a more likely cause of sudden and severe tooth pain is likely to be an abscess or infection of some sort.

For emergency relief oil of cloves remains one of the most popular and effective remedies. Apply a few drops of oil to cotton wool and apply to the gum. Clove oil is a potent anaesthetic and will provide temporary relief, although it can produce a stinging effect before numbing the area.

An abscess or infection can often be associated with more general feelings of being unwell or perhaps will follow a cold or low-grade 'flu. Herbal remedies, which stimulate the immune system and counter infections, can provide quite rapid relief in some cases, and may even help disperse abscesses quite effectively before dental treatment is necessary. Use of echinacea or garlic tablets will not provide instant pain relief but can help treat the cause while standard aspirin or paracetamol treatments tackle the ache.

Persistent toothache – with no obvious dental cause – can be associated with sinus problems and catarrh.
See Catarrh and sinus problems

Herbal remedies and supplements which may help

*Weleda Medicinal Gargle.
See clove, echinacea and garlic (Table 2) simples.

TRAVEL SICKNESS

Whether it occurs in trains, planes, ships or cars, travel sickness starts with pallor, sweating and nausea and soon leads to vomiting and faintness.

The problem is generally to do with the delicate balance mechanism in the inner ear leading to disturbances in what the eyes see and how the body responds to its position in space, so that eye and ear no longer agree on where and how the person is moving. Travel sickness can also be brought on by general stuffiness and lack of fresh air, mild claustrophobia, and the all-pervading smell of diesel and engine oil which once dominated cross-channel ferries.

Children's ears tend to be more sensitive to motion disturbances and travel sickness is thus more commonplace among the young and is often something they grow out of with time.

The best herbal remedy for nausea is ginger and there is a wide choice of powdered ginger capsules available over-the-counter. For children who cannot swallow capsules, use any ginger-based product they will tolerate: ginger beer, ginger biscuits, candied ginger sweets or a few drops of diluted ginger tincture (or ginger wine) on the tongue.

Herbal remedies and supplements which may help

*Frank Roberts Nervous Dyspepsia Tablets; *Weleda Melissa Comp.
See ginger simples

URTICARIA

Irritant weals which can suddenly appear on the skin are variously described as urticaria, hives and nettle rash. They usually fade within a few hours and are often associated with an allergic reaction to some substance – either something taken internally or with which there has been skin contact.

In severe cases there is also swelling of the hands, face, arms, eyelids or throat and there may be painful joints or breathing problems which can require emergency treatment.

Food allergy is a common cause: shellfish are frequently blamed as are strawberries. However, a reaction to strawberries can also suggest an intolerance of other foods containing salicylates (chemicals widely occurring in fruits, vegetables and many common herbs as well as forming the basis of aspirin). Identifying and avoiding allergenic foods is obviously important for sufferers. Lists of high salicylate foods are available in many popular books on nutrition and food allergy, while long-term use of aspirin (as is recommended for those suffering from high blood pressure) can sometimes trigger severe and persistent urticaria. Other drugs, including some antibiotics, can have a similar effect so always check with your GP if skin rashes follow a new prescription.

Contact irritants are equally numerous: insect stings especially bee stings and bee products, cosmetics, perfumes and a large number of common garden plants can cause urticaria. Hop plants, runner bean tendrils, borage, yarrow, chamomile and St John's wort have all been known to cause irritant skin rashes in sensitive individuals.

Stinging nettles are, of course, a common irritant. Their hairs actually contain histamine, a chemical normally present in the body, but one that can trigger the characteristic allergic response in excess. Orthodox remedies are thus generally based on antihistamines and will work quickly and effectively.

Herbal remedies usually take longer to restore order and tend to provide soothing relief rather than immediate cure: look for products containing chickweed, borage juice or distilled witch-hazel.

Herbal remedies and supplements which may help

External: Neal's Yard Hypericum and Urtica Ointment; *Lane's Number 44 Skin Ointment; *Rickard's Woodsap Ointment.

VARICOSE VEINS

Varicose veins are usually visible as tortuous, knotted veins on the surface of the legs. They can ache or the surrounding area can be prone to swelling. The flesh around the affected vein can often feel hot.

Veins, unlike arteries, have to help force blood back to the heart rather than depend on the impetus of this powerful pump. The muscles surrounding deep veins can help considerably, but the superficial veins in the legs often have little support for forcing blood back to the central pumping system and over the years they can become distended, lengthened and tortuous.

Deep breathing can help encourage the return of blood from the peripheries while a tendency for varicose veins can often be countered by alternatively hosing the legs with a hot and cold shower, several times, for 1–2 minutes each morning. Putting bricks under the end of the bed to aid venous return at night can also help.

A tendency for varicose veins is often hereditary and can also be associated with pregnancy, obesity, standing for long periods, constipation, tight clothing and lack of exercise.

Varicose ulcers generally occur in the elderly and are associated with poor circulation: the reduced blood flow to an area often making healing difficult. They require professional treatment.
See Piles

Herbal remedies and supplements which may help

Arkocaps Phytovarix; Bioforce Hyperisan; Full Potency Herbs Butcher's Broom Vegicaps; Potter's Buckwheat Tablets; Pure-fil Rutin; Reevecrest Nutrimental Plus; Rutivite.
External: Phytovarix; *Potter's Varicose Ointment.

WARTS AND VERRUCAS

Warts are benign lumps in the skin caused by a virus which makes the cells multiply abnormally quickly. Common warts are usually found on the hands, knees and face and are mildly contagious, spreading as the virus comes into contact with damaged skin or when flakes from the wart touch nearby moist skin areas. Although they can be unsightly and a nuisance, these sorts of warts are usually quite harmless and most will disappear of their own accord – eventually.

Like many common viruses, the one causing warts can remain dormant for some time, so they tend to reappear in sufferers although warts are usually commonest in younger people.

There is, of course, a wealth of folkloric traditions – some of them herbal – surrounding warts: warts could be charmed, "sold", tied off with horses hair, or rubbed with bacon fat which was then nailed to a door post and as it rotted, so the wart would disappear. The common garden weed, wood spurge (*Euphorbia amygdaloides*), is known in some country districts as wart weed from the tradition of using the juice to cure warts. More effective is dandelion juice or the yellow sap of the greater celandine, although great care is needed if applying drops to warts as these saps can be corrosive to unaffected skin.

Verrucas are plantar warts that occur on the soles of the feet. Because they are always being walked on the small growths can become painful and are often covered by thickened areas of skin or calluses. Readily available ring plasters and callous pads can provide some relief. The constant pressure also makes these warts grow inwardly rather than erupting outwards as with common warts and persistent cases usually need treatment from a chiropodist.

Venereal or genital warts are found around the genitals and anus. Again they will usually disappear of their own accord, but because of the contagious nature of viruses they can be transmitted during sexual intercourse. These warts need professional treatment and sufferers should not experiment with over-the-counter herbal remedies without first seeking advice.

Professional help is also needed for warts which appear to erupt on the site of moles or which start to bleed or change colour.

Herbal remedies and supplements which may help

Nelsons Tea Tree Cream; *Potter's Skin Clear Ointment; Thursday Plantation Antiseptic Cream.

WIND

See Flatulence

WORMS

There are three sorts of worms that can commonly affect the digestive system:
• tapeworms,
• threadworms or pinworms
• roundworms

Tapeworms are potentially dangerous parasites which breed in unsanitary conditions and require professional treatment, but the other two varieties can often be tackled with self-help medication, especially if infestations are treated before they become too firmly established.

Threadworms are about 1 cm/½ in long and are common in children. They live in the large intestine and the usual symptom is chronic rectal itching. The female migrates to the anal area to lay her eggs at night so it is often possible to see the worms on inspection. By scratching the area, the eggs are trapped in fingernails and thus transmitted. The problem is most common among toddlers and – by contact – to their mothers, so there tends to be a second peak in incidence among women in their late 20s and early 30s. Children suffering from threadworms often have a poor appetite, dark rings under the eyes, and show signs of irritability and sleeplessness with bad dreams. They often tend to reinfect themselves by sucking their fingers.

Threadworms have a life cycle of around two weeks so it can be important to repeat treatments cyclically to counter any reinfection. To prevent this nails should be kept short, biting nails must be forbidden and washing hands – and scrubbing nails – before meals is essential.

Roundworms (ascariasis) are fortunately much less common than thread-worms. They are around 20–35cm long and look rather like unsegmented earth-worms. They live in the gut developing via a complex process by way of the lungs; eggs being passed via the faeces. Infection occurs by eating food containing the eggs or embryos. In severe cases the worms can cause intestinal obstruction, although more usual symptoms are simply nausea, colicky pains and irregular motions. Occasionally roundworms are vomited up.

Eating foods that worms dislike can often help dislodge them: go for onions, raw carrots, garlic, cayenne pepper and pumpkin seeds. Herbal teas made from fennel, aniseed and peppermint can often help as can eating papaya fruit and raw carrots daily. At the same time avoid foods they like, especially sugars and refined carbohydrates.

As with any contagious condition scrupulous hygiene within the family is essential: never share towels, wash hands regularly and be particularly careful with laundry as worm eggs can often survive standard wash cycles.

Herbal remedies and supplements which may help

Full Potency Herbs Cayenne Capsules; Power Health Pumpkin Seed Oil.
See garlic simples (Table 2)

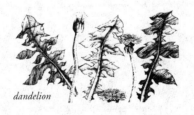

dandelion

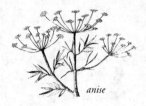

anise

A–Z of Herbs

All the herbs listed in this section can be found in over-the-counter herbal products currently on offer. Many other plants, popular with professional herbalists and in folk medicine, are not included simply because they do not occur in the OTC remedies and supplements reviewed. The basic actions and uses are given for each plant along with details of the remedies and supplements in which it is used. "Simples" are single herbs used on their own and details of any tinctures, capsules, tablets, juices or oils which can be bought over-the-counter are also given. Licensed products are indicated throughout with an asterisk (*).

ACEROLA

Malpighia punicifolia

Synonyms: Barbados cherry, West Indian cherry, Puerto Rica cherry

Parts used: berry

Known in the tropics as the "health tree", acerola berries are the richest known source of vitamin C. Each contains around 85 mg and they are widely used in nutritional supplements. It is estimated that 100 g/3½ oz of acerola juice contains some 3.4 g of vitamin C while the same amount of rosehip syrup would give only 0.3 g of the vitamin, and orange juice a paltry 50 mg. The tree is a native of the West Indies but is now cultivated in many areas of Central America and Florida. The juice has a tart flavour and so sugar is often added to preparations. Vitamin C is vital to maintain healthy connective tissues and bones. Without it wounds are slow to heal and blood will leak from tissues as happens in scurvy, once a major problem on long sea voyages. The vitamin is also believed to help the immune system and some regard it as an important cancer preventative.

Remedies and supplements
>   American Nutrition Acerola Plus 100 mg; BioCare NEF242; Melbrosia PLD

Simples
>   *Juice:* Schoenenberger Plant Juice

AGRIMONY

Agrimonia eupatoria

Synonyms: church steeples, cocklebur, sticklewort

Parts used: herb

Agrimony is a bitter herb that will stimulate bile flow and is also astringent so is useful for diarrhoea or to stop bleeding. It has a long tradition as a wound herb and was an ingredient of "arquebusade water" which was used in the fifteenth century for battlefield gunshot wounds. Agrimony is diuretic and contains silica which is a good healing remedy. Although herbalists use the plant for a range of ailments including cystitis, sore throats and gallstones, over-the-counter remedies tend to focus on its astringent action and it is included in a number of pile remedies. However, because of its astringency, agrimony is contraindicated in constipation, so most of these remedies also contain potent laxatives and only small amounts of agrimony.

Remedies and supplements
>   Absorb Plus; Colon Cleanse; Culpeper Pilewort Tablets; *Culpeper Rheumatic Tablets; *Frank Roberts Pilewort Compound Tablets – Orange Label; *Frank Roberts Pilewort Compound Tablets – Green Label; *Muir's Gastric-Ese; *Muir's Pick-Me-Up; *Potter's Piletabs

Simples
>   *Tincture:* Neal's Yard Remedies

ALDER BUCKTHORN

Rhamnus frangula

Synonyms: frangula bark

Parts used: bark

Alder buckthorn is a strong laxative generally given for chronic constipation. Fresh bark causes violent griping pains and nausea, so normally dried, seasoned bark (often two years old) is used. The herb contains anthraquinone glycosides which irritate the bowel and so should only be used for short periods. It also stimulates bile flow and has been used in jaundice and liver problems.

• Alder buckthorn should be avoided in pregnancy.

Remedies and supplements

Bioforce Linoforce; Herbulax; *Lusty's Herbalene; Ortilax; *Potter's Cleansing Herb

Simples

Capsules/tablets: Arkocaps Phytoclense (230 mg); *Heath & Heather Inner Fresh

ALFALFA

Medicago sativa

Synonyms: lucerne, purple medick

Parts used: herb

Alfalfa is an important fodder crop often used for hay or silage. It is also an extremely rich source of nutrients, including pro-vitamin A, several vitamins from the B group, and vitamins C, D, E, K, folic acid, biotin and several minerals. It can be helpful in convalescence and debility as a general tonic, or in anaemia. It also contains saponins which are thought to help reduce cholesterol levels and coumarins which act on the circulatory system reducing haemorrhage and strengthening blood vessel walls. Research suggests a hormonal action and it is sometimes used for menopausal problems and fibroids.

Remedies and supplements

BioCare NEF242; BioCare Phytosterol Complex; Bioforce Alfavena; Bioforce DBT; Herbcraft Burdock & Nettle Formula; Natural Flow Regular Ten Powder; Power Health Alfalfa, Kelp & Yeast

Simples

Capsules/tablets: Arkocaps Alfalfa (310 mg); Blackmores Alfalfa Tablets (380 mg); Lamberts Alfalfa Extract (450 mg); Power Health Alfalfa (500 mg); Solgar Alfalfa Tablets (600 mg)
Tincture: Neal's Yard Remedies

ALOE VERA

Aloe vera

Synonyms: *A. barbadensis*, Barbados aloe, Curaçao aloe

Parts used: sap, leaves

While "bitter aloes" is a purgative made from various species of *Aloe*, "aloe vera" is the name given to the mucilaginous gel from one particular type of aloe. The plant itself (like other aloes) is strongly purgative and is used for chronic consti-pation, but the gel is largely used externally as a wound healer and to relieve burns and inflammation. It can easily be applied fresh and it is an extremely useful plant to grow on the kitchen window sill to provide a readily available salve for minor burns. Aloe vera can also be used for eczema and can combat fungal infections such as ringworm and thrush.

Remedies and supplements

External: Herbcraft Aloe Lavender Spray

Simples

Juice: Neal's Yard Remedies, Power Health Aloe Vera 5000
Capsules: Full Potency Herbs Aloe Vera Leaf Vegicaps (520 mg)

ALOES

Aloe spp (including A. vera, A. ferox, A. perryi)

Synonyms: bitter aloes, Curaçao aloes, Cape aloes, Socotrine aloes, Zanzibar aloes

Parts used: liquid drained from the cut leaves

Aloes or "bitter aloes" is the name given to liquid drained from the cut leaves of various members of the *Aloe* family. The different species produce extracts of a slightly different colour and texture but all are potent laxatives. Although aloes has a long history of medicinal use, it is now restricted in some countries because of its toxicity: over-use can lead to gastritis, diarrhoea and kidney disorders. As a strong purgative, aloes can cause griping so most remedies also contain anti-spasmodics and carminatives. Over-the-counter remedies containing aloes are generally licensed and are recommended for more stubborn cases of constipation.
• Aloes should be avoided in pregnancy.

Remedies and supplements

Blackmores Cape Aloes and Cascara; *Box's Far Famed Indigestion Tablets; *Dorwest Natural Herb Tablets; *Frank Roberts B & L Tablets; Frank Roberts Constipation Tablets; *Gerard House Gladlax; *Lanes Dual-Lax Extra Strong; *Potter's Out of Sorts Tablets

AMACHAZURU

Gynostemma pentaphyllum

Synonyms: gospel herb

Parts used: herb

A member of the pumpkin family, this Chinese herb is well established as a folk cure for bronchitis, liver problems and ulcers. In the 1980s anti-cancer activity was identified in the plant and recent studies have also shown a high mineral and vitamin content as well as similar steroidal compounds to those found in ginseng. The plant also helps to improve heart function and stimulates the blood supply to the brain – rather like ginkgo. Amachazuru is thus promoted as a useful tonic for the elderly and for general fatigue as well as being used as an immune stimulant and sedative.

Simples

Tea: East West Amachazuru Tea

AMERICAN CRANESBILL

Geranium maculatum

Synonyms: alum root, storksbill, spotted cranesbill

Parts used: herb, root

All the geraniums are rich in tannins and highly astringent; they are thus generally used for treating diarrhoea, discharges, ulcers and sore throats. English cranesbill (*G. dissectum*) is very similar to its American cousin which is more widely used – largely due to the influence of US herbalists in the nineteenth century. American cranesbill also acts as a styptic to stop bleeding and it can be added to remedies for excessive menstruation and colitis. Externally it is used on varicose ulcers and piles.

Remedies and supplements

*Frank Roberts Cranesbill Compound Tablets; *Frank Roberts Pilewort Compound Tablets – Orange Label; *Gerard House Golden Seal Compound; *Gerard House Pilewort Compound Tablets; *Muir's Gastric-Ese

Simples

Capsules/tablets: *Gerard House Cranesbill Tablets
Tincture: Neal's Yard Remedies

AMERICAN GINSENG

Panax quinquefolius

Synonyms: Xi Yang Shen

Parts used: roots

American ginseng was first discovered in the eighteenth century by Jesuits who had become familiar with Korean ginseng from missionary work in China, and who believed that a similar plant may be found in the remote mountains of North America. Daniel Boone was reputedly an avid collector, amassing some 15 tonnes of the root in Ohio in 1787 and making far more money from collecting ginseng than he ever did from the fur trade. The herb has been used in China since 1765 and is regarded as a gentler tonic than Korean ginseng, rather more *yin* in character and more suited for young people and children whereas Korean ginseng is favoured by the elderly. It is useful in debility and chronic illness and can be helpful to counter stress and sleeplessness.

Remedies and supplements
Herbcraft Echinacea Formula; Herbcraft Liquorice Formula; Natural Flow Triple Ginseng

Simples
Capsules: Full Potency Herbs American Ginseng Root Vegicaps (520 mg); Health Aid American Ginseng (600 mg)
Tincture: Neal's Yard Remedies

AMERICAN VALERIAN

Cyprepedium parviflorum var. pubescens

Synonyms: lady's slipper orchid

Parts used: rhizomes

American valerian was listed in the US Pharmacopoeia until 1916 and was widely used as a tranquilliser, much as its European namesake still is. The orchid is now extremely rare in the wild and many herbalists prefer to use less endangered alternatives. It is a useful sedative and antispasmodic that also has a tonic effect on the nervous system.

Remedies and supplements
*Culpeper Head Cold and Throat Mixture

ANGELICA

Angelica archangelica

Parts used: leaves, essential oil, root, stem

Angelica is a sweet, pungent, warming plant which is familiar in candied form as a cake decoration. It is a carminative, antispasmodic, anti-inflammatory, diaphoretic, diuretic and expectorant, used for coughs and colds, in digestive remedies and to treat rheumatic disorders. As a uterine stimulant, the plant was once used to help prolonged labour and may be helpful for menstrual problems.

Over-the-counter remedies including the herb generally exploit its carminative and digestive actions.

• Angelica is a very sweet plant and should be avoided by diabetics. Large doses are also contraindicated in pregnancy. The plant is rich in furanocoumarins which can increase the photosensitivity of the skin.

Remedies and supplements
Bioforce Gastrosan; Gerard House Sooth-a-Tea; Health Aid FemmeVit; *Weleda Cough Drops; *Weleda Melissa Comp

Simples
>   *Oil:* Hartwood Aromatics
>   *Tincture:* Bioforce, Neal's Yard Remedies

ANISE

Pimpinella anisum

Synonyms: aniseed

Parts used: seeds, oil

Aniseed has been used as a spice since Egyptian times and is a popular flavouring for sweets and liqueurs. Medicinally it is carminative and expectorant and is included in various remedies for indigestion and flatulence as well as coughs, bronchial infections and sore throats. Like other similar carminatives it is occasionally included in laxative preparations to counter the griping pains these can cause. The oil has similar uses but is also antiseptic and can be applied topically for lice and scabies. Research suggests that anise may also have a tonic effect on the liver. It is mildly oestrogenic helping to increase milk flow in nursing mothers and traditionally used in childbirth and as a female aphrodisiac.

Remedies and supplements
>   BioCare Artemisia Complex; Bioforce Bronchosan; Bumbles Propolis, Aniseed & Liquorice Lozenges; *Culpeper Cough Relief Mixture; *Culpeper Herbal Mixture for Acidity, Indigestion and Flatulence; Frank Roberts Acidosis Tablets; *Hactos Cough Mixture; Herbcraft Peppermint Formula; *Lane's Cut-a-Cough; *Lanes Honey and Molasses Cough Mixture; Neal's Yard Echinacea & Mallow Linctus; Neal's Yard Horehound & Aniseed Linctus; Neal's Yard Horehound & Honey Lozenges; *Potter's Acidosis; *Potter's Lightning Cough Remedy; *Potter's Malted Kelp Tablets; *Potter's Vegetable Cough Remover; *Revitonil; *Weleda Carminative Tea; *Weleda Clairo Tea; *Weleda Cough Elixir; *Weleda Fragador Tablets; *Weleda Herb and Honey Cough Elixir; *Weleda Laxadoron Tablets

Simples
>   *Oil:* Neal's Yard Remedies

ANNUAL NETTLE

Urtica urens

Parts used: herb

The small annual nettle is very similar in action to its larger perennial relative, the stinging nettle. It is preferred for making homoeopathic remedies for burns often in combination with marigold or St John's wort extracts.

Remedies and supplements
>   *External:* *Nelsons Burns Ointment; *Weleda Comburdoron Ointment

ARISAEMA

Arisaema consanguineum

Synonyms: *Tian Nan Xing,* Jack-in-the-Pulpit

Parts used: tuber

Arisaema is used externally for abscesses and fungal problems. It is also an expectorant herb, taken internally in traditional Chinese medicine for coughs, fevers and convulsions.

Remedies and supplements
  External: Dr Shir's Liniment; Golden Yellow Ointment

ARNICA

Arnica montana

Synonyms: leopard's bane, mountain tobacco

Parts used: flowers

Arnica is primarily used in wound healing and to encourage tissue repair after traumatic injury. Recent work suggests that it may have immune-stimulant properties. Internally it is toxic and is generally used only in dilute homoeopathic doses. Arnica 6× tablets are an excellent way to speed recovery from any sort of accidents, trauma and surgery. Externally it is used on bruises, sprains, chilblains, or painful varicose veins. It should not be used on open wounds and may occasionally cause contact dermatitis.

Remedies and supplements
  Bioforce Arterioforce; Bioforce Hyperisan
  External: Bioforce Seven Herb Cream; Neal's Yard Arnica Ointment; Neal's Yard Sports Salve; *Nelsons Arnica Cream; *Nelsons Pyrethrum Spray; *Weleda Arnica Ointment; *Weleda Comburdoron Ointment; *Weleda Frost Cream; *Weleda Massage Balm with Arnica; *Weleda WCS Dusting Powder

Simples
  Capsules/tablets: Nelsons Arnica 6×; Weleda Arnica 6×
  Infused oil: Neal's Yard Remedies

ASAFOETIDA

Ferula assa-foetida

Synonyms: devil's dung

Parts used: oleo gum resin

Asafoetida is generally – and justifiably – described as the most foul smelling of all herbs. It is antispasmodic, expectorant and carminative and is used for nervous disorders and coughs. The plant also has a cleansing and strengthening effect on the digestive system and recent research suggests it may help to reduce blood pressure and have some anti-coagulant activity.

Remedies and supplements
   *Frank Roberts Nerfood Tablets; *Frank Roberts Pulsatilla Compound Tablets

ASPARAGUS

Asparagus officinalis

Parts used: young shoots, rhizomes

A number of asparagus species are used medicinally including *A. racemosus* which is an important tonic herb (known as *shatavari*) in Ayurvedic medicine. *A. officinalis* is the familiar vegetable which, asparagus eaters everywhere will know, has a fairly rapid effect on the urinary system. It is a diuretic and laxative and its constituents break down to form methylmercaptan which gives the urine a characteristic smell soon after eating asparagus as a vegetable.

As a cleansing herb, asparagus has been used for rheumatism, gout and to support liver function. Others recommend it as a slimming aid helping to accelerate the metabolism.

Simples
   Juice: Schoenenberger Plant Juice

ASPEN

Populus tremula

See Poplar

ASTRAGALUS

Astragalus membranaceus

Synonyms: *Huang Qi*, milk vetch

Parts used: root

Astragalus is one of the most important tonic herbs used in traditional Chinese medicine. It is a stimulant for the immune system and has a tonifying effect on lungs, stomach and kidneys. The plant is regarded as a more suitable tonic for younger people than ginseng and its strong immune-strengthening effects make it valuable for recurrent infections, slow healing wounds and general debility.

Remedies and supplements
  BioCare Buccalzyme

Simples
  Capsules/tablets: Full Potency Herbs Astragalus Root Vegicaps (520 mg)
  Tincture: Herbcraft; Neal's Yard Remedies

AUTUMN CROCUS

Colchicum autumnale

Synonyms: meadow saffron, naked ladies

Parts used: corm, seeds

The lovely autumn crocus was once a favourite medicinal herb used to relieve the pain of acute gout and other arthritic conditions. It is, however, extremely toxic and can be fatal even in very low doses. Its use is restricted and the plant is now really only used in homoeopathic dilutions. In these concentrations it is a valuable remedy for pain relief as well as for diarrhoea and nausea.
• Side effects of over-dose include gastro-intestinal pain, kidney damage and hair loss. It should not be taken by pregnant women or those with kidney problems. Its use in OTC preparations is confined to homoeopathic extracts.

Remedies and supplements
  Bioforce Imperthritica

BALM OF GILEAD

Populus candicans

Synonyms: Ontario poplar, balsam poplar

Parts used: leaf buds

Balm of gilead buds are collected from a small tree originally growing in the Middle East. The common name is slightly confusing as there are various aromatic shrubs also called "balm of gilead", largely because of similarities in the plants' smell rather than from any botanical reason. The buds have long been used in cough remedies and are cooling, expectorant, analgesic and stimulant. They have a pleasant taste and are popular in children's cough syrups. Externally the buds have been used in ointments for rheumatism, skin disorders and muscular aches and pains although such products are now rarely found commercially.

Remedies and supplements
  *Culpeper Balm of Gilead Cough Mixture; *Heath & Heather Balm of Gilead Cough Mixture; *Heath & Heather Balm of Gilead Cough Pastilles; Neal's Yard Balm of Gilead; *Potter's Balm of Gilead

BAMBOO

Bambusa arundinacea

Synonyms: spiny bamboo

Parts used: gum

Indian spiny bamboo is rich in silica and produces a milky deposit on the bark which is collected and used medicinally. This is known as *vamsha rochana* or bamboo manna in Ayurvedic medicine and is primarily used as a cooling remedy for the lungs. It is taken for feverish colds, asthma and in debilitated conditions and will also help to stop bleeding and clear coughs. Because the plant is rich in silica some suppliers suggest that it can be helpful for bone and joint disorders and may prevent bone loss after the menopause, although this is not at all how the plant is traditionally regarded.

Simples
>   *Capsules:* Arkocaps Phytosilica (270 mg)

BARBERRY

Berberis vulgaris

Synonyms: pipperidge bush

Parts used: stem and root bark, root, fruits

Various *Berberis* spp. are used medicinally in many parts of the world. In Ayurvedic medicine related plants are used as *daruharidra* for liver complaints and skin problems. *B. vulgaris*, the European variety, is similarly used as a bitter digestive remedy for a variety of liver and digestive problems. The plant contains a number of alkaloids, including berberine, which is strongly anti-bacterial and amoebacidal and it has been used for treating dysentery and similar digestive disorders. As a liver remedy, barberry is taken for hepatitis, gallstones and liver tumours.

Remedies and supplements
>   BioCare Candistatin; BioCare Eradicidin Forte; Blackmores Dandelion Complex;
>   *Muir's Gastric-Ese; Solgar Herbal Water Formula Capsules
>   *External:* *Weleda Catarrh Cream

Simples
>   *Tinctures:* Bioforce; Neal's Yard Remedies

BASIL

Ocimum basilicum

Parts used: leaves, oil

Although widely used as a culinary herb for pasta and tomato dishes, basil is regarded in India (where it originates) as an important and potent tonic. It is carminative, warming, antispasmodic, antibacterial and analgesic and has also been used to clear intestinal parasites, and improve digestion. In aromatherapy, the oil is used as a nerve tonic, anti-depressant and digestive remedy.

Simples
> *Oil:* Hartwood Aromatics; Neal's Yard Remedies; Tisserand
> *Tincture:* Bioforce

BAY

Laurus nobilis

Synonyms: bay laurel, sweet bay

Parts used: leaves, oil

A stimulating and aromatic herb, well known as a culinary flavouring, bay is also helpful for the digestion and is topically antiseptic. It can be used internally for colic and indigestion and is included in external rubs for rheumatism, sprains and bruising.

Remedies and supplements
> *External:* Chirali Old Remedy Strain & Sprain Cream

BAYBERRY

Myrica cerifera

Synonyms: candleberry, wax myrtle

Parts used: bark, root

Bayberry is another of the stimulating plants beloved of the physiomedicalists. It is highly astringent and tends to be used in catarrh remedies or as a warming, diaphoretic mix for colds and influenza. As an astringent it can be included in mixtures for both diarrhoea and heavy menstruation, but its main use in over-the-counter products is as a warming anti-catarrhal.

Remedies and supplements
> *Culpeper Influenza Mixture; *Culpeper Elder Flower and Peppermint Mixture; Neal's Yard Elderflower, Peppermint & Composition Essence; *Potter's Peerless Composition Essence; *Potter's Elderflowers, Peppermint and Composition Essence

Simples
> *Tincture:* Neal's Yard Remedies

BEANS

Phaseolus vulgaris

Synonyms: kidney bean

Parts used: husks, beans

Not surprisingly, beans are an important food source rich in trace elements and vitamins. The husks are used in slimming remedies on the basis that they can slow down absorption of sugars and reduce the activity of digestive enzymes thus helping with calorie intake. Beans are also hypoglycaemic so can be helpful to control blood sugar level in late-onset diabetes.

Remedies and supplements
Bioforce DBT (Diabetisan)

Simples
Capsules: Arkocaps Phytoslim (200 mg)
Juice: Schoenenberger Plant Juice

BEARBERRY

Arctostaphylos uva-ursi

Synonyms: uva-ursi, mountain box

Parts used: leaf

Bearberry is a small, ever-green shrub from Northern Europe and is a member of the heather family. It is an astringent, urinary antiseptic and is very widely used in herbal remedies for treating cystitis and similar complaints. It contains the hydroquinone, arbutin, which is anti-bacterial and very antiseptic for the entire urinary tract. The plant is generally considered as only mildly diuretic, but it still features in a number of remedies marketed for fluid retention and bloating.

Remedies and supplements
Bioforce Cystaforce; Blackmores Cornsilk Complex; Blackmores Cactus & Hawthorn; *Cantassium Boldo Aid; *Culpeper Parsley Piert Tablets; *Frank Roberts Buchu Backache Compound Tablets; Frank Roberts Parsley Piert Compound Tablets; *Frank Roberts Prickly Ash Compound Tablets; *Frank Roberts Sciatica Tablets; Frank Roberts Uva-Ursi Compound Tablets; *Gerard House Buchu Compound; *Gerard House Waterlex Tablets; Health Aid Boldo Plus; Health Aid Super Boldo; HRI Water Balance Tablets; Kordel's Women's Multi; Ladies Meno-Life Formula; LadyCare: For Women with Monthly Periods; *Lanes Cascade; *Muir's Sciatica;*Muir's Water-Ese; Neal's Yard Buchu Compound Capsules; *Potter's Antitis Tablets; *Potter's Backache Tablets;*Potter's Diuretabs; *Potter's Kas-Bah Herb; *Potter's Prementaid; *Potter's Sciargo Herb; *Potter's Tabritis; *Potter's Wellwoman Herbs; Professional Herbs Uva Ursi and Parsley; Solgar Herbal Water Formula Capsules; *Uvacin

Simples
> *Capsules:* Herbs of Grace Uva Ursi; Power Health Pure Uva-Ursi (200 mg)
> *Tincture:* Neal's Yard Remedies.

BENZOIN

Styrax benzoin

Parts used: gum resin

Astringent and expectorant, benzoin is regarded in aromatherapy as a soothing and relaxing herb for tired muscles. It is used in cough and cold remedies and may also be included in external treatments for sore throats, gum and mouth inflammations, itching skin rashes, wounds and ulcers. The Chinese regard it as a circulatory stimulant useful for colds and chills.

Remedies and supplements
> *External:* Arthur's Formula Bath and Massage Oil; *Lanes Heemex

Simples
> *Oil:* Hartwood Aromatics; Tisserand

BILBERRY

Vaccinium myrtillus

Synonyms: blueberry, huckleberry, whortleberry

Parts used: leaves, fruits

Bilberry fruits are a good source of vitamin C, highly astringent and anti-bacterial. They are used for diarrhoea and dysentery; in large quantities, however, the berries have a laxative effect so make an extremely palatable remedy for constipation. Externally the astringent fruits have been used in salves and ointments for piles, burns and skin complaints. The leaves will reduce blood sugar levels so are a useful support for late-onset diabetes that is under dietary control. Recent research also suggests that they can encourage insulin production.

Remedies and supplements
> BioCare Boswellic Acid Complex; BioCare Ginkgo Plus; BioCare Procydin; Bioforce DBT (Diabetisan); Full Potency Herbs Bilberry with Ginkgo Biloba Vegicaps; Herbcraft Echinacea, Eyebright and Bilberry Formula; Liquid Iron

Simples
> *Capsules:* Arkocaps Phytovainetone (230 mg)

BITTER CRESS

Cardamine pratensis

Synonyms: Meadow cress, lady's smock, cuckoo flower

Parts used: leaves

A member of the mustard family, bitter cress leaves can add a sharp flavour to salads. Medicinally the plant is tonic and expectorant: it is rich in vitamin C. It has been used for treating chronic skin complaints and asthma although rarely appears in herbal remedies these days.

Remedies and supplements
> Bioforce DBT (Diabetisan)

BITTER ORANGE

Citrus aurantium

Synonyms: bergamot, neroli, *Zhi Ke, Zhi Shi,* Seville orange

Parts used: fruit, peel, essential oil, flowers

The Seville orange – familiar from marmalade making – is also the source of a number of important medicinal products. The Chinese use both the unripe and ripe plants as carminative remedies for indigestion and coughs while neroli oil is distilled from the orange blossom. Bergamot oil, used for flavouring Earl Grey tea, is distilled from the peel. Neroli is used as an anti-depressant and sedative that can also be helpful for dry skin and digestive upsets, while bergamot is used by aromatherapists as a stimulating and uplifting massage oil. Bergamot can increase the photosensitivity of the skin and is added to tanning lotions. Petigrain oil, made from orange leaves, is also used in aromatherapy as a gentle astringent and skin tonic.

Simples
> *Oil:* Botanica; Hartwood Aromatics; Neal's Yard Remedies; Tisserand

BITTERSWEET

Solanum dulcamara

Synonyms: woody nightshade

Parts used: stems, root bark

Unlike its more poisonous namesakes, woody nightshade is a useful medicinal plant with little toxicity – except in excess. It is astringent, diuretic, sedative, expectorant and cleansing, with a characteristic bitter-sweet taste. It is largely used for skin complaints (including psoriasis) and to clear bronchial congestion. Bittersweet has also been used to treat jaundice and liver problems and is found in external preparations for ulcers, sores, skin rashes and rheumatism.

Remedies and supplements
*Weleda Dermatodendron Ointment

BLACK CATECHU

Acacia catechu

Parts used: leaves, young shoots

Black and pale catechu are very similar: both are astringent, very rich in tannins, and used for diarrhoea, chronic catarrh and dysentery. Black catechu is also used for haemorrhage and can be applied to sore gums and mouth inflammations.

Remedies and supplements
*Muir's Catarrh

BLACK COHOSH

Cimicifuga racemosa

Synonyms: black snakeroot, bugbane, rattlewort, squawroot

Parts used: rhizome

Black cohosh is another of the traditional North American herbs which entered the European repertoire in the nineteenth century. It has a wide range of attributes, although comparatively little is known of its constituents. Black cohosh is a sedative, anti-inflammatory, diuretic, anti-tussive and menstrual stimulant. It is used to treat ailments as diverse as period pain, whooping cough and rheumatism. Laboratory studies have shown that it can reduce blood pressure, lower blood sugar levels, and possibly act as a depressant on the central nervous system.

The herb's use in over-the-counter remedies is diverse: it appears in cough mixtures, tonics and menopausal preparations.
• Excess can cause nausea and vomiting and the herb should be avoided in pregnancy.

Remedies and supplements
*Gerard House Biophylin; Gerard House Fem-a-Tea; *Gerard House Helonias Compound; *Gerard House Ligvites; Kordel's Women's Multi; *Lanes Vegetex; *Muir's Rheumatic Pain; *Potter's Vegetable Cough Remover

Simples
Tincture: Neal's Yard Remedies

BLACK HAW

Viburnum prunifolium

Synonyms: stagbush

Parts used: stem bark, root bark

Like its relative, cramp bark (*V. opulus*), black haw is primarily a relaxant useful as an antispasmodic to relieve cramping pains and to calm the nerves. It seems more specific for the uterus than *V. opulus* and can be given for period pain, threatened miscarriage and related disorders.

Remedies and supplements
>   Blackmores Valerian Complex; Health Aid Tranquil Capsules with Viburnum; Ladies Meno-Life Formula.

BLACK NIGHTSHADE

Solanum nigra

Parts used: whole plant

Black nightshade is a poisonous plant which has traditionally been used for insomnia and to encourage sweating. Externally it was used in Arabic medicine for burns and ulcers and has been used to treat fungal skin diseases. Its appearance in an over-the-counter herbal product is a little surprising and could be a case of mistaken identify on the part of the supplier.

Remedies and supplements
>   Health Aid Liver Guard Forte

BLACK RADISH

Rhaphanus sativus

Parts used: root, whole plant

Black radish was used in Greek times to treat jaundice and digestive disorders and it is now known to stimulate bile flow and reduce gall bladder inflammation. The plant is mildly laxative.

Remedies and supplements
>   BioCare Silymarin Complex

Simples
>   *Juice:* Schoenenberger Plant Juice

BLACK ROOT

Veronicastrum virginicum

Synonyms: *Leptandra virginica*, Culver's root

Parts used: rhizome

Black root is another of the plants used by Native Americans which arrived in the UK in the nineteenth century and remains popular among traditional herbalists. The plant is a strong purgative and liver stimulant and is primarily used for chronic constipation associated with liver problems. and gall bladder inflammation. Its constituents have been little researched, although it is known to contain saponins, a volatile oil and a bitter substance called leptandrin.

Remedies and supplements
*Frank Roberts B & L Tablets; *Frank Roberts Black Root Compound Tablets; *Potter's GB Tablets

BLACK WILLOW

Salix nigra

See White willow

BLACKBERRY

Rubus villosus

Synonyms: dewberry, bramble

Parts used: root, root bark, leaves

The leaves and root of blackberry are rich in tannins, which make the herb an extremely astringent substance ideal for diarrhoea, piles and sore throats. The leaves are also added to herbal teas as a flavouring. The fruit is a good source of vitamin C.

Remedies and supplements
BioCare Procydin; *Potter's Spanish Tummy Mixture

BLACKCURRANT

Ribes nigrum

Synonyms: quinsy berry

Parts used: leaves, fruit, seed oil, buds

While blackcurrant leaves and fruits have a long history as medicinal herbs, the seed oil is a recent addition to the repertoire. Like evening primrose oil, blackcurrant oil contains *gamma*-linolenic acid (around 15–18%) and has started to join borage oil as an alternative to the more familiar evening primrose oil products. The leaves are largely used as a diuretic and anti-inflammatory, traditionally taken for sore throats and hoarseness. Infusions of both leaves and buds are also popular in parts of mainland Europe for rheumatism and urinary problems. The fruit is well-known as a source of vitamin C and is valuable for colds and influenza. Blackcurrant juice is rich in tannins and contains similar substances to those occurring in tormentil root, making it a valuable and pleasant tasting, remedy for diarrhoea.

Remedies and supplements
American Nutrition Acerola Plus; American Nutrition Super Acerola Plus; Ortis Fresh Devil's Claw Drink

Simples
Capsules: Glanolin 500.

BLACKTHORN

Prunus spinosa

Parts used: berries

Blackthorn fruits are more familiar, perhaps, as the sloes of sloe gin. The plant is very astringent and the fruits a useful tonic.

Remedies and supplements
Weleda Blackthorn Elixir
External: *Weleda Catarrh Cream

BLADDERWRACK

Fucus vesiculosis

Synonyms: kelpware, black tang, seawrack

Parts used: whole plant

Both bladderwrack and its relative *F. serratus* are included in numerous herbal remedies. Along with a number of other seaweeds, both are used to make kelp. They are salty, tonic, rich in iodine and trace metals, and are a good source of essential nutrients. The iodine content stimulates the thyroid and thus speeds up body metabolism – hence kelp's reputation as a slimming aid. This is, however, only effective in the long-term where an under-active thyroid is contributing to the obesity problem. Externally bladderwrack extracts and infused oils are used for rheumatic and arthritic problems and kelp tablets are also given as supplements in treatments for the same ailments.

• Bladderwrack concentrates toxic waste metals such as cadmium and strontium which pollute our oceans and should not be collected in contaminated areas.

Remedies and supplements
*Cantassium Boldo Aid; Culpeper Seaweed Tablets; *Frank Roberts Reducing (Slimming) Tablets; Health Aid Boldo Plus; Health Aid Super Boldo; *Heath & Heather Water Relief; *Potter's Boldo Aid to Slimming Tablets; *Rickard's Slimwell Herbal Anti-Fat Tablets

Simples
Capsules/tablets: *Dorwest Kelp Seaweed (190 mg); *Gerard House Kelp; Herbs of Grace Bladderwrack; Neal's Yard Bladderwrack (500 mg)
Tincture: Neal's Yard Remedies

BLOODROOT

Sanguinaria canadensis

Synonyms: red puccoon

Parts used: root

Listed in the US Pharmacopoeia until 1926, bloodroot was mentioned in 1612 by the early colonist, John Smith, as used by East Coast tribes to produce a red dye used for treating swollen joints and applied as skin decoration. It was later used as an emetic and purgative but is now mainly valued as a strong expectorant and diuretic which will also reduce fever and slow the heart rate. It can be included in cough remedies and gargles for throat inflammations as well as for topical preparations for warts and chilblains.
• Excess causes nausea and vomiting and it should not be taken by pregnant women.

Remedies and supplements
Herbcraft Mullein Formula

BLUE FLAG

Iris versicolor

Synonyms: wild iris

Parts used: rhizome

Blue flag has traditionally been used as a cleansing remedy for skin problems, included in preparations for psoriasis, acne and eczema. It is anti-inflammatory, laxative and diuretic and there have been some suggestions, following experiments with rats, that it might encourage a reduced food intake so could be used as a slimming aid.
• Blue flag should not be taken in pregnancy.

Remedies and supplements

Bioforce Usneasan Cough Lozenges; *Frank Roberts Kelp and Nettle Compound; *Frank Roberts Prickly Ash Compound Tablets; *Gerard House Blue Flag Root; *HRI Clear Complexion Tablets; *Potter's Catarrh Mixture; *Potter's Skin Eruptions Mixture

Simples

Tincture: Neal's Yard Remedies

BLUE VERVAIN

Verbena hastata

Parts used: herb

Blue vervain from North America is similar to the more familiar *V. officinalis*, acting as a nervine and liver remedy. It is generally regarded as rather more cleansing for the liver and is also used for chest infections and menstrual problems.

Remedies and supplements

Herbcraft Passiflora and Valerian Formula; Professional Herbs Cayenne & Ginger

BOGBEAN

Menyanthes trifoliata

Synonyms: buckbean, marsh trefoil

Parts used: leaves

Bogbean, which is an attractive, white flowered, water plant, is related to the gentian family and – like that group of herbs – is bitter and stimulating for the digestive system. The herb is diuretic and mildly laxative and is mainly taken as a cleansing remedy for rheumatism and arthritis. It can also be helpful for indigestion and anorexia but should be avoided by those suffering from chronic diarrhoea or irritable bowel syndrome.

Remedies and supplements

*Cantassium Rheumatic Pain; *Frank Roberts Rheumatic Pain Tablets; *Frank Roberts Sciatica Tablets; *Heath & Heather Rheumatic Pain; *Lanes Vegetex; *Muir's Rheumatic Pain; *Potter's Rheumatic Pain Tablets

Simples

Tincture: Neal's Yard Remedies

BOLDO

Peumus boldo

Parts used: leaves, bark

The boldo tree originates in Chile and was first investigated by French scientists in the 1870s. The plant is a liver and bile stimulant and diuretic, used for treating gall bladder problems and cystitis. It is also included in a number of proprietary slimming preparations and products aimed at solving "fluid retention" although it is certainly no more diuretic than many other herbs. Rudolf Weiss, a renowned German herb expert, is rather dismissive of the plant suggesting that "we can ignore boldo leaves for they achieve no more than our native cholagogues and choleretics".

Remedies and supplements
Bioforce Boldocynara; Blackmores Dandelion Complex; *Cantassium Boldo Aid; *Frank Roberts Reducing (Slimming) Tablets; *FSC Waterfall; Health Aid Boldo Plus; Health Aid FemmeVit; Health Aid Super Boldo; *Potter's Boldo Aid to Slimming Tablets

Simples
Tincture: Neal's Yard Remedies

BONESET

Eupatorium perfoliatum

Synonyms: thoroughwort, feverwort

Parts used: herb

Boneset takes its name, not from some ability to heal fractures, but from "boneset fever" probably a type of 'flu, prevalent in nineteenth century America. The herb is expectorant, diaphoretic, tonic and laxative, as well as reducing temperatures in fevers. It is a useful one for severe colds, influenza and bronchial congestion.

Remedies and supplements
*Cantassium Hay Fever; *Culpeper Influenza Mixture; *Muir's Catarrh; *Potter's Catarrh Mixture

BORAGE

Borago officinalis

Synonyms: starflower

Parts used: herb, seed oil

The old country saying of "borage for courage" is a rather apt description of the plant since it is now known to stimulate the adrenal glands to produce adrenaline – the "flight or fight" hormone which we make in moments of stress. The herb is also diuretic, diaphoretic, soothing for irritant tissues, mildly sedative and anti-depressant. Many old herbals focus on this last property describing the plant as one that will "lift the spirits".

Externally the juice can be used to sooth itching skin.

In recent years borage has come to the fore as a rich source of *gamma*-linolenic acid found in the pressed seed oil. Like evening primrose oil, borage has thus become a favourite with the health food industry. GLA is an essential fatty acid, a lack of which can lead to menstrual irregularities, skin problems, irritable bowel syndrome and arthritis. Borage oil contains substantially more GLA than evening primrose oil with figures of around 24% (compared with evening prim-rose's 9%) generally quoted. However, critics point to the traces of toxic erucic acid which are sometimes found in the oil. Similarly, borage is related to comfrey and traces of pyrrolizidine alkaloids, which in large quantities can cause liver cancer, have been found in its leaves. It has therefore been banned in some countries although most herbalists regard it as perfectly safe for regular use. The toxic alkaloids are not, of course, found in the pressed seed oil.

The "starflower" name is not traditional, but seems to have been adopted as a marketing ploy by suppliers.

Remedies and supplements

BioCare Candicin; Herbcraft Liquorice Formula; La Gelee Royale; Phoenix Nutri-tion Omega 3-6; Reevecrest Super Evening Primrose Oil and Borage Oil; Seven Seas Cod Liver Oil and Starflower; Seven Seas Evening Primrose and Starflower Oil; SX Formula

Simples

Capsules (oil): Arkofluid Mega GLA; Biocosmetics Starflower Oil; Lamberts High GLA; Power Health Borage Oil; Healthcrafts Starflower Oil; Seven Seas Pure Starflower Oil; Solgar Super GLA; Starflower Oil; Ultra Premium Starflower Oil
Juice: Schoenberger Plant Juice
Oil: Hartwood Aromatics

BRYONY

Bryonia dioica

Synonyms: white bryony, black bryony, English mandrake

Parts used: root

Bryony is a potent, highly toxic bitter purgative used in small quantities for rheumatic and respiratory disorders. In homoeopathic dilution it shows quite different properties and is used as a cold and catarrh remedy. Externally the plant is rubefacient and can be used in creams for muscular aches and pains or rheumatism.

Remedies and supplements
   External: *Nelsons Chilblain Ointment; *Weleda Catarrh Cream

BUCHU

Agathosma betulina

Synonyms: *Barosma betulina*

Parts used: leaves

Buchu is the name given to a number of closely related South African shrubs. "Oval", "long" and "round" forms are known, with the names descriptive of the leaf shapes, although all have identical medicinal uses. The herb contains a volatile oil with a smell reminiscent of blackcurrants, which helps to make it one of the more palatable herbs in the repertoire. As such it is sometimes included as a flavouring in OTC preparations. Buchu is diuretic, diaphoretic and stimulant. It is widely used in treatments for urinary infections and has a tonic, warming effect on the kidneys. Although it is generally regarded as a urinary antiseptic there is little scientific evidence of its actions in this area. It remains, however, one of the herbalist's favourites for cystitis. It appears in numerous over-the-counter remedies for fluid retention.

Remedies and supplements
   Blackmores Cornsilk Complex; *Culpeper Parsley Piert Tablets; Frank Roberts Black Willow Compound Tablets; *Frank Roberts Buchu Backache Compound Tablets; Frank Roberts Parsley Piert Compound Tablets; Frank Roberts Uva-Ursi Compound Tablets; *Gerard House Buchu Compound; Herbal Water Formula Capsules; HRI Water Balance Tablets; *Muir's Water-Ese; *Muir's Rheumatic Pain; Neal's Yard Buchu Compound Capsules; *Potter's Antitis Tablets; *Potter's Backache Tablets; *Potter's Diuretabs; *Potter's Kas-Bah Herb; *Potter's Skin Eruptions Mixture; *Potter's Stomach Mixture; *Potter's Watershed Mixture; Professional Herbs Uva Ursi and Parsley

Simples
   Tincture: Neal's Yard Remedies

BUCKWHEAT

Fagopyrum esculentum

Parts used: leaves, flowers, seeds

Buckwheat originates in the Middle East and was first brought to Europe by the Crusaders. It is still grown here as a cereal crop and used in making crêpes in Brittany and polenta in Italy. Buckwheat contains large amounts of the flavonoid rutin which has been shown to strengthen blood vessels, lower blood pressure and control bleeding. The herb can be helpful for such ailments as varicose veins, high blood pressure, bruising and retinal haemorrhage.

It is usually sold as a simple food supplement rather than being used in combination with other herbs.

Simples

Potter's Buckwheat Tablets; Pure-fil Rutin (180 mg); Reevecrest Nutrimental Plus; Rutivite

BURDOCK

Arctium lappa

Synonyms: beggar's buttons

Parts used: leaf, root, seeds

Burdock is a common European plant familiar for its hooked burrs which get caught in clothing and animal fur. It is a mild laxative and diuretic which has long been used as a cleansing herb for both skin and rheumatic problems – wherever, in fact, a sluggish digestion is contributing to a build-up of toxins. It is diaphoretic and the seeds are traditionally used in China for treating feverish colds, although modern research does suggest some antimicrobial activity. In the West the root is regarded as more potent and features in a number of over-the-counter remedies largely for skin and rheumatic complaints.

Remedies and supplements

Blackmores Celery Complex; Blackmores Echinacea Complex; *Gerard House Blue Flag Root; *Heath & Heather Water Relief; Heath & Heather Skin; Herbcraft Burdock & Nettle Formula; Herbcraft Dandelion Formula; *HRI Clear Complexion Tablets; *Lanes Cascade; *Lanes Kleer; Natural Flow Regular Ten Powder; *Potter's Catarrh Mixture; *Potter's GB Tablets; *Potter's Rheumatic Pain Tablets; *Potter's Skin Eruptions Mixture; *Potter's Tabritis

Simples

Capsules: Arkocaps Phytoderma (270 mg); Full Potency Herbs Burdock Root Vegicaps (520 mg)
Tincture: Neal's Yard Remedies

BURNET

Pimpinella saxifraga

Synonyms: small pimpernel, burnet saxifrage

Parts used: root

Burnet is a bitter herb that will stimulate the digestion and is also diuretic and expectorant. It is sometimes included in cough and catarrh remedies or may be taken for sore throats, cystitis and minor digestive upsets. The oil is used as a commercial flavouring for liqueurs and the leaves can give a cucumber-flavour to salads.

Remedies and supplements
Bioforce Bronchosan; *Ricola Swiss Herb Lozenges

BUTCHER'S BROOM

Ruscus aculeatus

Synonyms: Jew's myrtle, box holly

Parts used: whole plant

Currently used for venous insufficiency and piles, butcher's broom was once also recommended for jaundice, gout and kidney disorders. It is anti-inflammatory, diaphoretic and mildly laxative and has been used topically for piles and varicose veins.

Remedies and supplements
External: Phytovarix

Simples
Capsules: Full Potency Herbs Butcher's Broom Vegicaps (520 mg)

BUTTERBUR

Petasites hybridus

Synonyms: *P. officinalis*

Parts used: leaves, rhizome

Butterbur is a common European hedgerow plant with daisy-like flowers and dramatically large leaves. It was widely used in folk medicine as a cough remedy, although it has long-since fallen from use. More recent research has demonstrated considerable antispasmodic and pain-relieving properties making it suitable for tension headaches, migraine and period pain. Other researchers have shown that the plant can affect digestive function and it can be helpful for gastritis, gall bladder spasms and stomach upsets. Concentrates made from the fresh plant are believed to be most effective and a number of butterbur-based products are available from Swiss and German suppliers.

Remedies and supplements
Bioforce IMP (Imperthritica); Bioforce Petasan; Bioforce Petasan Syrup; Bioforce Tormentavena

Simples
Capsules: Bioforce Petaforce
Tincture: Bioforce

BUTTERNUT

Juglans cinerea

Synonyms: white walnut, lemon walnut, oilnut

Parts used: bark

Butternut is primarily used as a laxative having a gentler action than strong purgatives like senna and cascara sagrada. Unlike these it is safe to use in pregnancy. Butternut is often used as a cleansing remedy for skin problems related to an accumulation of toxins.

Remedies and supplements
> Natural Flow Colonite; *Potter's Boldo Aid to Slimming Tablets; Professional Herbs Cascara and Rhubarb

CABBAGE

Brassica oleracea

Parts used: Leaves

Jean Valnet, a notable French herbalist, has described cabbage as "the poor man's medicine chest" and it certainly has an impressive catalogue of applications in folk medicine. Leaves have been used as anti-inflammatory poultices to relieve a variety of complaints ranging from arthritic joints to mastitis. Cabbage lotions were once a regular household standby for skin problems, and juices and infusions are used for treating digestive problems including stomach ulcers. In Germany sauerkraut, a fermented cabbage mixture, is regarded as a preventative for cancer, rheumatism, gout and premature ageing.

Simples
> *Juice:* Schoenenberger Plant Juice

CAJUPUT

Melaleuca leucadendron

Synonyms: weeping tea tree, weeping paperbark

Parts used: essential oil

Long before tea tree became quite so fashionable as an antibacterial and antifungal oil its relative, cajuput, was used in aromatherapy as a painkiller and antiseptic. Taken internally the oil is expectorant and antispasmodic and has been used for bronchitis, sinusitis and gastric upsets. It has also been used to expel intestinal parasites.

Niaouli oil comes from a related plant – *M. viridiflora* – and is used in

aromatherapy in similar ways.
• Cajuput should not be used in pregnancy.

Remedies and supplements
*Box's Far Famed Indigestion Tablets
External: Bee Brand Massage Oil; Frank Roberts Cajuput Rub; *Olbas Oil

Simples
Oil: Botanica; Hartwood Aromatics; Neal's Yard Remedies; Tisserand

CALIFORNIAN POPPY

Eschscholzia californium

Synonyms: nightcap

Parts used: herb

Although a member of the poppy family, Californian poppy contains none of the alkaloids which depress the nervous system, that its more potent relatives do. It is a mild soporific, suitable even for sleepless children, and has also been used to relieve pain. It acts as a gentle diuretic and diaphoretic.

Simples
Capsules: Arkcaps Phytodream (240 mg)

CALUMBA

Jateorhiza palmata

Synonyms: colombo

Parts used: root

Used mainly as a bitter tonic and appetite stimulant, calumba will also reduce blood pressure and has anti-fungal properties. It has been given for morning sickness but is usually added to mixtures for sluggish digestion, poor appetite or diarrhoea.

Remedies and supplements
*Potter's Appetiser Mixture

CAMPHOR

Cinnamomum camphora

Parts used: crystallised distillate from the wood

Familiar as mothballs, camphor is also a circulatory stimulant, anti-inflammatory and mild analgesic. When applied topically, it helps to encourage blood flow to an area so is used in warming rubs for muscular aches and pains. It can soothe chilblains and cold sores and is included in balms for chapped and dried lips. Excess can cause vomiting and convulsions so, as it can be absorbed through the skin, large quantities should not be used. Internally, very small amounts are given for colds, catarrh and diarrhoea. The crystalline extract is generally further distilled to form an oil.

Remedies and supplements
> External: *Culpeper Healing Ointment; *Culpeper Head Cold and Throat Mixture; Dr Shir's Liniment; Frank Roberts Cajuput Rub; *Gerard House Dragon Balm Ointment; Power Health Head Clear; *Weleda Catarrh Cream

Simples
> Oil: Hartwood Aromatics

CAPERS

Capparis spinosa

Parts used: flower buds, root bark

Although more familiar as the main ingredient of tartar sauce, capers also have some medicinal action. The flower buds can be used for coughs while the bark is taken for digestive upsets, diarrhoea, gout and rheumatism. It is very rarely used in Western herbal medicine.

Remedies and supplements
> Health Aid Liver Guard Forte

CARAWAY

Carum carvi

Parts used: oil, seeds

Caraway seed is widely used in Middle Eastern dishes and for flavouring breads and cakes. Like many culinary herbs, it is has a calming effect on the digestion. Caraway is also an expectorant and antispasmodic. It is mainly used for stomach complaints in both adults and children but can help to relieve menstrual cramps and is occasionally found in cough remedies. Extracts are often added to laxative remedies to prevent griping and the seeds can also be chewed to relieve indigestion and wind.

Remedies and supplements
> Frank Roberts Acidosis Tablets; *Nurse Harvey's Gripe Water; *Potter's Acidosis; *Weleda Carminative Tea; *Weleda Laxadoron Tablets
> External: Bioforce Po Ho Oil

Simples
> *Oil:* Hartwood Aromatics

CARDAMOM

Elettaria cardamomum

Parts used: seed, oil

Popular in Ayurvedic medicine for treating bronchial and digestive upsets, cardamom – like other aromatic, culinary herbs – is a useful carminative, antispasmodic and expectorant. It is used, rather like dill or fennel, with laxative mixtures to ease griping and can also be given for indigestion and wind. It is good for productive coughs and also eases feelings of nausea.

Remedies and supplements
> Blackmores Cape Aloes and Cascara; Frank Roberts Acidosis Tablets; *Potter's Acidosis

Simples
> *Oil:* Neal's Yard Remedies

CASCARA SAGRADA

Rhamnus purshianus

Parts used: bark

Cascara sagrada is a potent laxative included in a number of proprietary preparations. It contains anthraquinones which irritate the lower bowel and increase peristalsis. As this can lead to griping pains, carminatives such as fennel or aniseed are generally included in the mix. Cascara also has a tonic effect on the liver and digestive system and is thus found in remedies aimed at stimulating the gall bladder, improving liver function or treating indigestion.

Remedies and supplements
> BioCare Colon Care; Blackmores Cape Aloes and Cascara; Culpeper Pilewort Tablets; *Dorwest Natural Herb Tablets; *Frank Roberts B & L Tablets; Frank Roberts Constipation Tablets; Frank Roberts Parsley Piert Compound Tablets; *Frank Roberts Pilewort Compound Tablets – Green Label; *Frank Roberts Reducing (Slimming) Tablets; *Gerard House Pilewort Compound; *Lanes Dual-Lax Extra Strong; *Lanes Pileabs; Natural Flow Regular Ten Powder; Neal's Yard Cascara Compound; *Potter's Out of Sorts Tablets; *Potter's Piletabs; *Potter's Skin Eruptions Mixture; Professional Herbs Cascara and Rhubarb

Simples
> *Tincture:* Neal's Yard Remedies

CASSIA

Cinnamomum cassia

See Cinnamon

CAT'S CLAW

Uncaria tomentosa

Parts used: inner bark

Cat's claw was discovered by a German researcher, Dr Klaus Keplinger, in the Peruvian rain forests in the 1970s. The plant is a vine with thorns resembling the claws of a cat – hence its name – and it is used by the local Ashaninka tribe for arthritis, gastritis, cancer and a wide range of disease. Tests have shown that it is anti-oxidant, anti-viral, anti-tumour and anti-inflammatory and it also has a cleansing and healing effect on the digestive system.

Extracts have been included in AIDS and cancer treatments and it has also been used successfully for genital herpes, chronic fatigue syndrome, asthma, diabetes and circulatory problems. Recommended dosage is 2–6 g daily and the plant could well emerge as one of the world's most important tonic herbs.

Remedies and supplements
   Full Potency Herbs Echinacea/Goldenseal/Cat's Claw Complex Vegicaps

Simples
   Capsules: Full Potency Herbs Cat's Claw Tablets (1000 mg); Higher Nature (350 mg)

CATUABA

Anemopaegma arvense

Parts used: tree bark

Catuaba is highly regarded in Brazil as an aphrodisiac. The name appears to be applied to a number of species including a tall tree growing to the North of the country and a more shrubby plant growing in central areas. The plant has been investigated by the World Health Organisation and is undergoing further research for possible anti-depressive activity. In Brazil it seems, there is a saying that "until a father reaches 60, the son is his, after that the son is catuaba's". The plant is also considered a stimulant for the nervous systems.

Simples
   Capsules: Rio D'Amor Catuaba

CAYENNE

Capsicum spp

Synonyms: chili, hot pepper, tabasco pepper

Parts used: fruit

The pepper generally used in medicine is *C. frutescens* although hot varieties of *C. annuum*, mainly grown for cooking, are just as good. The plants originated from South and Central America, India and south-east Asia and they have long been used medicinally. Although they were a favourite with the nineteenth century physiomedicalists, earlier herbalists were less enthusiastic: writing in 1597, John Gerard maintained that they were "enemies of the liver" and would also "killeth dogs".

Today cayenne is generally regarded as warming and stimulating: useful in chills and debility and also helpful for some digestive problems. Externally, cayenne ointments can be used to stimulate blood flow and may be used for treating chilblains, shingles, lumbago, muscle pain, and neuralgia. Many over-the-counter remedies contain small amounts of cayenne as a warming stimulant for a range of ailments.

Remedies and supplements

Blackmores Skullcap & Valerian; *Box's Far Famed Indigestion Tablets; *Cantassium Hay Fever; *Culpeper Elder Flower and Peppermint Mixture; *Culpeper Head Cold and Throat Mixture; *Culpeper Influenza Mixture; *Frank Roberts B & L Tablets; *Frank Roberts Black Root Compound Tablets; *Frank Roberts Cold Tablets; *Frank Roberts Drops of Life Tablets; Frank Roberts Parsley Piert Compound Tablets; *Frank Roberts Prickly Ash Compound Tablets; *Frank Roberts Rheumatic Pain Tablets; *Hactos Cough Mixture; Health Aid Herbal Booster; *Heath & Heather Indigestion & Flatulence; Herbcraft Peppermint Formula; Herbcraft Garlic and Horseradish Winter Formula; Herbcraft Liquorice Formula; Kordel's Quiet Time; La Gelee Royale; *Lane's Cut-a-Cough; *Lanes Herbelix Specific; *Lanes Honey and Molasses Cough Mixture; *Lanes Vegetex; *Muir's Rheumatic Pain; Nature's Plus Ginkgo Combo; Neal's Yard Horehound & Aniseed Linctus; Neal's Yard Elderflower, Peppermint & Composition Essence; *Potter's Antibron Tablets; *Potter's Catarrh Mixture; *Potter's Indian Brandee; *Potter's Life Drops; *Potter's Peerless Composition Essence; Professional Herbs Cascara and Rhubarb; Professional Herbs Cayenne & Ginger; Professional Herbs Uva Ursi and Parsley

External: Frank Roberts Cajuput Rub; Herbcraft Calendula & Goldenseal Spray; Herbcraft Liquorice and Propolis Spray

Simples

Capsules: Full Potency Herbs Cayenne Capsules (520 mg); Herbs of Grace Cayenne

Tincture: Neal's Yard Remedies

CEDAR

Cedrus libani subsp. *atlantica*

Parts used: essential oil

The cedar tree produces a very calming, relaxing oil that is also antiseptic and astringent. It is used in aromatherapy for a variety of respiratory and urinary complaint and also for skin diseases.

Simples

Oil: Hartwood Aromatics; Neal's Yard Remedies; Nelson & Russell; Tisserand

CELERY

Apium graveolens

Synonyms: smallage

Parts used: seed, essential oil

Celery seed is anti-inflammatory, anti-rheumatic, carminative and diuretic. It encourages the excretion of uric acid which is helpful in a number of arthritic conditions, especially gout. It also helps lower blood pressure and is a reputed aphrodisiac. Although the root was once used for urinary stones, the rest of the plant has markedly less medicinal action. Juice made from the whole plant and roots is regarded as a tonic for debilitated conditions and may also help with joint or urinary tract inflammations.

The essential oil, extracted from the seeds by steam distillation, is sometimes used in over-the-counter remedies and occasional use of the leaf is also recorded although it has little specific medical action.

Remedies containing celery are largely diuretic mixtures used for fluid retention, or else preparations for rheumatism and arthritis.

• Celery seed contains bergapten which can increase the photosensitivity of the skin. The oil and large doses of seed should be avoided in pregnancy.

Remedies and supplements

BioCare NEF242; BioCare Phytosterol Complex; Blackmores Celery Complex; *Cantassium Rheumatic Pain; *Dorwest Mixed Vegetable Tablets; *Frank Roberts Prickly Ash Compound Tablets; *Frank Roberts Rheumatic Pain Tablets; *Frank Roberts Sciatica Tablets; *FSC Waterfall; *Gerard House Celery; *Heath & Heather Rheumatic Pain; Kordel's Celery 3000 Plus; Kordel's Celery and Juniper; Kordel's Kalm-Ex; *Lanes Vegetex; SX Formula

Simples

Capsules/tablets: BioCare Celery Seed (580 mg); *Heath & Heather Celery Seed (600 mg); Power Health Pure Celery Seed (200 mg)
Juice: Schoenenberger Plant Juice
Oil: Hartwood Aromatics
Tincture: Neal's Yard Remedies

CENTAURY

Centaurium erythraea

Synonyms: feverwort, *Erythraea centaurium*

Parts used: herb

An aromatic, bitter herb used mainly as a bitter digestive stimulant for indigestion, liver and gall bladder problems and to stimulate the appetite, centaury has also been used to reduce fevers. The plant is closely related to yellow gentian and has very similar constituents and properties. It is used in small amounts in a few over-the-counter preparations.

Remedies and supplements
Blackmores Dandelion Complex; Bioforce Gastrosan; *Lanes Digest; *Weleda Laxadoron Tablets

Simples
Tincture: Bioforce, Neal's Yard Remedies

CHAMOMILE

Matricaria recutita

Synonyms: *Chamomilla recutita*, German chamomile, mayweed

Parts used: flowers, essential oil

Both German chamomile and its relative, Roman chamomile (*Chamaemelum nobile*) are among the most widely used medicinal herbs. Their actions are very similar with Roman chamomile having a slightly more bitter taste and German chamomile greater anti-inflammatory and analgesic properties. While herbalists may have their individual favourites the plants are extremely close in action and almost interchangeable. They are sedative, antispasmodic, carminative and anti-inflammatory and are used for nervous stomach upsets, nausea and insomnia. Externally, chamomile creams are used for eczema, wounds, nappy rash, sore nipples and piles.

The flowers are readily available in tea bags or loose for infusions and, although the flavour can be something of an acquired taste, chamomile tea is probably one of the most popular herbal drinks on the market.

Chamomile is also used in homoeopathy and Chamomilla 3× is a valuable standby for babies, used to treat both colic and teething. It is one of the safest herbs for children and babies and some mothers use weak infusions as a nighttime drink to encourage restful sleep. The infusion can also be added to baby's bath water.

On steam distillation, chamomile yields a deep blue essential oil which is very relaxing and useful in skin care. The oil is also used for a range of digestive disorders, inflammations, emotional problems, muscle aches and pain.

Remedies and supplements

*Bio-Strath Chamomile Formula; *Bio-Strath Liquorice Formula; *Cantassium Quiet Nite Sleep; Colon Cleanse; Frank Roberts Golden Seal Compound Tablets; Herbcraft Passiflora and Valerian Formula; *HRI Calm Life Tablets; *Kordel's Quiet Time; *Lanes Biobalm; *Lanes Digest; *Potter's Appetiser Mixture; *Weleda Carminative Tea; *Weleda Chamomilla 3× Pillules and Drops

External: Bioforce Seven Herb Cream; Gerard House Chamomile Ointment; Health Aid Eczem Oil

Simples

Capsules/tablets: Full Potency Herbs Chamomile Vegicaps (520 mg)
Juices: Schoenenberger Plant Juice
Oil: Botanica; Hartwood Aromatics; Neal's Yard Remedies; Nelson & Russell; Tisserand
Tincture: Herbcraft; Neal's Yard Remedies

CHAPARRAL

Larrea tridentata

Synonyms: creosote bush

Parts used: leaves, twigs

Chaparral, related to the *Guaiacum* spp, was once widely used as a remedy for infections, skin problems, urinary disorders, respiratory complaints, muscular inflammations and in cancer treatment. Something, in fact, of a cure all. Chaparral was originally used by the Papago and Maricopas tribes in the American south-west for stomach problems, diarrhoea and wounds while the Pimas Indians used it to relieve toothache by sharpening a young branch to a point and inserting it into the cavity. Western medicine discovered the herb in the 1840s and until 1945 extracts from chaparral were included in the US Pharmacopoeia as an expectorant.

The herb remained popular in the USA until 1992 when a series of hepatitis cases, among patients taking chaparral tablets, led the US Food and Drug Administration to issue a formal warning about the risks of using the plant and its potential toxicity, declaring that the herb was a health risk to the public. While many herbalists believed that chaparral had been wrongly maligned, suppliers voluntarily withdrew it from use.

However, in 1995 after a thorough investigation, the American Herbal Products Association concluded that the patients involved in the 1992 incident probably had prior liver disease and chaparral was not to blame. They rescinded the voluntary ban but set up a telephone line, in conjunction with the FDA, for reporting any further incidents involving the herb. The plant was never quite so popular in the UK as it was in America but it may be reintroduced here again following the AHPA decision.

Remedies and supplements
    Absorb Plus

CHASTETREE

Vitex agnus-castus

Synonyms: agnus castus, monk's pepper

Parts used: berries

The chastetree reputedly takes its name from its action as a male anaphrodisiac, used by medieval monks to reduce libido and lascivious thoughts. It is an important hormonal herb, acting on the pituitary gland to increase the production of female sex hormones which are involved in ovulation. It is thus extremely useful for menstrual irregularities and menopausal problems. In southern Europe, where it originates, chastetree is regarded as a female aphrodisiac.

Remedies and supplements
    BioCare PT208; Gerard House Fem-a-Tea

Simples
    Capsules/Tablets: Cantassium Agnus Castus (500 mg); Frank Roberts Agnus Castus Tablets; Gerard House Agnacast; Herbs of Grace Agnus Castus; Power Health Pure Agnus Castus (200 mg)
    Tinctures: *Agnolyt; Bioforce; Galen Herbal Supplies; Herbcraft; Neal's Yard Remedies

CHERRY STALKS

Prunus avium

Synonyms: Prunus cerasus

Parts used: stalks

Stalks of the wild cherry were traditionally used as a diuretic for cystitis and problems of fluid retention although they are rarely found in proprietary remedies today.

Simples
    Capsules: Arkocaps Phytosistitus

CHICKWEED

Stellaria media

Parts used: herb

Chickweed, as the name suggests, is a favourite food for domestic fowl. It is an extremely common garden weed and one that can be easily gathered and made into ointments for home use. It makes a useful remedy for irritant skin rashes and eczema and can also be used in the first aid box for burns, boils and drawing splinters. Internally it can sometimes be found added to remedies for rheumatism and was once regarded as a significant source of vitamin C with sprigs added to salads or cooked as a vegetable.

Remedies and supplements
External: Gerard House Chickweed Ointment; Neal's Yard Stellaria Ointment; *Potter's Eczema Ointment; *Potter's Herbheal Ointment

Simples
Tincture: Neal's Yard Remedies

CHICORY

Chicorium intybus

Synonyms: succory

Parts used: leaves. roots

Chicory is a bitter herb, stimulating for liver and gall-bladder, diuretic and slightly laxative. It is mainly used as a cleansing remedy in rheumatism and gout or for liver disorders. In Ayurvedic medicine it is regarded as cooling and "anti-*pitta*".

Remedies and supplements
Health Aid Liver Guard Forte

CHINESE DATE

Zizyphus jujuba

Synonyms: French jujube, Indian plum

Parts used: fruit, seeds

The Chinese regard the jujube date as a useful harmonizer for complex prescriptions helping to modify actions. The seeds are seen as sedative and tranquillizing and are given for insomnia and palpitations, as well as night sweats.

Remedies and supplements
Equillence

CHINESE FOXGLOVE

Rehmannia glutinosa

Synonyms: *Shu Di Huang; Sheng Di Huang*

Parts used: root

Rehmannia root is highly prized in Chinese tradition as a blood and energy tonic. The root is used raw as a blood cooling remedy and is also cooked for use as a liver and kidney tonic. It features in a number of preparations for menstrual and menopausal disorders which can be found in Chinese herb shops.

Externally the plant can help to stop bleeding.

Remedies and supplements
Equillence
External: Spring Wind Ointment

Simples
Tincture: Neal's Yard Remedies

CHINESE GOLD THREAD

Coptis chinensis

Synonyms: *Huang Lian*

Parts used: rhizome

Chinese gold thread is extremely bitter to taste and is largely used in traditional medicine for digestive problems including diarrhoea, gastroenteritis and dysentery. It stimulates bile flow and is also anti-inflammatory, astringent and is used for mouth inflammations and fever.

Remedies and supplements
External: Golden Yellow Ointment, Spring Wind Ointment

CHRYSANTHEMUM

Dendranthema × grandiflorum

Synonyms: *Ju Hua*

Parts used: flowers

Popular as a cooling and calming tea in China, chrysanthemum flowers will also help to reduce high blood pressure and relax the coronary artery so can be beneficial in angina pectoris. As a cooling herb the tea is also given for feverish colds. In traditional Chinese theory the plant is believed to help clear liver stagnation.

Simples
Tea: East West Ju Hua Tea

CINNAMON

Cinnamomum zeylanicum

Parts used: bark, oil

Cinnamon is widely used as a flavouring in cooking and perfumery and also has a long tradition as a medicinal plant. It is astringent, stimulant and carminative and is regarded as warming so can be helpful for all sorts of "cold" conditions including chills, rheumatic aches and pains.

Cinnamon has been used for centuries to treat nausea and vomiting and is also helpful for many digestive problems including diarrhoea and gastroenteritis. It shows some anti-fungal activity and is thus used in products for candidiasis. Because of its pungent and pleasant flavour, cinnamon is added to a number of remedies to disguise the less palatable herbs.

C. cassia, Chinese cinnamon, is used in similar ways and is sometimes found in over-the-counter products as cassia oil. The Chinese use cassia twigs for treating colds and chills and believe it encourages circulation to the peripheries.
• Cinnamon should be avoided in pregnancy.

Remedies and supplements
*Culpeper Elder Flower and Peppermint Mixture; *Culpeper Influenza Mixture; Frank Roberts Acidosis Tablets; Neal's Yard Elderflower, Peppermint & Composition Essence; Neal's Yard Slippery Elm Tablets; *Potter's Acidosis; *Potter's Slippery Elm Stomach Tablets; *Weleda Cough Drops; *Weleda Melissa Comp
External: *Gerard House Dragon Balm Ointment; Herbcraft Fresh Breath Cinnamint Spray

Simples
Oil: Hartwood Aromatics; Neal's Yard Remedies

CITRON

Citrus medica

Parts used: peel, oil

Citron is the major source of candied peel and is believed to be one of the earliest cultivars of the *Citrus* genus, which has been extended by hybridisation for centuries. Lemon, for example, is believed to be a cross between citron and lime. Citron oil is used in some over-the-counter products and is very similar in character to lemon oil.

Remedies and supplements
External: Bioforce Po Ho Ointment

CLARY SAGE

Salvia sclarea

Parts used: essential oil

Clary sage produces a tonic oil with an attractive scent which is widely used in aromatherapy. It is considered to be antispasmodic, carminative, sedative and a useful digestive remedy, and is used in massage treatments for depression, period pain, kidney disorders, and skin complaints.

Simples

> *Oil:* Botanica; Hartwood Aromatics; Neal's Yard Remedies; Nelson & Russell; Tisserand

CLIVERS

Galium aparine

Synonyms: cleavers, goosegrass, sticky Willie

Parts used: herb

Most gardeners regard clivers as a rampant weed as it scrambles through shrubberies threatening to choke the prize specimens. The plant is, however, a valuable lymphatic tonic – an astringent with mild laxative and diuretic effects. It has largely been used as a cleansing herb for skin problems and externally is effective in ointments for psoriasis.

As a lymphatic remedy it can also be helpful for tonsillitis, glandular fever, benign cysts and swollen lymph glands. Although it is only mildly diuretic (the fresh juiced herb is more effective) it is included in a large number of over-the-counter remedies for "fluid retention" and similar problems.

Remedies and supplements

> *Cantassium Boldo Aid; Frank Roberts Uva-Ursi Compound Tablets; *Gerard House Buchu Compound; *Heath & Heather Water Relief; Health Aid Boldo Plus; Health Aid Super Boldo; *Lanes Athera; *Lanes Cascade; *Muir's Sciatica; *Potter's Antitis Tablets; *Potter's Kas-Bah Herb; *Potter's Sciargo; *Potter's Sciargo Herb; *Potter's Tabritis; *Potter's Watershed Mixture; Professional Herbs Uva Ursi and Parsley; *Rickard's Slimwell Herbal Anti-Fat Tablets
> External: *Potter's Parasolv Ointment

Simples

> *Tincture:* Neal's Yard Remedies

CLOVE

Syzygium aromaticum

Parts used: flower buds, oil

Familiar as a culinary spice, clove is also carminative, warming, anodyne, antiseptic, antispasmodic and will relieve feelings of nausea. The oil makes a valuable emergency first aid remedy for toothache and is included in a number of proprietary toothpastes and dental preparations. The pungent aroma and pleasant taste of cloves make it ideal for flavouring less palatable brews and it is used like this in a number of mixtures. However, as it is also a suitable herb for chills and digestive upsets its presence is not always totally irrelevant. The Chinese regard clove as a good kidney tonic helpful for the reproductive organs.

Remedies and supplements
BioCare Candicidin; *Culpeper Elder Flower and Peppermint Mixture; *Culpeper Influenza Mixture; *Hactos Cough Mixture; *Lane's Cut-a-Cough; Natural Flow Colonite; Natural Flow Regular Ten Powder; Neal's Yard Elderflower, Peppermint & Composition Essence; Neal's Yard Slippery Elm Tablets; *Olbas Pastilles; *Potter's Slippery Elm Stomach Tablets; *Revitonil; *Weleda Clairo Tea; *Weleda Cough Drops; *Weleda Laxadoron Tablets; *Weleda Melissa Comp
External: Bee Brand Massage Oil; *Olbas Oil; *Potter's Nine Rubbing Oils; *Weleda Medicinal Gargle

Simples
Oil: Hartwood Aromatics; Neal's Yard Remedies

COFFEE

Coffea arabica

Parts used: seeds

Coffee is well known as a stimulant and diuretic, thanks to its high caffeine content, and as regular coffee drinkers know well, excess can lead to palpitations and sleeplessness. In homoeopathic medicine it is used to treat these sorts of ailments and is given for restlessness and nervous agitation.

Remedies and supplements
*Weleda Avena Sativa Comp.

COLA

Cola vera

Synonyms: bissy nuts, kola, goora nut

Parts used: seed

Cola contains up to 2.5% caffeine with traces of theobromine making it a rather more effective stimulant than coffee (which contains up to around 0.3% caffeine). Like coffee, it is also diuretic and acts as a heart stimulant and anti-depressant. The nuts are astringent and can be helpful in diarrhoea.

Like other caffeine sources, cola essentially provides a short-term energy boost rather than acting as a more deep-seated energy tonic. It is included in a large number of tonic preparations usually promoted as remedies for fatigue and tiredness. It was, of course, once used in the original Coca Cola recipe – the "coca" being provided by cocaine leaves – although less potent synthetic substitutes have long been used.

Remedies and supplements
Blackmores Cactus & Hawthorn; *Culpeper Herbal Tonic for Digestive Disorders; *Dorwest Damiana and Kola tablets; *Fo Ti Tieng; *Frank Roberts Strength Tablets; *Frank Roberts Supa-Tonic Tablets; Health Aid Herbal Booster; Herbatone; *Muir's Pick-Me-Up; *Potter's Chlorophyll Tablets; *Potter's Strength Tablets

Simples
Tincture: Neal's Yard Remedies

COLTSFOOT

Tussilago farfara

Synonyms: horsehoof

Parts used: flowers, leaves

Once one of our most popular remedies for coughs and catarrh, use of coltsfoot has declined in recent years due to the discovery of pyrrolizidine alkaloids in the plant. While there is no firm evidence to suggest that coltsfoot can cause liver damage its use has been restricted in a number of countries and many herbalists prefer to keep it for occasional short term use. It is, however, an extremely effective expectorant, demulcent and anti-catarrhal, helpful for irritating and spasmodic coughs including whooping cough, asthma and bronchitis.

Remedies and supplements
Neal's Yard Horehound & Honey Lozenges; *Potter's Antibron Tablets

Simples
Tincture: Neal's Yard Remedies
Juice: Schoenenberger Plant Juice

COMFREY

Symphytum officinalis

Synonyms: knitbone

Parts used: root, leaves

Comfrey has undergone a chequered history in recent years: alternately acclaimed as a panacea and banned as a health hazard.

The plant has long been used as a wound herb helping to repair damaged tissues both internally and externally. Its action is due to the presence of a chemical called allantoin which encourages proliferation of various cells and thus accelerates healing. Its old country name of knitbone testifies to its traditional role in treating fractures and severe strains. Internally, comfrey was used by herbalists for stomach ulceration and digestive upsets and was highly regarded as a soothing anti-inflammatory.

During the 1960s and 1970s the plant was over-hyped as a cure-all for arthritis and over-the-counter products proliferated. These were soon followed by reports of liver damage attributed to the plant and research studies – which involved feeding huge amounts of comfrey to rats – purported to demonstrate that comfrey could cause liver cancer. The problem is a group of chemicals called pyrrolizidine alkaloids (known carcinogens) which are present in the herb. Opponents of the various bans on the plant which followed, argue that these alkaloids are not absorbed in digestion and may even be destroyed in processing the herb. They also point out that the rat-feeding experiment involved enormous amounts of comfrey leaving the animals with very little else in their diets so the creatures also had to cope with malnutrition.

Comfrey is banned in the US and Australia and in parts of Europe its use is restricted to external applications which must not be used on broken skin. In the UK comfrey ointments are readily available and although some suppliers similarly recommend avoiding use of the herb on broken skin this is not a statutory requirement. Many internal comfrey preparations have disappeared from sale although the leaf can still be used and tablets occasionally found. Internal products using the root are no longer available.

Remedies and supplements
Potter's Comfrey Tablets
External: Bioforce Comfrey Comfrey Cream; *Culpeper Comfrey Ointment; Frank Roberts Comfrey Ointment; Gerard House Comfrey Ointment; Herbcraft Aloe Lavender Spray; Neal's Yard Comfrey Ointment; Neal's Yard Sports Salve; *Potter's Comfrey Ointment

Simples
Infused oil: Neal's Yard Remedies
Tincture: Bioforce; Neal's Yard Remedies

COMMON PLANTAIN

Plantago major

Synonyms: white man's foot, rat-tail plantain, greater plantain

Parts used: leaves

Common plantain can be used fresh as a wound herb or for insect stings. The plant is astringent, anti-inflammatory and diuretic and is generally recommended for gastric inflammations, cystitis and diarrhoea. Like ribwort plantain it contains aucubin and is antimicrobial. It can be used for respiratory problems and catarrh although ribwort plantain is traditionally preferred. Ointments containing the herb can be used for slow healing wounds, burns and piles.

Remedies and supplements
Gerard House Eez-a-Tea

Simples
Capsules: Arkocaps Phytodesensatine (200 mg)

CORDYCEPS

Cordyceps sinensis

Synonyms: *Dong Chong Xia Cao*, Chinese caterpillar fungus, deer fungus

Parts used: whole fungus

This parasitic fungus grows on certain sorts of caterpillar, feeding on the animal and then fruiting in the spring. Today, the fungus is cultivated rather more pleasantly on a grain base. It is highly regarded in Chinese medicine as an energy tonic, especially for lungs and kidney, and the herb has been shown to have anti-cancer and antibacterial action.

Remedies and supplements
Mycoherb Myco Forte; Mycoherb Tri Myco Gen

Simples
Tincture: Mycoherb Cordy-Gen (East West Herbs)

CORIANDER

Coriandrum sativum

Parts used: seed, oil

Like other traditional aromatic culinary herbs, coriander is carminative and antispasmodic and can be helpful for minor digestive upsets. It is sometimes added to laxative mixtures to ease griping. The seeds are also expectorant and figure in some cough remedies.

Remedies and supplements
*Weleda Cough Drops; *Weleda Melissa Comp

Simples
Oil: Hartwood Aromatics; Neal's Yard Remedies

CORNSILK

Zea mays

Parts used: stamens

Cornsilk comprises the long, silky stamens from maize plants which dry to form a crinkled mass often described as resembling red beard clippings. It is used as a diuretic and demulcent, useful for irritant and inflamed bladder and urinary tract disorders including prostate problems. The herb also contains allantoin (the same cell proliferant found in comfrey) so is very healing. Although a diuretic, it can be helpful for bedwetting in children where this is associated with bladder irritation.

Remedies and supplements

Absorb Plus; Frank Roberts Black Willow Compound Tablets; Natural Flow Colonite; *Potter's Elixir of Damiana and Saw Palmetto; *Potter's Protat; Professional Herbs Uva Ursi and Parsley

Simples

Tincture: Neal's Yard Remedies

COUCHGRASS

Elymus repens

Synonyms: twitch, *Agropyron repens*

Parts used: rhizome

Regarded, rightly, by gardeners as an invasive weed, couchgrass is valued by herbalists as a urinary antiseptic and soothing diuretic. It is mainly used for cystitis, prostate problems and kidney infections but may also be added to remedies for gout and rheumatism.

Remedies and supplements

Blackmores Cornsilk Complex; Frank Roberts Uva-Ursi Compound Tablets; *Potter's Antitis Tablets; *Potter's Kas-Bah Herb

Simples

Tincture: Neal's Yard Remedies

COUGH ROOT

Lomatium dissectum

Parts used: root

Cough root comes from the North and Western parts of America where it was traditionally boiled and used in cough remedies by Native Americans. It is still used in US folk medicine and may be occasionally found in over-the-counter products formulated in the United States.

Remedies and supplements
Herbcraft Echinacea Formula

COWSLIP

Primula veris

Parts used: root, flower

Cowslip roots are rich in saponins making the plant a potent expectorant effective for harsh, difficult coughs with sticky mucous that is difficult to shift. The root also contains salicylates and has been used for arthritis. The flowers contain neither of these chemicals and are mainly used as a relaxing nervine for insomnia and tension. Traditional herbals often describe cowslip flowers as ideal for treating "frenzies" and they can also be used in feverish chills and headaches.

Remedies and supplements
*Bio-Strath Thyme Formula;*Bio-Strath Willow Formula; *Ricola Swiss Herb Lozenges

CRAMP BARK

Viburnum opulus

Synonyms: guelder rose

Parts used: bark

Cramp bark is a useful relaxant for both muscles and nerves. It can relieve the spasms of cramp and colic and forms a useful addition to remedies for constipation, as well as being included in products to calm the nerves. As a relaxant it is sometimes included by herbalists in blood pressure remedies to relax and dilate blood vessels. Externally it is used in creams to relieve muscle cramps.

Cramp bark may also be used for period pain and pain following childbirth, although many herbalists prefer its close relative black haw for these conditions.

Simples
Capsules: Gerard House Cramp Bark
Tincture: Neal's Yard Remedies

CRANBERRY

Vaccinium oxycoccus

Parts used: fruits

Research in the early 1990s in the USA, based on a six-month trial involving elderly women, indicated that cranberry juice has an effect on urinary bacteria and it is thus starting to be recommended for urinary infections and cystitis. The berries are a useful vitamin C source and are sometimes included as such in food supplements.

Remedies and supplements
BioCare CP227; BioCare UR 228; Cantassium Concentrated Cranberry; FSC Cranberry Concentrate Tablets; Solgar Natural Cranberry Extract with Vitamin C Vegicaps

Simples
Capsules: Power Health Cranberry Juice (140 mg)

CREEPING JENNY

Lysimachia nummularia

Synonyms: moneywort

Parts used: herb

Creeping jenny was once widely used as a wound herb in compresses and lotions for sores and injuries. The plant is slightly astringent and will stop bleeding. In the past it was also regarded as a specific for whooping cough.

Remedies and supplements
*Weleda Dermatodendron Ointment

CYPRESS

Cupressus sempervirens

Parts used: essential oil

The essential oil distilled from the cypress tree is widely used in both perfumery and aromatherapy. It is regard as antiseptic, antispasmodic, astringent, diuretic, sedative and a liver stimulant and is used in massage treatments for asthma, whooping cough and influenza. Cypress is calming and can be helpful at the menopause. It is used in France for varicose veins and piles and French *phytotherapists* also give the oil internally for coughs, colds and menopausal problems.

Remedies and supplements
Neal's Yard Horehound & Honey Lozenges
External: Phytovarix

Simples
Oil: Botanica, Hartwood Aromatics; Neal's Yard Remedies; Nelson & Russell; Tisserand

DAMIANA

Turnera diffusa var. aphrodisiaca

Parts used: leaves

Damiana is a popular stimulant and aphrodisiac included in a number of remedies aimed at countering fatigue and giving energy. The plant is an aromatic shrub largely found in Central and South America and acts as a tonic for the nervous system and anti-depressant. It is also stimulating for the digestion and urinary system and can be helpful in convalescence and general debility, both as a tonic and to encourage the appetite.

Damiana can be helpful for menstrual problems, loss of libido, impotence and prostate problems. Aromatherapists use the oil as an uplifting tonic.

Remedies and supplements
*Dorwest Damiana and Kola Tablets; *Frank Roberts Strength Tablets; *Frank Roberts Supa-Tonic Tablets; Gerard House Vig-a-Tea; La Gelee Royale; *Potter's Elixir of Damiana and Saw Palmetto; *Potter's Strength Tablets; SX Formula

Simples
Capsules/tablets: Arkocaps Phytophrodisiac (250 mg); *Gerard House Curzon
Oil: Tisserand
Tincture: Neal's Yard Remedies

DANDELION

Taraxacum officinale

Parts used: root, leaves

Dandelion is a comparative newcomer to Western herbalism, first mentioned in the fifteenth century. The plant is strongly diuretic while the root is also a good liver tonic: bitter and stimulating to improve the digestion. Long-term use of diuretics can often deplete the body's supply of potassium which can affect normal cell function and heart rate. Dandelion leaves are, however, an extremely rich source of potassium so by using the whole plant the body's natural balance is maintained.

Dandelion also shows anti-inflammatory action and is used as a cleansing remedy in rheumatism, although it is mainly included in over-the-counter remedies for kidney and liver problems. Its use in slimming preparations is largely as a diuretic and mild laxative, and these products should really not be used long term in an attempt to lose body fluids and thus reduce weight.

Remedies and supplements
*Aqualette; BioCare Liv243; Bioforce Boldocynara; Bioforce Gastrosan; Blackmores Dandelion Complex; *Cantassium Boldo Aid; *Cantassium Rheumatic Pain; Colon Cleanse; *Culpeper Herbal Mixture for Acidity, Indigestion and Flatulence; *Culpeper Parsley Piert Tablets; *Dorwest Natural Herb Tablets; *Frank Roberts Nervous Dyspepsia Tablets; *Frank Roberts Reducing (Slimming) Tablets;

FSC Milk Thistle Tablets; *Gerard House Buchu Compound; *Gerard House Golden Seal Compound; *Gerard House Waterlex Tablets; Health Aid Boldo Plus; Herbcraft Dandelion Formula; *Herbulax; HRI Water Balance Tablets; Neal's Yard Buchu Compound Capsules; *Potter's Boldo Aid to Slimming Tablets; *Potter's Out of Sorts Tablets; *Potter's Stomach Mixture; *Uvacin

Simples

Capsules/tablets: Arkocaps Dandelion (250 mg); Full Potency Herbs Dandelion Root Vegicaps (520 mg); Herbs of Grace Dandelion Root; Power Health Pure Dandelion (250 mg)
Tincture: Bioforce; Herbcraft; Neal's Yard Remedies

DANG GUI

Angelica polymorpha var. sinensis

Synonyms: *A.sinensis*, Chinese angelica, *Tong Kwai*

Parts used: root

Dang Gui is generally regarded in China as the most important tonic herb after ginseng. It is used, in Chinese terminology, to "nourish the blood" and may be helpful for anaemia, menstrual problems or as a tonic after childbirth. It is also included in general purpose tonic preparations usually targeted at women. It is a painkiller, mild laxative – especially suitable for the elderly – and has some anti-bacterial action.

A comparative newcomer to the Western herbal repertoire, Chinese angelica is often marketed as "*Tong Kwai*," – a name derived from older systems of transliterating Chinese characters.

Remedies and supplements

Equillence
External: Amber Massage Salve; Dr Shir's Liniment; Golden Yellow Ointment; Spring Wind Ointment

Simples

Capsules/tablets: Cantassium Tong Kwai; Full Potency Herbs Dong Quai Vegicaps; Herbs of Grace Angelica S.
Tincture: Herbcraft; Neal's Yard Remedies

DEADLY NIGHTSHADE

Atropa belladonna

Synonyms: dwale

Parts used: herb, root

Deadly nightshade is a highly toxic plant which was once used both as a primitive anaesthetic before surgery and in eye drops to dilate the pupils and make the eyes more attractive – hence "belladonna".

The plant is a narcotic and antispasmodic used in pain relief; it contains the alkaloid, atropine, which reduces bodily secretions of the mouth, bronchi and stomach. This is used in orthodox medicine in a number of critical and chronic conditions, such as Parkinson's disease. In the UK, use of the plant is restricted to qualified practitioners. It is rarely used in OTC remedies.

Remedies and supplements
Bioforce Cystaforce

DEVIL'S CLAW

Harpagophytum procumbens

Parts used: tuber

Devil's claw grows in the Kalahari Desert in South Africa and takes its name from the shape of its seed pods. It was reputedly introduced into Western medicine by a South African farmer who noticed bushmen using it in decoctions for a number of ills – notably digestive upsets and rheumatism. The plant was sent to Germany for investigation and by the late 1950s its anti-inflammatory and anti-rheumatic properties were well established. Researchers found that constant use of the herb for at least six weeks significantly improved the movement of arthritic joints and reduced swelling. Devil's claw is now also known to be analgesic and sedative although precise constituents have yet to be identified so the whole plant extract is always used. It is also a bitter herb and can be used as a digestive stimulant, as well as externally for muscle and joint pains.

Like other recently introduced herbs, it is often sold as a simple rather than in complex preparations.
• Devil's claw is believed to stimulate uterine contractions and should be avoided in pregnancy.

Remedies and supplements
Arthur's Formula; FSC Devil's Claw Plus; Health Aid Devil's Claw with Royal Jelly; Imuno-Strength; Kordel's Celery 3000 Plus; Ortis Fresh Devil's Claw Drink
External: Harpago Gel; Phytorhuma

Simples
Capsules/tablets: Arkocaps Phytorhuma (330 mg); Frank Roberts Devil's Claw Tablets (820 mg); Full Potency Herbs Devil's Claw Vegicaps (520 mg); Gerard House Devil's Claw; Harpago; Power Health Pure Devils Claw (250 mg)
Tincture: Bioforce, Neal's Yard Remedies

DILL

Anethum graveolens

Parts used: seeds

Dill is the classic ingredient of baby's gripe water: it is carminative and soothing for the stomach and is an ideal remedy for colic and wind.

Remedies and supplements
*Herbcraft Peppermint Formula; Nurse Harvey's Gripe Water; *Woodward's Gripe Water

Simples
Oil: Hartwood Aromatics

DOG'S MERCURY

Mercurialis perennis

Parts used: whole plant

A toxic plant which can be fatal for animals when eaten fresh, dog's mercury has been used in external ointments for sores, warts and inflammations since the days of Hippocrates. Culpeper suggested the juice for ear disorders and this has also been used as a douche for nasal catarrh. The herb is rarely used today, although it is found in anthroposophical ointments for boils, abrasions and nappy rash.

Remedies and supplements
External: *Weleda Balsamicum Ointment

DRAGON'S BLOOD

Daemonorops draco

Synonyms: *Xue Jie*

Parts used: resin

The rather exotically named dragon's blood is a resin collected from an oriental variety of rattan. It is used in traditional Chinese medicine in pain relief for sprains, fractures and other contusions, and can also help to stop bleeding. Although the remedy can be used internally for chest and abdomen problems, it tends to be more widely used externally, often as a powder, although it is included in a number of proprietary ointments.

• Dragon's blood should be avoided in pregnancy.

Remedies and supplements
External: Amber Massage Salve; Dr Shir's Liniment

ECHINACEA

Echinacea spp

Synonyms: purple cone flower

Parts used: root

Several species of echinacea have been used by Native Americans, who regarded the plant as a valuable cure-all, for centuries. European interest in the plant started in Germany in the 1930s when its potent antibiotic actions were first identified: it is antibacterial, anti-viral and anti-fungal and is used for a broad spectrum of infections and now regarded as one of the most useful herbs in the repertoire.

Echinacea is most usually recommended for common colds, kidney and urinary infections and skin complaints such as acne, boils and carbuncles. It also aids wound healing and has been used for septicaemia. *Echinacea purpurea* and *E. angustifolia* are most commonly used, with *E. pallida*, which is rather harder to grow successfully in cultivation, less often found.

Echinacea is often sold as a simple, although it does feature in a number of combinations mainly for skin complaints and colds.

Remedies and supplements

BioCare Artemisia Complex; BioCare Buccalzyme; BioCare Salicidin; Bioforce Cystaforce; Bioforce Prostasan; Blackmores Celery Complex; Blackmores Echinacea Complex; Cantassium Didamega; *ColdEeze; *Frank Roberts Catarrh Tablets; *Frank Roberts Cranesbill Compound Tablets; Frank Roberts Golden Seal Compound Tablets; *Frank Roberts Sinus and Hay Fever Tablets; Full Potency Herbs Echinacea/Goldenseal/Cat's Claw Complex Vegicaps; *Gerard House Echinacea & Garlic; Health Aid Herbal Booster; Health Aid Liquid Herbal Booster; Herbcraft Calendula & Goldenseal Spray; Herbcraft Echinacea, Eyebright and Bilberry Formula; Herbcraft Echinacea Formula; Herbcraft Liquorice and Propolis Spray; Imuno-Strength; *Lanes Kleer; *Lanes Sinotar; *Muir's Catarrh; Nature's Plus ImmunForte; Neal's Yard Echinacea & Mallow Linctus; Neal's Yard Lemon & Honey Lozenges; Phoenix Nutrition Echinacea ACES; *Potter's Antifect; *Revitonil
External: Bioforce Echinacea Cream; Neal's Yard Echinacea and Propolis Ointment; *Nelsons Burns Ointment; *Nelsons Pyrethrum Spray; *Weleda Catarrh Cream; *Weleda WCS Dusting Powder

Simples

Capsules/tablets: Arkocaps Phytokold (250 mg); Bioforce Echinaforce Tablets; Cantassium Echinacea 500 (200 mg); *Frank Roberts Echinacea Tablets; Full Potency Herbs Echinacea Vegicaps; FSC Organic Echinacea (500 mg); *Gerard House Echinacea; Herbs of Grace Echinacea Angustifolia; *Muir's Echinacea (250 mg); Neal's Yard Echinacea Capsules; *Potter's Skin Clear Tablets; Power Health Echinacea Standardised; Pure-fil Echinacea Root (400 mg)
Juice: Schoenenberger Plant Juice
Tinctures: Bioforce (Echinaforce); Echinex; Galen Herbal Suppliers; Herbcraft; Neal's Yard Remedies

ELDER

Sambucus nigra

Parts used: flowers, berries, leaves, bark

The elder tree was once regarded as a complete medicine chest since all parts of the plant could be used in some way. The leaves formed the basis of a "green ointment" for sprains and strains, and, like the bark, are a strong purgative. The berries – a good source of vitamin C – acted as a prophylactic against colds and infections, while the flowers are strongly anti-catarrhal.

Today only the flowers are widely used, although berry juice is still available and the leaves are occasionally found in laxative products.

The flowers are also topically anti-inflammatory, diaphoretic and expectorant. They appear to strengthen the mucous membrane so, although some argue that they cause hay fever, they can also help to increase resistance to irritant allergens. Elder flowers are included in a wide range of cold, catarrh and hay fever products.

Remedies and supplements
*Culpeper Elder Flower and Peppermint Mixture; *Frank Roberts Cold Tablets; *Frank Roberts Drops of Life Tablets; *Frank Roberts Sinus and Hay Fever Tablets; *Lanes Sinotar; *Lusty's Herbalene; Neal's Yard Elderflower, Peppermint & Composition Essence; *Potter's Elderflowers, Peppermint and Composition Essence; *Potter's Life Drops; *Potter's Tabritis; *Ricola Swiss Herb Lozenges; *Weleda Herb and Honey Cough Elixir

Simples
Juice: Schoenenberger Plant Juice (berries)
Tincture: Neal's Yard Remedies

ELECAMPANE

Inula helenium

Synonyms: scabwort, yellow starwort

Parts used: root, flowers

Elecampane was regarded as a magical herb by the Anglo-Saxons and figures in numerous eighth century remedies for elf-shot and evil eye. Modern medicine regards it as an important expectorant and lung tonic which is mainly used in cough and catarrh remedies. It is also diaphoretic and diuretic and has some antibacterial and anti-fungal properties.

Elecampane also helps to stimulate the immune system and, with its bitter taste, also has a tonic effect on the digestive system. It is a useful herb for the lingering coughs and debility that can follow bouts of influenza. Although the root is used in Western herbalism, the Chinese use the flowers of a related species in a number of similar ways.

Remedies and supplements

Bioforce Drosinula Cough Syrup; *CatarrhEeze; *CoughEeze; Neal's Yard Horehound & Aniseed Linctus; *Potter's Horehound and Aniseed Cough Mixture;
*Potter's Vegetable Cough Remover

Simples

Tincture: Neal's Yard Remedies

EUCALYPTUS

Eucalyptus globulus

Synonyms: blue gum

Parts used: leaves, oil

The many species of eucalyptus originate from Australia where they were used in
Aboriginal medicines to treat fevers, dysentery and sores. The plant was introduced into Europe in the nineteenth century and is now a common garden ornamental as well as being commercially cropped in parts of Southern Europe.
Eucalyptus is antiseptic, antispasmodic, expectorant, stimulating and will reduce
fevers. The herb is mainly used in external preparations as the essential oil
(extracted by steam distillation) which is included in rubs for muscle aches, steam
inhalations for catarrh and colds, or added in small quantities to throat pastilles.
The leaf is also available over-the-counter.

Other varieties of eucalyptus have similar properties and are sometimes
found in herbal remedies: they include lemon-scented eucalyptus (*E. citriodora*)
and Australian peppermint (*E. dives*).

• Excess may cause headache and delirium.

Remedies and supplements

Bioforce Bronchosan; Bumbles Propolis, Menthol & Eucalyptus; Neal's Yard Euca-
lyptus & Menthol Lozenges; *Lane's Cut-a-Cough; *Olbas Pastilles; *Revitonil
External: Bioforce Po Ho Oil; Chirali Old Remedy Strain & Sprain Cream;
*Culpeper Healing Ointment; *Gerard House Dragon Balm Ointment; Herbcraft
Calendula & Goldenseal Spray; *Lanes Kleer Ti-Tree and Witch Hazel Cream;
*Olbas Oil; *Potter's Nine Rubbing Oils; Power Health Head Clear; *Rickard's
Woodsap Ointment; Weleda Catarrh Cream; *Weleda Medicinal Gargle*; *Weleda
Oleum Rhinale

Simples

Capsules: Arkocaps Phytoseptik (230 mg)
Oil: Botanica; Hartwood Aromatics; Neal's Yard Remedies; Nelson & Russell;
Tisserand

EVENING PRIMROSE

Oenetheris biennis

Parts used: seed oil

Evening primrose is a North American plant, traditionally taken in standard infusions of the leaves and stems as a remedy for asthma and digestive disorders.

During the 1970s researchers identified that its seeds were actually rich in an essential fatty acid called *gamma*-linolenic acid (GLA). GLA is an essential building block for various prostaglandins: these are hormone-like chemicals essential for health. A healthy metabolism can convert *cis*-linoleic acid (widely found in leafy vegetables and seed oils, as well as abundant in evening primrose oil) into GLA, but this process can be affected by poor diet and high cholesterol levels. Some individuals are also unable to complete this metabolic pathway: a deficiency which has been related to disorders like chronic psoriasis and rheumatoid arthritis.

The result has been a massive growth in the market for evening primrose oil which has become a major cash crop in many parts of the world and has set the plant breeders an on-going task of producing strains which contain ever more GLA in the seeds. Naturally occurring evening primrose oil seeds usually average around 9% of GLA, while new strains and extraction techniques have been recorded as producing as much as 24% of the essential acid. Suppliers differ in their views of the importance of the percentage of GLA but the acid is essential to normal bodily function and is found in very few foods. Lack of GLA has been associated with various systemic rheumatic and skin disorders, and it is also reputed to ease menstrual and menopausal problems, strengthen the circulatory system and boost the immune system.

Recommendations on dosage vary: clinical trials have used quantities as high as 3–5 g a day to treat irritable bowel syndrome associated with the menstrual cycle and similar doses are used for treating severe eczema. The oil can also be used neat on the skin for eczema and similar problems.

Most evening primrose oil products are unlicensed, but Efamol has two licensed brands which are thus available on prescription.

Since the 1980s GLA has also been found in borage and blackcurrant seeds in higher proportions than in evening primrose. However, supporters of evening primrose argue that the GLA it contains is more efficient in production of the important PGE_1 series prostaglandins than other varieties and also that evening primrose contains none of the potentially toxic fatty acids (such as erucic acid found in borage oil).

An enormous number of evening primrose products are now available: most are sold as simples (see Table 1) although the oil is also contained in multivitamin preparations and skin creams.

Remedies and supplements

Efalex; Efamol with Safflower and Linseed Oils; Hartwood Aromatics Especially Yours' Kordel's Women's Multi; Man Power; Phoenix Nutrition Omega 3-6; Seven Seas Evening Primrose and Starflower Oil; Super Garlic Perles for Women

External: Arthur's Formula Cream; Chirali Old Remedy Strain & Sprain Cream; Health Aid Eczem Oil; Nelsons Evening Primrose Cream.

Simples

Capsules: See Table 1

Oil: Cantassium Evening Gold; Efamol Original; Hartwood Aromatics Evening Primrose Oil; Neal's Yard Evening Primrose Oil Drops.

Table 1: Evening primrose oil products

Product	Capsule content (mg)	%age GLA (where specified)	Additives
Arkofluids EPO	n/a	n/a	
BioCare EPO 2509%			
Culpeper Evening Primrose Capsules	n/a	n/a	
Dorwest Herbs	500	n/a	
Efacal	400	9%	100 mg calcium 44 mg fish oil.
Efamol High Strength Original	1000	9%	Vitamin E
Efamol High Strength Pre-Menstrual Pack	1000	9%	Multi- vitamin/ mineral tablets also included
Efamol Marine	430	9%	107 mg fish oil 10 mg vitamin E
Efamol Original	500	9%	Vitamin E
Efamol Plus CoQ10	356	9%	218 mg fish oil; 10 mg vitamin E; 10mg Co-enzyme Q10
Efamol Plus Multi	250	9%	Multivitamin & mineral mix
Frank Roberts Eprimoil Silver	500	8%	
Frank Roberts Eprimoil Gold	500	10%	
FSC Pure Evening Primrose Oil Cool Pressed	250	n/a	Vitamin E
FSC Pure Evening Primrose Oil Cool Pressed	500	n/a	Vitamin E
FSC Pure Evening Primrose Oil Cool Pressed	1000	n/a	Vitamin E

continued

Product	Capsule content (mg)	%age GLA (where specified)	Additives
Gammaoil Premium	500	n/a	10 IU vitamin E
Gammaoil Premium	1000	n/a	10 IU vitamin E
Gerard House Evening Primrose	500	n/a	
Hartwood Aromatics	500	n/a	
Hartwood Aromatics	100	n/a	
Health Plus Evening Primrose Oil	500	n/a	
Healthcrafts Evening Primrose Oil	250	n/a	
Healthcrafts Evening Primrose Oil	500	n/a	
Healthcrafts Evening Primrose Oil	1000	n/a	
Healthwise Evening Primrose Oil	500	n/a	
Lamberts Evening Primrose	250	8%	
Lamberts Evening Primrose	500	8%	
Lamberts Evening Primrose	1000	8%	
Natural Flow Evening Primrose Oil	500	10%	
	1000	10%	
Neal's Yard Evening Primrose Oil Capsules	500	n/a	
Omega 3	250	n/a	250 mg fish oil; 50 IU vitamin E
Power Health Evening Primrose Oil	250	n/a	
Primrosa	600	20%	
Primrosa	1200	20%	
Primrosa Marine	600	20%	Fish lipid concentrate
Pure-fil Evening Primrose Oil	500	n/a	
Seven Seas Evening Primrose Oil	250	9%	
Seven Seas Evening Primrose Oil	500	9%	
Seven Seas Evening Primrose Oil	1000	9%	

continued

Product	Capsule content (mg)	%age GLA (where specified)	Additives
Seven Seas Cod Liver Oil and Evening Primrose Oil	n/a	n/a	Cod liver oil
Solgar Evening Primrose Oil	500	n/a	15 IU vitamin E
Solgar Evening Primrose Oil	1300	n/a	10 IU vitamin E
Ultra Premium Evening Primrose	500	10%	Vitamin E

EYEBRIGHT

Euphrasia officinalis

Parts used: herb

Eyebright is a tiny, semi-parasitic plant which grows in grassy meadows. It has been regarded as a remedy for eye problems since at least the fourteenth century and is useful in eye baths for conjunctivitis, eye injuries and to relieve the eye irritation of hay fever. Internally the plant is an effective anti-catarrhal, astringent and tonic. It can help a variety of upper respiratory tract problems including allergic rhinitis, hay fever and sinusitis.

Remedies and supplements

Herbcraft Echinacea, Eyebright and Bilberry Formula; Kordel's I-Vista

Simples

Capsules: Full Potency Herbs Eyebright Vegicaps (520 mg)
Tincture: Bioforce, Neal's Yard Remedies

FENNEL

Foeniculum vulgare

Parts used: seeds

Familiar as a vegetable and culinary herb, fennel is also a valuable medicinal plant. It is carminative and anti-inflammatory and will stimulate the appetite. It is largely used for indigestion, wind or colic and is often added to laxative mixtures to ease the griping pains that strong purgatives can cause.

Fennel can help to increase milk flow in nursing mothers and is also used as a mouthwash and gargle for gum disease and sore throats; it is sometimes added to herbal toothpastes and is a component in gripe water used for infant colic. The essential oil is primarily used in the food and perfumery industries but can be in external rubs for bronchial congestion. The oil is used in cleansing and tonifying massage rubs.

Remedies and supplements

Absorb Plus; Colon Cleanse; *Gerard House Gladlax; *Heath & Heather Indigestion & Flatulence; Herbcraft Dandelion Formula; Herbcraft Peppermint Formula; *Lusty's Herbalene; Neal's Yard Cascara Compound; *Potter's Out of Sorts Tablets; *Potter's Senna Tablets; *Revitonil; St Hildegard-Posch Galangal and Fennel Tablets; *Weleda Carminative Tea

External: Bioforce Po Ho Oil

Simples

Juice: Schoenberger Plant Juice

Oil: Hartwood Aromatics; Neal's Yard Remedies; Tisserand

FENUGREEK

Trigonella foenum-graecum

Synonyms: hilba

Parts used: seeds, herb

The potent aroma and taste of fenugreek are familiar from Indian and Middle Eastern cookery and the herb gives a spicy flavour to curries, pickles and garnishes. The seeds are mainly used in herbal medicine as a warming remedy for stomach and kidney chills and weakness.

Fenugreek is a digestive tonic, anti-inflammatory and expectorant and has been shown to reduce blood sugar and cholesterol levels. It can thus help dietary control of late-onset diabetes. The herb is used as a tea in modern Egypt as a remedy for spasmodic abdominal pain – due to both digestive upsets and menstruation – while the Chinese associate its action on the kidney with increasing reproductive energy and use the seeds for impotence and loss of libido. It is also used externally for skin problems and cellulitis

Remedies and supplements

*Dorwest Garlic and Fenugreek Tablets; *Gerard House Fenulin; Kordel's Horseradish, Odourless Garlic and Vitamin C

Simples

Capsules: Full Potency Herbs Fenugreek Vegicaps

FEVERFEW

Tanacetum parthenium

Synonyms: featherfew, midsummer daisy

Parts used: leaves

Writing in 1640, the herbalist John Parkinson suggested that feverfew leaves were too bitter and unpleasant to actually eat: to treat headaches they should, he recommended, be made into a poultice and placed on the crown of the head. Today, rightly or wrongly, it is one of the most popular over-the-counter herbs for treating migraines, although the bitter substances it contains do have a tendency to cause mouth ulcers in a significant number of users.

The plant has been extensively researched since the 1970s and contains parthenolide and similar compounds which are believed to account for its action in easing the symptoms of both migraine and chronic arthritis. The plant is analgesic, antispasmodic and relaxes peripheral blood vessels as well as reducing fevers and stimulating the digestion. As an antispasmodic it can be helpful for period pain and is useful for minor fevers. Interestingly the common name is believed to derive, not from its ability to lower body temperature but from a corruption of "featherfew" which describes the shape of its leaves.

Clinical trials have well demonstrated its efficacy as a migraine remedy and many sufferers happily eat a couple of leaves a day as a prophylactic. The herb does, however, have anti-platelet activity reducing the blood's ability to clot so should not be taken by those on blood thinning drugs, like warfarin or heparin.
• Migraine sufferers should stop taking regular doses of feverfew if side effects (skin rashes or mouth ulceration) occur.

Remedies and supplements
Cantassium Didamega; Herbcraft Passiflora and Valerian Formula; Kordel's Celery 3000 Plus; Kordel's Feverfew and Willow

Simples
Capsules/tablets: Arkocaps Phytofeverfew (200 mg); Bare Foot Feverfew Tablets; Culpeper Feverfew Tablets (200 mg); FSC Feverfew (150 mg); Full Potency Herbs Feverfew Vegicaps (520 mg); Gerard House Feverfew; Heath & Heather Feverfew; Neal's Yard Feverfew Capsules (500 mg); Power Health Pure Feverfew (200 mg); Professional Herbs Feverfew (150 mg); Pure-Fil Feverfew Leaf (100 mg); Reevecrest Feverfew Forte (150 mg)
Tincture: Herbcraft; Neal's Yard Remedies

FIELD MINT

Mentha arvensis

See Peppermint

FIG

Ficus carica

Parts used: fruit, leaves

Fig syrup is an old household standby for constipation often used in combination with senna and carminative herbs. Medicinally, the fig is also considered a demulcent to soothe irritated tissues and can be taken for sore throats, coughs and bronchial problems.

Remedies and supplements
Ortisan; Ortis Fruit & Fibres; Ortisan Liquid

Simples
Juice: Schoenenberger Plant Juice

FRANKINCENSE

Boswellia sacra

Parts used: gum resin

Frankincense has been prized for its aromatic resin for at least 3,500 years and images of the plant growing in pots can be seen on the funerary temple to Queen Hatshepsut's temple near Luxor. The herb is a stimulant for the circulation, is antiseptic, expectorant and sedative. It is used in inhalants for catarrh and colds and is taken internally for respiratory and urinary problems. An essential oil is distilled from the resin which is an important aromatherapy remedy for anxiety and tension.

Remedies and supplements
BioCare Boswellic Acid Complex
External: Neal's Yard Cellulite Oil

Simples
Oil: Hartwood Aromatics; Nelson & Russell; Tisserand

FRINGE TREE

Chionanthus virginianum

Synonyms: snowdrop tree

Parts used: root bark

Fringe tree was used for malaria and as a wound herb by Native Americans for centuries before the settlers arrived, but was very soon absorbed into Pioneer medicine – not as a wound herb but as a highly effective liver and gall bladder remedy. The active constituents are largely unknown, but the plant is effectively used for jaundice, gall stones, hepatitis and poor liver function. It can also help bilious headaches and migraines which can be related to liver congestion.

Remedies and supplements
BioCare Liv243; *Frank Roberts Black Root Compound Tablets

Simples
Tincture: Neal's Yard Remedies

GALANGAL

Alpinia galanga

Synonyms: Siamese ginger, *Gao Liang Jiang*

Parts used: rhizomes

Like its relative ginger, galangal is a carminative and stimulant largely used in Western medicine for indigestion and stomach upsets. Hildegard of Bingen believed that the plant could be effective for angina pectoris and it is still used in this way by some German therapists. The Chinese consider it useful in abdominal pain and gastroenteritis while in Ayurvedic medicine it is regarded as diaphoretic and useful for rheumatic disorders.

Remedies and supplements
St Hildegard-Posch Galangal and Fennel Tablets
External: Bee Brand Massage Oil

GARLIC

Allium sativa

Parts used: bulb, oil

Garlic has been used in medicine for at least 5,000 years and a recipe based on the herb survives in the cuneiform script of ancient Babylon. Its main use has always been as an antiseptic, effective against a wide range of bacteria and fungi and used for colds, chest infections and digestive upsets, including amoebic dysentery. Its characteristic smell is due to a group of sulphur-containing compounds, notably allicin.

As well as its anti-bacterial action, garlic also affects the blood and it is now known to reduce cholesterol levels and prevent the development of arteriosclerosis, which is caused by a build-up of fatty deposits on the inner walls of blood vessels. Studies in recent years among heart attack patients have demonstrated that taking the herb can significantly reduce the risk of a second attack.

In the East, garlic has long been regarded as an important tonic for the elderly helping to improve weak digestive function and researchers have now shown that low doses of garlic do indeed have a tonifying effect on the intestine, improving peristalsis and performance.

Recommendations on dosage vary considerably with some authors suggesting consumption of up to 1 kg/2 lbs a day although most research has involved doses of around 7-15 g/¼–½ oz daily. These sorts of levels are needed in serious conditions: to counter the risks of arteriosclerosis or heart attack, for example, although the small amounts used in cooking can often be sufficient to improve digestion.

Suppliers of garlic capsules and tablets usually suggest a daily intake of the equivalent of 2 g of fresh garlic is sufficient and many people balk at the high doses needed therapeutically because of the smell. Some capsules are supplied with enteric coatings so that they only dissolve in the stomach which avoids the initial smell. However, since the pungent chemicals in garlic are mainly excreted through the skin and lungs there will still be some odour later. Some fully "de-odourised" capsules only achieve this status by removing the allicin completely which, since this is a main active constituent, considerably reduces the therapeutic properties of the garlic.

Eating parsley can help to reduce garlic odour and this is included in a few OTC products.

Remedies and supplements

BioCare Candistatin; Bioforce Arterioforce; Cantassium Didamega; *ColdEeze; *Culpeper Rheumatic Tablets; *Dorwest Garlic and Fenugreek Tablets; *Frank Roberts Sinus and Hay Fever Tablets; *Gerard House Echinacea & Garlic; Herbcraft Garlic and Horseradish Winter Formula; Höfels One-a-Day Cardiomax Garlic Pearles; Kordel's Horseradish, Odourless Garlic and Vitamin C; *Lane's Sage and Garlic Catarrh Remedy; *Lanes Garlodex; Natural Flow Regular Ten Powder; *Potter's Antifect; Power Health Circulating Compound; Super Garlic Perles for Men; Super Garlic Perles for Women; Three G's

External: Arthur's Formula; Bee Brand Massage Oil; Gerard House Garlic Ointment

Simples

Capsules/Tablets: See Table 2
Juice: Schoenenberger Plant Juice

Table 2: Garlic simples

Brand	Garlic content/ Dosage equivalent		Notes
Arkocaps Phytoimune	330 mg powdered garlic	2 capsules, 3 times a day	
BioCare Garlicin	400 mg freeze dried garlic concentrate	1 capsule with evening evening meal	
BioCare Garlicin Plus	n/a	n/a	also contains 200 µg of biotin
Bioforce Garlic Capsules	270 mg garlic extract	1–3 capsules, 3 times a day	
Blackmores Garlix	2000 mg of freeze dried garlic in an enteric coating	1 a day	
Blackmores Odourless Garlic	10 mg garlic	1 tablet, 3 times a day	also contains 20 mg parsley
Cantassium Garlimega 2000	equivalent to 2 g of fresh garlic	1 tablet a day	
Cantassium Garlimega 2000	equivalent to 2 g of fresh garlic	1 tablet a day	

continued

Brand	Garlic content/ Dosage equivalent		Notes
Cantassium Micro Garlic	n/a	n/a	Mini-size tablets for those who find pills difficult to swallow
Culpeper Garlic Capsules	garlic oil	3 capsules a day	
*Frank Roberts Garlic Oil Capsules	garlic oil	1 capsule 3 times a day	
FSC Garlic Gems	2mg odourless garlic oil	1 per day	
FSC Whole Bulb Garlic	300 mg Pure-Gar™ powder equivalent to 750 mg	1–2 capsules per day	
*Gerard House Garlic Perles		1 capsule, 3 times a day or 2–3 at night	
Health Aid Mega Garlic Oil	2 mg garlic oil	1 per day	
Health Aid Organic Garlic Oil	n/a	1 per day	
Healthcrafts Garlic	2mg odourless garlic extract	1 per day	
Healthwise Garlic Pearls	n/a	1 per day	
Heath & Heather Garlic Perles One a day	2 mg odourless garlic extract	1 per day	
Heath & Heather Odourless Garlic	0.66 mg odourless garlic extract	3 a day	
Höfel's One-a-Day Neo-garlic Pearles	2mg of garlic oil	1 a day	
*Höfel's One-a-Day Garlic with Parsley	2 mg garlic oil/ equivalent to 2 g	1 a day	also contains 15mg of parsley
*Höfel's Original One-a-Day Garlic Pearles	2 mg garlic oil/ equivalent to 2 g	one a day	
*HRI Herbal Catarrh and Rhinitis Tablets	150 mg garlic plus 1 mg garlic oil	1 tablet, three 3 times a day children over 8, 1 tablet, twice a day	
Cantassium Garlic Oil Capsules	equivalent to 660 mg	n/a	
Kordel's Garlic 3000	n/a	n/a	Enteric coating with lemon grass oil

continued

Brand	Garlic content/ Dosage equivalent		Notes
Kwai	300 mg garlic	2 tablets 3 times a day	
Kwai One a Day		1 a day	
Kyolic	300 mg	1-4 a day	
Kyolic	350 mg	1-4 a day	
Kyolic	600 mg	1-4 a day	
Lamberts Garlic Oil	2mg garlic oil (equivalent 1g garlic)	1–3 daily	
Lamberts Garlic & Parsley	574 mg	1–3 daily	Also contains 110 mg parsley
Lamberts Pure-Gar™	500 mg Pure-Gar™	1–3 daily	
Lanes Shen	equivalent to 300 mg of fresh garlic	1–2 tablets, 3 times a day children (over 7) one table, three times a day.	
*Lusty's Garlic Perles	0.66 mg garlic oil	1 capsule, 3 times a day; children (5–12) 1 capsule twice a day.	
Nature's Plus Garlite	500mg	n/a	
Neal's Yard Garlic Capsules	n/a	1 capsules, 3 times a day	
*Potter's Garlic Tablets		2 tablets, 3 times a day; children (over 8) 1 tablet, 3–4 times a day	
Power Health Garlic Oil	250 mg	1–2 capsules daily	
Pure-fil Low Odour Whole Garlic Concentrate	250mg/equivalent to 2g fresh	n/a	
Seven Seas Odourless Garlic Perles	n/a	one a day	
Seven Seas Garlic Oil Perles	n/a	one a day	
Solgar Certified Organic Garlic Oil Vegicaps	equivalent to 500 mg	n/a	
Solgar Garlic Oil Softgels	equivalent to 500 mg	n/a	
Solgar MaxGar Garlic Softgels	equivalent to 672 mg		
Wassen Garlic Tablets	Equivalent of 968 mg	1 a day	

GINGER

Zingiber officinale

Parts used: root, oil

Ginger has been valued as a culinary and medicinal plant since ancient times. It was mentioned by the Romans, listed in some of the earliest Chinese herbals and is regarded in Ayurvedic medicine as a universal medicine. The plant is carminative, antispasmodic, and can control nausea and coughing. It has a pungent, aromatic flavour and is widely used in the food industry as well as included in medicines to disguise the taste of less palatable plants.

Ginger is warming and will increase perspiration so makes a useful tea for colds and chills. It is included in a number of digestive remedies as well as preparations for colds and influenza. Externally the oil is heating and will encourage blood flow so is useful for muscular stiffness, aches and pains. In Chinese medicine the fresh and dried roots are regarded rather differently with the dried believed to be more helpful for abdominal pain and diarrhoea and the fresh more suitable for feverish chills, coughs and vomiting.

As a remedy for nausea, ginger is ideal for travel sickness and has been very successfully tested in clinical trials for severe morning sickness. Ginger in capsules is ideal, but ginger biscuits or ginger beer can also prove effective – especially with children – if nothing else is available.

Remedies and supplements

BioCare Boswellic Acid Complex; BioCare Candicidin; Bioforce Linoforce; Blackmores Cape Aloes and Cascara; Blackmores Euphorbia Complex; *Box's Far Famed Indigestion Tablets; *Culpeper Elder Flower and Peppermint Mixture; *Culpeper Influenza Mixture; *Dorwest Digestive Tablets; *Frank Roberts B & L Tablets; *Frank Roberts Black Root Compound Tablets; *Frank Roberts Nervous Dyspepsia Tablets; FSC Bromelain Plus; FSC Ginger and Turmeric; Health Aid FemmeVit; Health Aid Herbal Booster; Herbcraft Garlic and Horseradish Winter Formula; Herbcraft Mullein Formula; Herbcraft Peppermint Formula; *HRI Golden Seal Digestive; *Lanes Herbelix Specific; Neal's Yard Elderflower, Peppermint & Composition Essence; Neal's Yard Lemon & Honey Lozenges; *Nurse Harvey's Gripe Water; *Potter's Indian Brandee; Professional Herbs Cascara and Rhubarb; Professional Herbs Cayenne & Ginger; SX Formula

External: Bee Brand Massage Oil; Neal's Yard Ginger and Juniper Warming Oil; Neal's Yard Sports Salve

Simples

Capsules/tablets: Arkocaps Phytotravel (280 mg); Blackmores Ginger Tablets (Travel Calm) (400 mg); *Cantassium Travel Sickness (250 mg); Culpeper Ginger Root Capsules (300 mg); Full Potency Herbs Ginger Root Vegicaps (520 mg); *Gerard House Ginger; Herbs of Grace Ginger; Höfels Ginger Pearles; Potter's Ginger Root Tablets; Power Health Pure Ginger (280 mg); Pure-fil Travellers Friend (500 mg)

Oil: Hartwood Aromatics; Neal's Yard Remedies; Tisserand

Tincture: Herbcraft; Neal's Yard Remedies

GINKGO

Ginkgo biloba

Synonyms: maidenhair tree

Parts used: leaves

Although ginkgo seeds have been used to treat asthma and urinary problems in Chinese medicine for many centuries, it is only in the past few years that the herb has been used medicinally in the West. The tree is a fossil survivor – a deciduous conifer which has been unchanged since before the evolution of mammals. It was brought to Europe in 1727 and grown as an ornamental in many botanical gardens. Research in the past decade has highlighted its action as a platelet activating factor (PAF) which counters the allergic response reinforcing its traditional use as an anti-asthmatic.

More significantly the plant has been shown to improve cerebral circulation. In Germany, ginkgo has been tested on patients recovering from brain surgery following strokes and found to have dramatic effects on recovery. Its action in strengthening the cerebral circulation has led many to regard it as an anti-ageing remedy, since hardening of the arteries in the brain is a common cause of apparent confusion in the elderly. Equally its action as a circulatory stimulant has spawned a range of commercial products, some of which imply cosmetic effectiveness for varicose veins and similar problems.

Essentially, ginkgo has been shown to help cerebral insufficiency and is known to have anti-allergenic effects. Some of its other reported actions (to help tinnitus, for example) have not fully stood up to scientific scrutiny.

In general, ginkgo preparations are sold as simple food supplements although a number of combinations, largely emphasising tonic properties, are available.

Remedies and supplements

BioCare Ginkgo Plus; Full Potency Herbs Bilberry with Ginkgo Biloba Vegicaps; Kordel's Women's Multi; Nature's Plus Ginkgo Combo; Red Kooga Ginseng and Ginkgo Biloba; Three G's

Simples

Capsules/tablets: Arkocaps Phytomemo (180 mg); Cantassium Ginkgo 2000; Frank Roberts Ginkgo Biloba (200 mg); Full Potency Herbs Ginkgo Biloba Vegicaps; Full Potency Herbs Super Ginkgo Vegicaps; (520 mg); Gerard House Ginkgo Biloba; Ginkyo; Healthwise Ginkgo Biloba; Idoloba; Lamberts Ginkgo Biloba Extract (40 mg); Power Health Pure Ginkgo Biloba (180 mg); Seredrin
Juice: Schoenenberger Plant Juice
Tincture: Bioforce; Herbcraft; Neal's Yard Remedies

GINSENG

Panax ginseng

Synonyms: Korean ginseng, red ginseng, *Ren Shen*

Parts used: root

Ginseng has been used in China for more than 5,000 years and is believed to strengthen the vital energy – *Qi* – of the body. It has always been an expensive and highly prized herb that had, ideally, to be gathered in the wild using roots that were several years old. Today most ginseng is cultivated and it is an important cash crop.

The plant is rich in steroidal compounds which are very similar to human sex hormones, hence its reputation as an aphrodisiac. It is, however, a rather more all-round tonic helping the body adapt to stressful situations and especially valuable for the elderly. In some Chinese traditions, ginseng should only be taken by those over 40 while astragalus is prefered as a tonic for younger people. The Chinese believe ginseng acts on the lungs and spleen and can be helpful during recovery from chest problems – such as asthma – and digestive disorders. As a general tonic it is ideally taken for a month in late autumn when the weather is changing from hot summer to cold winter – from *yang* to *yin* – and the body needs to adapt to the new environment. Although the herb can, of course, obviously also be taken whenever there are problems due to tiredness and overwork.

Many simples containing only ginseng are available over-the-counter (Table 3) while several products also incorporate vitamins, royal jelly and other energy-giving herbs.
• Ginseng is best avoided in pregnancy although it may be taken for short periods then. Other herbal stimulants, such as caffeine-containing drinks, should be avoided while taking ginseng.

Remedies and supplements
Bioforce Ginsavena; Bioforce Ginsavita; Bioforce Neuroforce; HealthAid Ginseng; Healthcrafts Korean and Siberian Ginseng; Herbatone; Honeyrose Herbal Cigarettes; La Gelee Royale; Man Power; Melbrosia Executive; Natural Flow Triple Ginseng; Nature's Plus ImmunForte; Ortis Fresh Ginseng in Solution; Ortis Ginseng + E; Ortis Panax Ginseng and Royal Jelly; Panax Ginseng and Royal Jelly; Red Kooga Betalife Capsules; Red Kooga Ginseng and Ginkgo Biloba; SX Formula; Three G's

Simples
Capsules/Tablets: See Table 3
Tincture: Galen Herbal Supplies; Neal's Yard Remedies

Table 3: Korean ginseng simples

Product	Extract or equivalent of dried herb	Dosage
Cantassium Red Ginseng 600	600 mg	1–2 tablets daily
Cantassium Red Panax Ginseng	500 mg	1–2 tablets daily
Culpeper Ginseng Capsules	460 mg	1 tablet daily
Frank Roberts Ginseng Capsules	n/a	2 tablets daily
FSC Korean Ginseng	600 mg	one a day
Full Potency Herbs Korean Ginseng Vegicaps	520 mg	1 a day
Gerard House Korean Ginseng	n/a	n/a
Ginseng Slices	n/a	Honey soaked slices to be chewed daily
Health Aid Korgin Korean Ginseng	250mg	2–3 a day
Health Aid Korean Ginseng Extract	600 mg	1 a day
Healthcrafts Korean Ginseng	600 mg	1–2 daily
Healthcrafts Korean Ginseng	1200mg	1 a day
Herbs of Grace Ginseng	n/a	n/a
Neal's Yard Ginseng Capsules	500 mg	n/a
Ortis fresh Ginseng	liquid	5 ml a day
Power Ginseng	n/a	n/a
Pure-fil Super Panax Korean Ginseng	500 mg	1 a day
Red Ginseng in Honey	10ml phials	1 a day
Red Kooga Elixir	liquid	10 ml daily
Red Kooga Ginseng Capsules	600 mg	1 a day
Red Kooga Ginseng Tablets	600 mg	1 a day
Reevcecrest Ginseng- Red Roots	n/a	n/a
Seven Seas Korean Ginseng	250 mg	1 a day

GLOBE ARTICHOKE

Cynara scolymus

Parts used: leaves, roots, flowerheads

Artichoke is primarily regarded as a liver remedy: a bitter, cleansing herb that can help to detoxify the liver and encourage regeneration. The herb also has a cleansing effect in the kidneys and can help to reduce blood cholesterol levels; the flowerheads make an excellent vegetable served with melted butter.

Medicinal use of artichoke is more widespread in mainland Europe than in the UK, although it is included in a number of over-the-counter remedies for the liver which are available here. Other preparations focus on the herb's ability to lower cholesterol levels.

Remedies and supplements
BioCare Liv243; BioCare Silymarin Complex; Bioforce Boldocynara; *Bio-Strath Artichoke Formula

Simples
Capsules/tablets: Arkocaps Phytodigest (150 mg)
Juice: Schoenenberger Plant Juice
Tincture: Bioforce.

GLOSSY PRIVET

Ligustrum lucidum

Synonyms: *Nu Zhen Zi*

Parts used: Berries

Glossy privet berries are seen in traditional Chinese medicine as an energy tonic for liver and kidney. Falling kidney energy is associated with ageing and menopausal problems so the berries are often prescribed for associated problems including hearing and failing eyesight as well as general menopausal difficulties.

Remedies and supplements
Equillence

GOLDEN ROD

Solidago vigaurea

Parts used: leaves and flowering tops

Writing in 1597, the great herbalist John Gerard lamented the fact that because golden rod grew so abundantly on Hampstead Heath, Londoners despised it as a medicine, preferring instead to buy exotic and expensive remedies and ignoring the treasures so freely available.

Golden rod is largely used as a diuretic and urinary antiseptic for treating kidney and bladder problems. It is also diaphoretic and anti-inflammatory and has been included in various catarrhal and cough remedies. It is also a gentle liver stimulant and mildly sedating so may be found in remedies for indigestion or nervous dyspepsia. Externally it is used for sores and ulcers.

Remedies and supplements
> Bioforce Golden Grass Tea; Bioforce IMP (Imperthritica); Bioforce Nephrosolid; Bioforce Prostasan

Simples
> *Tincture:* Bioforce; Neal's Yard Remedies

GOLDEN SEAL

Hydrastis canadensis

Synonyms: yellow root, orange root

Parts used: rhizome

Golden seal was once used by the Cherokee for digestive problems and to make an insect-repellent ointment. It soon became popular among the settlers and was listed in the official US Pharmacopoeia until 1936. The root has an extremely bitter taste and acts as a digestive stimulant. It is also mildly laxative, anti-microbial, anti-inflammatory and will check bleeding. It is largely used as a digestive remedy and occurs as such in a number of over-the-counter preparations.

It can also be useful for a range of menstrual and menopausal problems and has been used to stop post-partum haemorrhage. It can affect the beneficial gut flora as well as invading bacteria, so should not be taken continuously for long periods.
• Golden seal is best avoided in pregnancy .

Remedies and supplements
> BioCare Artemisia Complex; BioCare Candistatin; BioCare Colon Care; BioCare Salicidin; *Dorwest Digestive Tablets; Frank Roberts Black Willow Compound Tablets; Frank Roberts Golden Seal Compound Tablets; *Frank Roberts Nervous Dyspepsia Tablets; Full Potency Herbs Echinacea/Goldenseal/Cat's Claw Complex Vegicaps; *Gerard House Fenulin; *Gerard House Golden Seal; *Gerard House Papaya Plus Tablets; *HRI Golden Seal Digestive; *Muir's Gastric-Ese; Neal's Yard Eucalyptus & Menthol Lozenges
> External: Herbcraft Calendula & Goldenseal Spray; Herbcraft Liquorice and Propolis Spray

Simples
> *Capsules:* Full Potency Herbs Goldenseal Root Vegicaps (520 mg); Herbs of Grace Golden Seal
> *Tincture:* Herbcraft; Neal's Yard Remedies

GOTU KOLA

Centella asiatica

Synonyms: Fo Ti; *Hydrocotyle asiatica*, Indian pennywort

Parts used: herb

Known in India as *brahmi*, gotu kola is one of the most important Ayurvedic tonic herbs long established as a rejuvenating remedy, to counter the problems of old age and improve failing memory. In the East it is also used to treat leprosy and has been successfully applied to a range of skin conditions and scar tissue. Although it has been used for conditions as diverse as malaria and venereal disease, gotu kola tends to be mainly regarded as a nervine and tonic in the West and features in stimulating, energy-giving formulations.

Remedies and supplements

BioCare AD206;*Fo Ti Tieng; Health Aid Herbal Booster; Health Aid Liquid Herbal Booster; Herbcraft Liquorice Formula; Nature's Plus Ginkgo Combo

Simples

Capsules: Arkocaps Phytoexcel (240 mg); Full Potency Herbs Gotu Kola Vegicaps (520 mg)
Tincture: Herbcraft

GRAPEFRUIT

Citrus × paradisis

Parts used: seed, essential oil

Work in the 1980s identified grapefruit seeds as anti-parasitic, anti-fungal and supportive for the gut flora. Preparations including the seeds are used in anti-candida treatments and the oil is regarded by aromatherapists as tonifying with an elevating effect on the emotions.

Remedies and supplements

BioCare Biocidin; BioCare Eradicidin Forte; BioCare Salicidin

Simples

Oil: Botanica; Hartwood Aromatics; Neal's Yard Remedies; Tisserand

GRAVEL ROOT

Eupatorium purpureum

Synonyms: Joe Pye weed, queen of the meadow

Parts used: root

Like its close relative boneset, gravel root is a North American herb. The "Joe Pye" of its country name is believed to refer to a nineteenth century medicine man who peddled preparations containing the plant. It is a bitter, diuretic herb used mainly for urinary tract problems, although it can also be helpful for period pain or to ease a difficult labour. As the name suggests, it was also used to clear kidney and urinary stones (gravel).

Remedies and supplements
*Potter's Backache Tablets; Professional Herbs Uva Ursi and Parsley

Simples
Tincture: Neal's Yard Remedies

GREATER CELANDINE

Chelidonium majus

Synonyms: swallow wort, tetterwort

Parts used: herb, sap

Greater celandine is mainly used as a liver herb, cleansing the gall bladder and stimulating bile flow, in hepatitis and jaundice. It is diuretic and has also been used for skin conditions where liver stagnation is a contributing factor. The fresh plant produces a yellow sap which can be used to clear warts. Its alternative name of swallow wort derives from an ancient tradition that swallows fed the seeds to their young to improve the chick's eyesight, and the plant was widely recommended until the seventeenth century for eye complaints.
• Excess can cause skin irritation, dry mouth, dizziness and drowsiness and its use in the UK is restricted under the 1968 Medicines Act.

Remedies and supplements
BioCare Liv243; Blackmores Sarsparilla Complex

Simples
Tincture: Bioforce

GREY ATRACTYLODES

Atractylodis lancea

Synonyms: *Cang Zhu*

Parts used: rhizome

A bitter, warming herb, grey atractylodes is used in Chinese medicine for arthritic problems, poor appetite and nausea.

Remedies and supplements
External: Golden Yellow Ointment

GROUND IVY

Glechoma hereacea

Synonyms: alehoof

Parts used: herb

Variegated ground ivy is often found in garden centres as a suitable plant for hanging baskets and containers, while the plain green variety tends to be regarded as a rather invasive weed (although it does make good ground cover!). The herb was used in brewing in the sixteenth century, hence its common name, and is used medicinally as an anti-catarrhal, astringent, expectorant and diuretic. It can be helpful for sinus and ear problems as well as for soothing gastritis and cystitis. Lotions containing ground ivy can be used externally for piles and throat inflammations.

Remedies and supplements
> *Heath & Heather Water Relief

Simples
> *Tincture:* Neal's Yard Remedies

GUAIACUM

Guaiacum officinale

Synonyms: lignum vitae, guaiac

Parts used: wood raspings, resin

Guaiacum is generally sold as wood shavings or raspings and is extracted from the heartwood of a tree growing in the West Indies and Florida. The herb is a circulatory stimulant, diaphoretic, diuretic and anti-inflammatory and is primarily used for rheumatism, arthritis and gout. It is sometimes given for upper respiratory tract infections and was once a regular treatment for syphilis.

It is popular in over-the-counter rheumatism remedies.

Remedies and supplements
> Blackmores Celery Complex; *Cantassium Rheumatic Pain; *Culpeper Rheumatic Tablets; *Frank Roberts Prickly Ash Compound Tablets; *Frank Roberts Rheumatic Pain Tablets; *Frank Roberts Sciatica Tablets; *Gerard House Ligvites; *Heath & Heather Rheumatic Pain; *Potter's Rheumatic Pain Tablets; *Rheumasol

GUARANA

Paullinia cupana

Synonyms: Brazilian cocoa, zoom

Parts used: seed

Guarana seeds are used by Amazonian tribes to make a stimulating, tonic drink – much as we would take tea or coffee in Europe. The seeds are rich in guaranine, which is a caffeine-like compound but is slower to metabolize thus giving a gentler, more sustained stimulant effect. Nowadays, the seeds are included in tonic drinks and confectionery as well as a number of stimulant and tonic remedies.

• Like other caffeine-containing plants, guarana can cause sleeplessness if taken in excess.

Remedies and supplements
Health Aid Herbal Booster; Health Aid Liquid Herbal Booster

Simples
Capsules/tablets: Arkocaps Phytoenergyze (340 mg); Herbs of Grace Guarana; Power Health Pure Guarana (500 mg); Reevecrest Bom-Dia (500 mg); Rio Amazon Guarana (500 mg); Rio Amazon Guarana Buzz Gum; Rio Amazon Guarana Jungle Elixir (1 g)

GUGULON

Commiphora mukul

Synonyms: guggulu

Parts used: oleo-gum resin

The gugulon tree grows in dry areas of the Indian sub-continent and its resin is one source of myrrh. More recently, resinous gugulon extracts have been shown to contain guggulipids which have an anti-inflammatory effect and will also reduce blood cholesterol levels improving the ratio of high-density lipids (thought to have a protective action), while reducing the low-density lipids which are regarded as harmful.

Simples
Capsules: Arkocaps Phytochol (340 mg)

GUMPLANT

Grindelia camporum

Synonyms: gumweed, tarweed

Parts used: herb

A bitter, aromatic herb, gumplant is antispasmodic and expectorant and is largely used in remedies for asthma and bronchial congestion. It can also be useful for relieving the discomfort of cystitis. Lotions containing the plant have been used for skin problems including eczema.

Remedies and supplements
Blackmores Euphorbia Complex; Blackmores Liquorice Complex; *Culpeper Cough Relief Mixture; Herbcraft Mullein Formula

HART'S TONGUE

Scolopendrium vulgare

Parts used: leaves

Hart's tongue was regarded as a good liver remedy by Culpeper who also suggested that a distilled water made from it was "good against the passion of the heart and to stay the hiccoughs". It was largely used for digestive upsets and diarrhoea while an ointment made from the plant was a folk remedy for piles in the Scottish Highlands. Hart's tongue is rarely used today, although it does figure in anthroposophical digestive remedies and some German products based on the writings of Hildegard of Bingen.

Remedies and supplements

St Hildegard-Posch Hart's Tongue Elixir; *Weleda Digestodoran Tablets

HAWTHORN

Crataegus laevigata; C. monogyna

Synonyms: may, quickset, *C. oxycantha*

Parts used: flowers, berries

Hawthorn is currently one of the herbalist's favourite heart remedies regarded as an important cardiac tonic which will also improve peripheral circulation, regulate heart rate and blood pressure, and improve coronary blood flow. The plant is also astringent and was once used for sore throats and diarrhoea.
• Although hawthorn is non-toxic, its use for heart disorders should really be confined to professional practitioners.

Remedies and supplements

Bioforce Arterioforce; Bioforce Cardiaforce; Blackmores Cactus & Hawthorn; Health Aid Herbal Booster; Health Aid Tranquil Capsules with Viburnum; Jay-Vee Tablets; Power Health Circulating Compound

Simples

Capsules/tablets: Full Potency Herbs Hawthorn Berry Vegicaps (520 mg); Gerard House Hawthorn; Power Health Pure Hawthorn Tablets
Juice: Schoenenberger Plant Juice
Tincture: Bioforce, Herbcraft; Neal's Yard Remedies

HEARTSEASE

Viola tricolor

Synonyms: wild pansy

Parts used: herb

Well known as an attractive garden flower, heartsease is expectorant, diuretic and anti-inflammatory. It is added to cough remedies, especially for bronchitis and whooping cough, and can soothe eczema and skin inflammations (both taken internally and used as a cream). It is rich in flavonoids (including rutin) so can also help to strengthen capillary walls. As a generally healing and cleansing plant, it also finds a role in the treatment of rheumatism and arthritis.

Remedies and supplements
> Bioforce Golden Grass Tea; Bioforce Nephrosolid; Heath & Heather Skin Tablets
> *External:* Bioforce Echinacea Cream

Simples
> *Tincture:* Bioforce (Violaforce); Neal's Yard Remedies

HEATHER

Calluna vulgaris

Synonyms: ling

Parts used: herb

Heather, like its relative bearberry, is valued as a remedy for the urinary system. It is an astringent, urinary antiseptic, mildly sedative and diuretic. As an astringent it may be added to cough and cold remedies and also used for diarrhoea.

Remedies and supplements
> Gerard House Sooth-a-Tea

HELONIAS

Chamaelirium luteum

Synonyms: false unicorn root, starwort, devil's bit, blazing star

Parts used: rhizome

Another of the traditional Native American herbs, helonias was used by tribes in Arkansas for treating ulcers, diarrhoea and urinary problems. The early settlers found that it was also helpful for threatened miscarriage and it is now largely used for menstrual irregularities and menopausal problems. It is bitter and diuretic with a hormonal action, stimulating the ovaries and uterus. Again, like a number of other North American plants, little research has been carried out on its pharmacology.

Remedies and supplements
> Frank Roberts Alchemilla Compound; Frank Roberts Black Willow Compound Tablets; *Gerard House Helonias Compound

Simples
> *Tincture:* Neal's Yard Remedies

HEMLOCK SPRUCE

Tsuga canadensis

Synonyms: *Pinus canadensis*, pinus bark

Parts used: bark

The hemlock spruce is a North American tree originally used by northern forest tribes for a variety of infections and wound healing. The Menominees used the bark to make a tea for colds and abdominal pain, while the MicMac Indians also took it for coughs. Several also used the leaves to increase perspiration in "sweat lodges" and it was added to various medicines to disguise unpleasant flavours. Like other Native American herbs it has been little researched and its inclusion in UK products dates back to the influence of the physiomedicalists. It is known to be astringent, diaphoretic, antiseptic and diuretic and can be used for diarrhoea, cystitis and colitis or as a gargle for sore throats. It is largely found in products derived from Potter's Composition Essence – a warming brew often added to mixtures for colds and chills.

Remedies and supplements
> *Culpeper Elder Flower and Peppermint Mixture; *Culpeper Influenza Mixture; Neal's Yard Elderflower, Peppermint & Composition Essence; *Potter's Elder-flowers, Peppermint and Composition Essence; *Potter's Peerless Composition Essence

HEMP NETTLE

Galeopsis segetum

Parts used: herb

Although rarely used in the UK, hemp nettle is an established medicinal herb in other parts of Europe. The plant is a common weed in cereal crops but is rich in silica and has diuretic, astringent and expectorant properties. It is primarily used for chronic bronchitis and other chest complaints.

Remedies and supplements
> Bioforce Tormentavena

Simples
> *Tincture:* Bioforce

HOLY THISTLE

Cnicus benedictus

Synonyms: blessed thistle, *Carbenia benedictus*

Parts used: herb

Although once widely used to treat the plague, holy thistle is best known today as a bitter, digestive remedy for indigestion, poor appetite and stomach upsets. It is also expectorant, antiseptic and will stop bleeding and can be used externally on wounds and sores. Over-the-counter remedies focus on its digestive properties.

Remedies and supplements

Bioforce Gastrosan; Discovery Coliclens; *Gerard House Gladlax; Natural Flow Colonite

HOPS

Humulus lupulus

Parts used: female flowers (strobiles), leaves, shoots

Hops have been used in brewing in Germany since the eleventh century, although they were not introduced to England until the sixteenth century when contemporary herbalists condemned them as encouraging melancholy. Certainly hops have a sedative effect and should be avoided in depression. They are also diuretic and anaphrodisiac: excessive consumption can lead to a loss of libido – a factor which beer drinkers may be aware of.

Hops are bitter tasting and can be used as a digestive stimulant; and they are also a good restorative for the nervous system so find a use in many over-the-counter remedies for stress, irritability and anxiety as well, of course, as insomnia. The female flower or strobile is generally used.

• Hops should not be taken by those suffering from depression.

Remedies and supplements

BioCare Phytosterol Complex; Bioforce Dormeasan; Bioforce Hyperiforce; Blackmores Skullcap & Valerian; Blackmores Valerian Complex; *Cantassium Quiet Days; *Cantassium Quiet Nite Sleep; *Cantassium Quiet Tyme; *Frank Roberts Calmanite Tablets; *Frank Roberts Pulsatilla Compound Tablets; FSC Valerian Formula; Gerard House Sooth-a-Tea; *Gerard House Valerian Compound Tablets; *Gerard 99; *Healthcrafts Night Time; *Heath & Heather Quiet Night; *Heath & Heather Becalm; *HRI Calm Life Tablets; HRI Night Tablets; Jay-Vee Tablets; Kordel's Kalm-Ex; Kordel's Quiet Time; *Lanes Kalms; *Lanes Quiet Life Tablets; *Natrasleep; *Potter's Anased Pain Relief Tablets; *Potter's Newrelax; *Potter's Nodoff Mixture; Professional Herbs Valerian; *Valerina – Night-Time; *Weleda Avena Sativa Comp

Simples
> *Capsules/tablets:* Arkocaps Phytopremenstrual (150 mg)
> *Tincture:* Herbcraft; Neal's Yard Remedies

HORSE CHESTNUT

Aesculus hippocastanum

Parts used: bark, seeds

Horse chestnut is anti-inflammatory, astringent and will reduce body temperature in fevers. Extracts are used in remedies for rheumatism, piles and varicose veins. The main active component is aescin, a potent anti-inflammatory saponin, and this is sometimes used in OTC remedies in preference to the whole plant; it is used both internally and externally.

Remedies and supplements
> Bioforce Hyperisan
> *External:* *Nelsons Haemorrhoid Cream; Phytovarix; *Weleda Medicinal Gargle

Simples
> *Tincture:* Bioforce, Neal's Yard Remedies

HORSERADISH

Armoracia rusticana

Synonyms: *Cochlearia armoracia*

Parts used: root

The pungent, mustard-like taste of horseradish is familiar to those who eat it in sauces for roast beef or smoked fish. It is a very hot herb – warming and stimulating – which will increase perspiration and is also diuretic. Topically horseradish is irritant and encourages local circulation: it can cause blisters if applied directly to the skin for long periods. Horseradish has been used medicinally for arthritis and rheumatism (often regarded as "cold" complaints that respond to hot treatments) as well as for colds and some types of catarrh
• Excessive use of horseradish can cause vomiting and allergic reactions. It should be avoided by those with stomach ulcers

Remedies and supplements
> *Dorwest Mixed Vegetable Tablets; Kordel's Horseradish, Odourless Garlic and Vitamin C; *Lanes Vegetex; *Weleda Fragador Tablets

Simples
> *Juice:* Schoenenberger Plant Juice
> *Tinctures:* Bioforce

HORSETAIL

Equisetum arvense

Synonyms: shave grass, bottlebrush

Parts used: herb

Horsetails have grown since prehistoric times and their decayed remains form much of the world's coal seams. The plants are rich in silica and have a rough abrasive texture – so rough that they were used for scouring pewter bowls until well into the eighteenth century. Silica is a very healing substance and horsetail can be used to control bleeding, both internally and externally, and as an astringent. The plant features in remedies for urinary tract problems, including prostate disorders, and can also be helpful in deep-seated lung problems, such as chronic bronchitis.

Remedies and supplements

*Aqualette; BioCare NEF242; Bioforce Golden Grass Tea; Bioforce Imperthritica; Bioforce Nephrosolid; Frank Roberts Uva-Ursi Compound Tablets; *Gerard House Waterlex Tablets; Herbcraft Burdock & Nettle Formula; Kordel's Celery and Juniper; Kordel's Women's Multi; *Potter's Antiglan Tablets; *Potter's Antitis Tablets; *Potter's Kas-Bah Herb

Simples

Capsules: Full Potency Herbs Vegital Silica Vegicaps (520 mg)
Juice: Schoenenberger Plant Juice
Tincture: Bioforce, Neal's Yard Remedies

HYDRANGEA

Hydrangea arborescens

Synonyms: wild hydrangea, seven barks

Parts used: root

Hydrangea is a useful remedy for prostate and urinary problems. It is diuretic and soothing for the urinary tract and can be helpful for both kidney and urinary stones. Its diuretic action means that it is also sometimes included in cleansing remedies for arthritis and gout.

Remedies and supplements

*Potter's Antiglan Tablets; *Potter's Backache Tablets

Simples

Tincture: Neal's Yard Remedies

HYSSOP

Hyssopus officinale

Parts used: herb, oil

The purgative hyssop of the Bible (Psalm 51, v. 7) is thought unlikely to be the plant we call by that name but more probably a Middle Eastern variety of marjoram. Hyssop belongs to the same family (the mints) and is certainly a bitter digestive tonic, useful in cooking; its prime use is, however, in cough remedies. The herb is anti-inflammatory and expectorant; useful for upper respiratory tract infections, congestion, coughs and feverish chills.

As a digestive remedy it can be relevant for wind and colic and is quite safe to use with children.

The essential oil is also available and can be included in chest rubs for congestion and coughs. Hyssop is mildly sedative so the oil can be added to relaxing baths.

Remedies and supplements
BioCare Artemisia Complex; *Potter's Catarrh Mixture; *Potter's Vegetable Cough Remover

Simples
Oil: Hartwood Aromatics
Tincture: Bioforce, Neal's Yard Remedies

ICELAND MOSS

Cetraria islandica

Parts used: lichen

Lichens have long been used medicinally as soothing demulcents and expectorants helpful for gastric inflammations and dry coughs. More recent research suggests that the acids contained in Iceland moss are also antibiotic, active against bacteria like *Trichomonas vaginalis* which infects the vagina causing discharge and discomfort. Iceland moss is included in throat pastilles for dry coughs and sore throats.

Remedies and supplements
Bioforce Usnean Cough Lozenges; *Weleda Herb and Honey Cough Elixir

INDIAN TOBACCO

Lobelia inflata

Synonyms: pukeweed, asthma weed, lobelia

Parts used: herb

Indian tobacco is another of the physiomedicalist's favourites which found its way into the European repertoire in the nineteenth century. The plant contains a number of potent alkaloids, one of which is a depressant for the central nervous system and another causes vomiting. So while overdose of the plant is potentially life-threatening it is rather difficult to achieve. In the UK its use is restricted to professional practitioners and it is mainly used as a respiratory stimulant to ease asthma, bronchitis and whooping cough. Externally it can be used in muscle relaxant creams and as a poultice for boils and ulcers.

Lobeline, one of its alkaloids, is similar to nicotine and may help to relieve symptoms of withdrawal by those trying to give up smoking.

Remedies and supplements

*Cantassium Hay Fever; *Culpeper Balm of Gilead Cough Mixture; *Culpeper Head Cold and Throat Mixture; *Frank Roberts Catarrh Tablets; *Frank Roberts Rod-Bron Tablets; *Gerard House Lobelia Compound; *Heath & Heather Balm of Gilead Cough Mixture; *Heath & Heather Balm of Gilead Cough Pastilles; *Lanes Herbelix Specific; Neal's Yard Balm of Gilead; Neal's Yard Horehound & Aniseed Linctus; *Potter's Antibron Tablets; *Potter's Antismoking Tablets; *Potter's Balm of Gilead; *Potter's Chest Mixture; *Potter's Horehound and Aniseed Cough Mixture

IPECACUANHA

Cephaelis ipecacuanha

Synonyms: matto grosso, rio, ipecac

Parts used: root, rhizome

Ipecacuanha originates from South America where it was used as a cough and diarrhoea remedy by native peoples before being introduced into Europe in the seventeenth century. Like many expectorants it acts by irritating the gastric mucosa so in large doses can cause nausea and vomiting, especially in children. It is also an amoebacide – hence its traditional role in treating dysentery.

Ipecacuanha still features in a number of prescription cough mixtures as well as over-the-counter herbal cough preparations.

Remedies and supplements

Bioforce Drosinula Cough Syrup; *CoughEeze; *Frank Roberts Cold Tablets; *Frank Roberts Rod-Bron Tablets; *Lanes Honey and Molasses Cough Mixture; Neal's Yard Balm of Gilead; *Potter's Vegetable Cough Remover; *Weleda Cough Elixir

IRISH MOSS

Chondrus crispus

Synonyms: caragheen

Parts use: whole plant

Irish moss is a common seaweed found on the Atlantic coasts of Europe and North America. It is a mucilaginous plant used for dry coughs and gastric inflammations, and is also mildly laxative and expectorant. As well as its medicinal properties, Irish moss is used extensively in the food industry as a stabiliser (E407) and for a number of industrial processes in brewing, tanning and paint production.

Remedies and supplements
*Lanes Biobalm; Professional Herbs Cascara and Rhubarb

ISPHAGHULA

Plantago psyllium; P. ovata

Synonyms: psyllium, flea seeds, fleawort

Parts used: husks, seeds

Isphaghula is widely used as a bulking laxative: *P. ovata* seeds are pinkish brown while *P. psyllium* seeds are blackish brown, but both have the same action. The seeds swell when moistened to form a glutinous mass which encourages peristalsis and lubricates the bowel. Although primarily used for constipation, the resulting bulky mass can help to soothe diarrhoea and is sometimes recommended in irritable bowel syndrome.

The seeds are often sold loose and need to be soaked in water before use. If taken in capsule form they should be accompanied by a large glass of water to prevent over absorption of gut fluids as they swell. Isphaghula is sometimes recommended as a slimming remedy and research has shown that if the seeds are taken before a meal they will reduce consumption of fats and create a feeling of fullness which discourages overeating.

Remedies and supplements
BioCare Colon Care; Discovery Coliclens; Natural Flow Regular Ten Powder; *Potter's Cleansing Herb

Simples
Capsules/tablets: Arkocaps Phytofibre (350 mg); *Fybogel; Natural Flow Psyllium Husks; Power Health Pure Isphaghula (350 mg); *Regulan; Solgar Psyllium Seed Husks; Trimulina Isphaghula.

IVY

Hedera helix

Parts used: young leaves

Ivy is a bitter, cathartic herb with a nauseating taste which has been used to clear worm infestations (and liver flukes in sheep), and is liable to cause vomiting and destroy red blood cells. In homoeopathic doses is it rather more friendly and is used in mainland Europe to treat catarrh and colds. Externally it is included in cosmetics and used for a range of skin problems.

It appears in a few herbal preparations in the UK in homoeopathic guise.

Remedies and supplements
Bioforce Bronchosan; Bioforce Drosinula Cough Syrup

JAMAICA DOGWOOD

Piscidia erythrina

Synonyms: fish poison tree

Parts used: bark

As both its botanical and alternate common name imply, Jamaica dogwood is not ideal for fish. It is added to streams by Caribbean fisherman to stupefy the fish which then float to the surface and can easily be caught. Its sedating effect is, fortunately, not quite so dramatic on warm-blooded creatures. The plant is also analgesic and antispasmodic and can be used for period pain, neuralgia, migraine and asthma. It is mainly included in over-the-counter products for tension and stress.
• Jamaica dogwood should not be used in pregnancy

Remedies and supplements
*Frank Roberts Valerian Compound; *Gerard House Biophylin; *Gerard House Valerian Compound Tablets; Herbcraft Passiflora and Valerian Formula; *HRI Calm Life Tablets; *Muir's Head-Ese; *Muir's Stress-Ese; *Potter's Anased Pain Relief Tablets; *Potter's Nodoff Mixture

JAPANESE QUINCE

Cydonia japonica

Parts used: seeds

The Japanese quince, with its attractive orange spring flowers and autumn fruits, is popularly grown as a garden ornamental. It is not usually regarded as a medicinal plant, but in anthroposophical medicine it is used to relieve the symptoms of hay fever and allergic rhinitis.

Remedies and supplements
*Weleda Gencydo Ointment

JASMINE

Jasminum officinale

Synonyms: jessamine

Parts used: essential oil

The heavy scent of jasmine makes it a favourite garden flower and a popular oil in perfumery. It is used in aromatherapy as an anti-depressant, an antispasmodic helpful as a uterine tonic, and for period pains. It also acts as an aphrodisiac for both men and women.

Simples
Oils: Hartwood Aromatics; Neal's Yard Remedies; Tisserand

JERUSALEM ARTICHOKE

Helianthus tuberosus

Parts used: tuber

Jerusalem artichoke is one of many vegetables which can help to reduce blood sugar levels and can sometimes be useful in the treatment of late onset diabetes.

Simples
Tincture: Bioforce

JUNIPER

Juniperis communis

Parts used: berries, oils

Juniper berries, and the steam-distilled oil extracted from them, are both used medicinally. The berries are diuretic, antiseptic and anti-inflammatory and are generally used for cystitis and other urinary tract infections. Prolonged use can, however, irritate the kidneys and it is better not to take any preparation containing juniper for longer than four to six weeks. The oil is used externally and can provide relief from muscular aches and pains and arthritis.

Cade oil is made by dry distillation of the heartwood of various species of juniper; it contains phenol and is mildly disinfectant. Cade is included in external preparations for chronic skin conditions, such a scaling eczema and psoriasis.
• Juniper should not be taken internally by those suffering from kidney disease. High doses should be avoided in pregnancy.

Remedies and supplements
Bioforce Nephrosolid; Frank Roberts Parsley Piert Compound Tablets; *FSC Waterfall; Health Aid FemmeVit; *Lane's Sage and Garlic Catarrh Remedy; Kordel's Celery and Juniper; *Muir's Sciatica; *Muir's Water-Ese; Neal's Yard Ginger and Juniper Warming Oil; *Olbas Pastilles; *Potter's Diuretabs; *Potter's Sciargo; *Potter's Sciargo Herb; *Potter's Watershed Mixture; Professional Herbs Uva Ursi and Parsley; Solgar Herbal Water Formula Capsules; St Hildegard-Posch Wacholder Elixir
External: Arthur's Formula Bath and Massage Oil; Bioforce Po Ho Oil; Frank Roberts Cade Oil Ointment; Harpago Gel; Heloderm CT Ointment; Heloderm CT Shampoo; Neal's Yard Cellulite Oil; *Olbas Oil; *Potter's Varicose Ointment

Simples
Oil (Juniper): Botanica; Hartwood Aromatics; Neal's Yard Remedies; Nelson & Russell; Tisserand
Tincture: Neal's Yard Remedies

KAVA KAVA

Piper methysticum

Synonyms: kava

Parts used: root

Kava kava is a pungent tasting herb that smells slightly of lilac. It originates in the South Sea Islands and a drink made from the fermented root was used in Melanesian rituals as a calming potion to increase mental awareness. Medicinally it is regarded as a diuretic and stimulating tonic generally given for urino-genital infections or as a tonic for these organs in middle age. It has also been used as a gall bladder stimulant, taken for gout and included in external rubs for rheumatism.
• Kava kava should not be taken in pregnancy.

Remedies and supplements
Ladies Meno-Life Formula; *Potter's Antiglan Tablets; *Potter's GB Tablets; *Potter's Protat
External: Arthur's Formula Cream

KELP

Ascophyllum nodosum; Laminaria spp; Macrocysris pyrfera

Parts used: whole plant

Various seaweeds are used to make kelp tablets. They all tend to be rich in iodine which acts as a stimulant for the thyroid gland and can thus increase metabolism. Kelp is sometimes recommended as a slimming aid but it will really only be effective if a sluggish thyroid is part of the problem. Misuse and excess can lead to thyrotoxicosis. Kelp is also useful in general debility and is highly nutritious.
• Kelp should not be taken by those with thyroid problems or before going to bed at night.
See bladderwrack

Remedies and supplements
Culpeper Seaweed Tablets; *Frank Roberts Kelp and Nettle Compound; Healthcrafts Kelp Plus; Kelp Plus 3; Ladies Meno-Life Formula; Gerard House Seaweed and Sarsparilla Tablets; *Potter's Malted Kelp Tablets; Power Health Alfalfa, Kelp & Yeast; Professional Herbs Cayenne & Ginger; Professional Herbs Uva Ursi and Parsley

Simples
>   *Capsules/tablets:* Bioforce Kelpasan; Healthcrafts Kelp; Lamberts Kelp Tablets;
>   Neal's Yard Kelp Tablets; Power Health Kelp; Pure-fil Aqua-Vite Super Kelp

KNOTWEED

Polygonum aviculare

Synonyms: knotgrass

Parts used: herb

Knotweed is an astringent herb, rich in tannins, flavonoids and silica. It is a common weed with pink flowers found widely across Europe and is used as a diuretic, wound herb and diarrhoea remedy. Like many tannin-rich astringents it will help to stop bleeding and is added to cough and bronchitis medicines largely for this reason.

Remedies and supplements
>   Bioforce Golden Grass Tea; Bioforce IMP (Imperthritica); Bioforce Nephrosolid;
>   Bioforce Tormentavena

KUDZU

Pueraria lobata

Synonyms: Ge Gen, Ge Hua

Parts used: root, flowers

Although kudzu vine is regarded as a pernicious weed in parts of North America, recent research has highlighted its importance as a remedy for alcoholism. The plant is a traditional Chinese medicinal herb used for colds, influenza, fevers, gastritis and muscle stiffness. It is also antispasmodic and diaphoretic. In Chinese folk medicine the root has long been considered as a convenient remedy for reducing alcoholic intake and this property has now been confirmed. Its constituents daidzin and daidzein both help to suppress the desire for alcohol and it is being used to help addicts.

Simples
>   *Tincture:* Herbcraft

LADY'S MANTLE

Alchemilla xanthoclora

Synonyms: A. vulgaris, lion's foot

Parts used: herb

Like other members of the rose family, lady's mantle is rich in tannins and is thus highly astringent. It can be used in the treatment of diarrhoea and sore throats and externally for sores and weeping dermatitis. Like many plants with "lady" or "mother" in their names, it is long-established as a gynaecological herb. In parts of Europe it is used as a menstrual regulator for heavy menstrual flow and in ointments for vaginal itching.

Remedies and supplements
Frank Roberts Alchemilla Compound; *Ricola Swiss Herb Lozenges

Simples
Tincture: Neal's Yard Remedies

LARCH

Larix decidua

Parts used: bark

Larch is a bitter, astringent, diuretic herb used to relieve bronchitis and congestion. It makes a soothing remedy for urinary inflammation.
• Larch is best avoided by those suffering from kidney disease.

Remedies and supplements
Bioforce Usneasan Cough Lozenges
External: *Weleda Larch Resin Lotion

LAVENDER

Lavandula angustifolia

Synonyms: *L. officinalis*, English lavender

Parts used: flowers, oil

Widely used in perfumes and toiletries, lavender has long been prized for its scent. The plant is antispasmodic and carminative so is helpful for digestive upsets. It is also uplifting and anti-depressant so makes a valuable addition to remedies for tension and emotional upsets.

Lavender is generally regarded as cooling, so can be helpful for the sort of migraines and headaches which are eased by the use of an ice pack. It may be taken internally as a tea made from the flowers, or used externally by massaging the diluted oil into the neck and temples.

Despite this range of applications, the herb is rarely used in over-the-counter internal remedies although lavender oil features in a number of external rubs. Added to bathwater, it is relaxing and soothing for nervous tensions and insomnia; in massage oils it can be helpful for muscular aches and pains, strains and some rheumatic problems.

Remedies and supplements

External: Arthur's Formula Cream; Arthur's Formula Bath and Massage Oil; Herbcraft Aloe Lavender Spray; Neal's Yard Ginger and Juniper Warming Oil; Neal's Yard Sports Salve; Phytovarix; *Weleda Larch Resin Lotion; *Weleda Medicinal Gargle

Simples

Oil: Botanica; Hartwood Aromatics; Neal's Yard Remedies; Nelson & Russell; Tisserand
Tincture: Neal's Yard Remedies

LEMON

Citrus limon

Parts used: juice, oil

Taken internally, lemon is diuretic, anti-inflammatory and cooling; it can improve the peripheral circulation and is useful for piles and varicose veins. In folk medicine it is a popular remedy for feverish chills and is widely used as a decongestant in numerous honey and lemon cough mixtures. The oil can ease sore throats and insect stings as well as the pain of neuralgia.

Remedies and supplements

Neal's Yard Lemon & Honey Lozenges; Neal's Yard Eucalyptus & Menthol Lozenges; Neal's Yard Cellulite Oil; *Weleda Melissa Comp; *Weleda Cough Drops
External: Thursday Plantation Walkabout; *Weleda Gencydo Ointment

Simples

Oil: Hartwood Aromatics; Neal's Yard Remedies; Nelson & Russell; Tisserand

LEMON BALM

Melissa officinalis

Synonyms: balm, sweet balm

Parts used: leaves, oil

Lemon balm was regarded by the ancient Greeks as something of a cure-all, closely associated with bees and the healing power of honey (hence the botanical name, from the Latin for honey – *mel*). It is mostly used in over-the-counter remedies as a carminative and sedative, although the plant is also valuable in fever management as a diaphoretic to help lower body temperature.

Lemon balm is a gentle herb useful for treating nervous tummy upsets in adults and children, but is also potent enough to help with depression, anxiety and tension headaches.

Externally, lemon balm creams can be used on insect bites, sores and slow-healing wounds although they are not generally available from UK suppliers. The essential oil is used in aromatherapy for nervous problems and is valuable, well-diluted in sprays, for keeping insects away.

Remedies and supplements
Bioforce Cardiaforce; Bioforce Cystaforce; Bioforce Dormeasan; Bioforce Gastrosan; Bioforce Hyperiforce; Gerard House Sooth-a-Tea; Jay-Vee Tablets; Ricola Swiss Herb Lemon Mint Lozenges; Thursday Plantation Throat Lozenges; *Valerina – Day-Time; *Valerina – Night -Time; *Weleda Cough Drops; *Weleda Melissa Comp
External: Nature's Vyrbrit

Simples
Juice: Schoenenberger Plant Juice
Oil: Hartwood Aromatics; Neal's Yard Remedies; Tisserand
Tincture: Bioforce; Neal's Yard Remedies

LEMONGRASS

Cymbopogon citratus

Parts used: essential oil

Lemongrass leaves are widely used in Thai cookery giving a fresh, characteristic lemon flavour to dishes. Medicinally the oil is used primarily as an insect repellent, thanks to the high levels of citronellal it contains. It can also be used externally for treating lice, insect bites and fungal infections.

Remedies and supplements
Bee Brand Massage Oil

Simples
Oil: Botanica; Hartwood Aromatics; Neal's Yard Remedies; Tisserand

LIFE ROOT

Senecio aureus

Synonyms: squaw weed

Parts used: rhizome

Life root is one of a number of traditional Native American plants used for treating gynaecological problems, that found their way into the European repertoire in the nineteenth century. It is a menstrual regulator and was also traditionally used to ease childbirth, menopausal symptoms and vaginal discharge. The plant is now known to contain pyrrolizidine alkaloids which can cause liver damage, so its use is restricted in some countries and it is gradually falling from favour.

Remedies and supplements
Ladies Meno-Life Formula

LIME

Tilia cordata

Synonyms: linden

Parts used: flowers

Lime flowers – known as *tilleul* in France – are a popular after-dinner tisane taken to encourage relaxation as well as improve the digestion after a meal. The plant is calming for the nerves and will help to reduce high blood pressure. It is believed to help lower the build-up of fatty deposits in the blood vessels that can lead to arteriosclerosis. Lime flowers are also antispasmodic, diaphoretic and a gentle tonic. The herb is mainly included in mixtures aimed at lowering blood pressure which is raised either due to stress or because of menopausal upsets, although it can also be suitable for digestive problems associated with nervous tension and in feverish colds or influenza.

Remedies and supplements

Frank Roberts BP Tablets; *Frank Roberts Motherwort Compound Formula; *Frank Roberts Valerian Compound; *Gerard House Motherwort Compound; Health Aid Tranquil Capsules with Viburnum; *Muir's Pick-Me-Up; *Potter's Wellwoman Herbs; *Potter's Wellwoman Tablets

Simples

Oil: Tisserand
Tincture: Neal's Yard Remedies

LINSEED

Linum usitatissimum

Synonyms: flax seed

Parts used: seeds, oil

Flax is well known both as a source of fibre used to make linen and for the oil expressed from its seeds, which is widely used in the paint industry. This same oil and the seeds are both used medicinally. The seeds have long been regarded as a bulk laxative, rather like isphaghula, and are taken crushed with water for chronic constipation and diverticulitis. They are demulcent and expectorant, used to soothe gastritis and chronic bronchial conditions and to ease sore throats.

The oil is now known to be rich in both *cis*-linoleic acid and *alpha*-linolenic acid which are both essential in the production of prostaglandins. Like evening primrose oil it thus contains chemicals vital for maintaining healthy cell structure and hormonal function. It may be helpful for those suffering from chronic skin and rheumatic disorders and menstrual problems. The oil is soon oxidized and will produce toxins on long exposure to air so needs to be fresh.

Remedies and supplements

BioCare CoQ10 Plus; BioCare EFA Complex; BioCare Linseed Oil 500 mg; Bio-Care Linseed Oil 1000 mg; Bioforce Linoforce; Efamol EPO with Linseed and Saf-flower.
External: *Potter's Nine Rubbing Oils

Simples

Capsules: Lamberts Flax Seed Oil (1000 mg); Power Health Omega Oil (250 mg); Solgar Linseed Oil (1250 mg)

LIQUORICE

Glycyrrhiza glabra

Parts used: root, stolons (underground stem)

Liquorice is one of the most widely researched medicinal herbs and is anti-inflammatory, antispasmodic, expectorant and controlling for coughs; it also has a hormonal effect, stimulating the adrenal cortex. This hormonal action is due to glycyrrhizin, which is some 50 times sweeter than sucrose, and which encourages production of hormones like hydrocortisone.

The plant is very soothing and demulcent and is used to treat gastric ulcer-ation. Liquorice is also a digestive stimulant and laxative and is included in many remedies for constipation.

The plant is regarded in China as an energy tonic and pieces of root are often given to children to chew to promote muscle growth. It is used in a range of herbal products – primarily cough mixtures and remedies for stomach disor-ders.

• Excessive liquorice can cause fluid retention and increase blood pressure and it should therefore be avoided by those suffering from hypertension. It should not be taken by those on digoxin-based drugs.

Remedies and supplements

BioCare AD206; BioCare Artemisia Complex; BioCare Buccalzyme; BioCare Phy-tosterol Complex; BioCare Salicidin; Bioforce Bronchosan; Bioforce Usnean Cough Lozenges; *Bio-Strath Liquorice Formula; Blackmores Euphorbia Complex; Blackmores Liquorice Complex; Bumbles Propolis Aniseed & Liquorice; *Culpeper Cough Relief Mixture; *Culpeper Herbal Mixture for Acidity, Indigestion and Flat-ulence; East West Shi Hu and Gan Cao Tea; *Frank Roberts Althaea Compound Tablets; *Frank Roberts Rod-Bron Tablets; Health Aid Herbal Booster; Herbcraft Liquorice Formula; Herbcraft Mullein Formula; *Lane's Sage and Garlic Catarrh Remedy; *Muir's Gastric-Ese; *Natraleze; *Potter's Antibron Tablets; *Potter's Lightning Cough Remedy; *Potter's Vegetable Cough Remover; *Revitonil
External: Golden Yellow Ointment; Spring Wind Ointment

Simples

Capsules: Full Potency Herbs Liquorice Root Vegicaps (520 mg)
Tincture: Herbcraft; Neal's Yard Remedies

LITHOSPERMUM

Lithospermum erythrorhizon

Synonyms: *Zi Cao*

Parts used: root

Used to reduce fevers and improve circulation internally, this Chinese herb is also anti-bacterial and healing. Externally it is used in skin remedies, both as a wound herb and for burns and frostbite. Internally the Chinese include the plant in remedies for measles and other feverish conditions.

Remedies and supplements
    External: Amber Massage Salve; Spring Wind Ointment

LUNGMOSS

Lobaria pulmonaria

Synonyms: oak lungs, lungwort

Parts used: lichen

Like other lichens, lungmoss is astringent and demulcent. It can improve appetite and is also expectorant. It is rarely used these days but may still be found in cough remedies and is helpful for asthma and bronchitis.

Remedies and supplements
    Neal's Yard Balm of Gilead

LUNGWORT

Pulmonaria officinalis

Synonyms: Jerusalem cowslip

Parts used: leaves

The speckled green leaves of lungwort were once regarded, under the Doctrine of Signatures, as resembling a diseased lung, hence the plant's initial use as a cough cure. It is a member of the borage family, and like comfrey, contains pyrrolizidine alkaloids so has been restricted in some countries. It is a mucilaginous herb and – also like comfrey – contains allantoin which encourages cell growth. It is expectorant and is still used for treating coughs, especially bronchitis, and can also be helpful for catarrh and laryngitis. Lungwort can also soothe diarrhoea and piles, and has been used in eye lotions and as a wound herb.

Remedies and supplements
    *Culpeper Balm of Gilead Cough Mixture; *Culpeper Cough Relief Mixture;
    *Potter's Balm of Gilead

MAITAKE

Grifola frondosa

Synonyms: *Bai Mo Gu*, hen of the woods, sheep's head

Parts used: fruiting body

Maitake means "dancing mushrooms" in Japanese. Some say this is because the fruiting body of the fungus resembles a butterfly while others suggest, more prosaically, that the name stems from the fact that collectors could exchange the mushrooms for their weight in silver and thus danced for joy on finding them. The fungus is a strong immune stimulant and has been widely used as an anticancer remedy. It will lower blood sugar, may be helpful in late-onset diabetes and has also been used in AIDS therapy.

Remedies and supplements
 Mycoherb Myco Forte

Simples
 Capsules: Mycoherb Grifo-Gen (East-West Herbs)
 Tincture: Mycoherb Grifo-Gen (East-West Herbs)

MALABAR TAMARIND

Garcinia cambogia

Synonyms: goraka, garcinia

Parts used: rind

A tree from southern Asia where the fruit is used for flavouring curries and "to make meals more filling": the tamarind resembles a small yellow or reddish pumpkin and the rind is dried and extracted to make a patented product known as CitriMax*.

Research by pharmaceutical company Hoffmann-La Roche has identified a substance called (-)-hydroxycitric acid (HCA) in the rind which has been shown to curb appetite and thus reduce food intake. HCA is said to inhibit an enzyme (ATP-citrate lyase), responsible for converting carbohydrates into fat for storage, through competitive inhibition. The HCA binds to the ATP-citrate lyase thus preventing it from storing fat and so surplus is instead converted to glycogen. This increase in glycogen production sends a satiety signal to the brain suppressing the appetite.

HCA is thus promoted as an appetite suppressant and slimming aid.

Orthodox appetite suppressants include a number of prescription drugs (such as amphetamines) and OTC products like phenylepropanolamine. However, these tend to act on the central nervous system to suppress food cravings and critics suggest that in the long-term this can cause depression, nervousness, insomnia or increased heart rate. By acting purely on the digestive system's chemistry proponents of HCA argue that it is a safer and more effective slimming remedy. *CitriMax™ is a trademark of Interhealth Co which markets the preparation to other herbal product manufacturers worldwide.

Remedies and supplements
BioCare CitriMax Forte; Citri-Trim; Natural Flow CitriMax Fat Control Nutritional Complex; Phoenix Nutrition CitriMax; Weight Logic

MALE FERN

Dryopteris filix-mas

Synonyms: *Aspidium filix-mas*

Parts used: rhizomes

The male fern is an extremely potent herb once used for intestinal parasites and guaranteed to kill just about any worm (including tapeworms) and liver fluke. It is toxic and overdose can lead to heart failure and its use in conventional herbal medicine is restricted. In anthroposophic medicine very small amounts are used to stimulate the digestion.

Remedies and supplements
*Weleda Digestodoran Tablets

MALLOW

Malva sylvestris

Synonyms: blue mallow, common mallow

Parts used: flowers, leaves

Like its relative, marshmallow, the common mallow is a good demulcent – soothing and anti-inflammatory for irritated tissues. It is slightly astringent and expectorant and is largely used for coughs, sore throats, catarrh and stomach inflammations. In large doses it has a laxative action and can be used externally on sores and boils. The flowers were once popular in cough syrups.

Remedies and supplements
*Ricola Swiss Herb Lozenges

MARIGOLD

Calendula officinalis

Synonyms: Marybud, calendula, pot marigold

Parts used: petals, flowerheads, oil

In the twelfth century simply looking on the golden colour of the marigold was supposed to lift the spirits and encourage cheerfulness, and the plant has been a favourite with herbalists ever since. It is astringent, antiseptic, anti-fungal and anti-inflammatory. Taken internally it can help to regulate the menstrual cycle and help various gynaecological disorders. Marigold is also a bitter herb and stimulates bile production and improves the digestion.

Very few internal over-the-counter remedies include marigold, and the plant largely features in external preparations for dry skin and eczema. As an anti-fungal it is used in thrush remedies and it also makes a valuable all-purpose wound cream for minor cuts, grazes and burns.

Remedies and supplements

BioCare Buccalzyme

External: Arthur's Formula Cream; Bioforce Po Ho Ointment; Bioforce Seven Herb Cream; Galen Calendula and Vitamin E Cream; Gerard House Calendula Ointment; Herbcraft Aloe Lavender Spray; Hartwood Aromatics Calendula Ointment; Herbcraft Calendula & Goldenseal Spray; Herbcraft Fresh Breath Cinnamint Spray; Neal's Yard Calendula Ointment; Neal's Yard Hypercal Ointment; *Nelsons Burns Ointment; *Nelsons Calendula Cream; *Nelsons Hypercal Cream; *Nelsons Haemorrhoid Cream; *Nelsons Healing Ointment; *Nelsons Hypercal Tincture; *Nelsons Pyrethrum Spray; *Weleda Calendula Lotion; *Weleda Calendolon Ointment; *Weleda Hypericum/Calendula Ointment; *Weleda Oleum Rhinale; *Weleda WCS Dusting Powder; *Weleda Massage Balm with Calendula

MARJORAM

Origanum spp

Synonyms: oregano

Parts used: herb, essential oil

Marjoram (*O. majorana*) and oregano (*O. vulgare*) are very closely related with numerous cultivars largely grown for their culinary flavour. Medicinally the two are also similar, used internally for colds and minor digestive upsets, while marjoram oil is used in aromatherapy to ease digestive spasms and period pains as well as being included in rubs for rheumatic aches and pains.

Like other members of the mint family (notably thyme and rosemary) marjoram has recently been investigated for anti-oxidant properties. Researchers suggest that it can prevent premature ageing of cells and could have a role in geriatric medicine. Marjoram can combat "free radicals" which are chemical groups produced as by-products of various metabolic processes which can oxidize and damage healthy cells.

Remedies and supplements

BioCare Candicidin; Neal's Yard Anti-Oxidant Herbs Elixir; Pure-fil Romagen Herbal Antioxidant

External: Arthur's Formula Cream

Simples
> *Oil:* Hartwood Aromatics; Nelson & Russell; Tisserand

MARSHMALLOW

Althea officinale

Parts used: leaves, roots

Marshmallow is a sweet, highly mucilaginous plant that is softening and soothing. It is also expectorant and diuretic and is used for bronchitis, irritating coughs and cystitis. The root is especially soothing for the gastric membranes and can be used for gastritis, heartburn and other inflammations of the digestive tract.

Most over-the-counter remedies containing marshmallow exploit this property and are suggested for indigestion, heartburn and similar digestive upsets. However, marshmallow is also a soothing expectorant and as such is included in various preparations for coughs and colds.

Marshmallow is used externally in softening preparations for various skin problems and is included in drawing ointments for splinters and boils.

Remedies and supplements
> BioCare Gastroplex; Blackmores Liquorice Complex; *Culpeper Herbal Mixture for Acidity, Indigestion and Flatulence; *Frank Roberts Althaea Compound Tablets; *Frank Roberts Cranesbill Compound Tablets; Frank Roberts Golden Seal Compound Tablets; Gerard House Marshmallow and Peppermint; *Gerard House Golden Seal Compound; Honeyrose Herbal Cigarettes; Kordel's Horseradish, Odourless Garlic and Vitamin C; *Lanes Biobalm; *Lanes Digest; *Lanes Garlodex; *Lanes Sinotar; Neal's Yard Echinacea & Mallow Linctus; *Ricola Swiss Herb Lozenges; *Weleda Cough Elixir; *Weleda Herb and Honey Cough Elixir
> *External:* *Potter's Herbheal Ointment; *Rickard's Woodsap Ointment

Simples
> *Tincture:* Neal's Yard Remedies

MATÉ

Ilex paraguariensis

Synonyms: Paraguay tea, yerba maté

Parts used: leaves

Maté is generally used as a pleasant tasting alternative to tea. Like tea it contains caffeine (up to 2%) and theobromine so has a stimulant and mildly diuretic effect. It has been used for mild depression, nervous tension, migraines and neuralgia and can also be combined in remedies for rheumatism. It is sometimes included in herbal product to improve the flavour.

Remedies and supplements
>   Gerard House Sleek-a-Tea; Gerard House Vig-a-Tea; *Lusty's Herbalene

MEADOWSWEET

Filipendula ulmaria

Synonyms: queen of the meadow

Parts used: herb

Perhaps meadowsweet's best known claim to fame is that under its old botanical name of *Spiraea ulmaria*, it gave its name to the drug aspirin which was patented by Bayer in the 1890s. The plant contains salicylate compounds which have a similar action to those used in the familiar drug. Meadowsweet is astringent, antacid, anti-rheumatic and anti-inflammatory. It is used internally for gastritis, indigestion and heartburn as well as easing arthritic and rheumatic aches and pains. It is often combined with marshmallow and lemon balm and is used in a number of over-the-counter remedies for indigestion and gastric upsets.

• Meadowsweet is best avoided by those sensitive to salicylates and aspirin.

Remedies and supplements
>   *Culpeper Herbal Mixture for Acidity, Indigestion and Flatulence; *Fo Ti Tieng;
>   *Frank Roberts Althaea Compound Tablets; Frank Roberts Acidosis Tablets;
>   *Natraleze; *Potter's Acidosis; *Potter's Indigestion Mixture

Simples
>   *Tincture:* Neal's Yard Remedies

MILK THISTLE

Silybum marianum

Synonyms: Carduus marianus, Marian thistle

Parts used: seed

Today, milk thistle is usually regarded as a protective remedy for the liver. It contains silymarin which has been shown to prevent toxic chemicals from damaging the liver. It has also been successfully used for liver cirrhosis and hepatitis. In the past the plant was popular for encouraging milk flow in nursing mothers – hence it name – and was also considered a bitter digestive tonic.

Remedies and supplements
>   BioCare Candistatin; BioCare Silymarin Complex; *Bio-Strath Artichoke Formula;
>   Bioforce Boldocynara; Colon Cleanse; FSC Milk Thistle Tablets; Herbcraft Dande-
>   lion Formula; Lamberts Silymarin Extract

Simples
>   *Capsules:* Full Potency Herbs Milk Thistle Vegicaps (520 mg); Power Health Pure

Milk Thistle (100 mg capsules)
Tincture: Herbcraft; Neal's Yard Remedies

MISTLETOE

Viscum album

Parts used: leafy twigs

The parasitic mistletoe was a source of fascination to the ancients, fruiting in mid-winter and associated with fertility and religious rites. The Druids cut it from oak trees with golden sickles and lovers have kissed underneath it at mid-winter festivals for millennia. In recent years it has been associated with anti-cancer therapies and is also an important heart tonic, immune-stimulant and sedative.

Mistletoe is used in remedies to reduce blood pressure or improve the circulation and it can also calm irregular heart beats.

Remedies and supplements

Bioforce IMP (Imperthritica); Bioforce Petasan; Power Health Circulating Compound

Simples

Juice: Schoenenberger Plant Juice
Tincture: Bioforce; Neal's Yard Remedies

MOTHERWORT

Leonurus cardiaca

Synonyms: lion's tail

Parts used: herb

Motherwort is mainly used as a heart tonic and sedative. It reputedly takes its name from a traditional use of calming anxiety in childbirth and recent research also suggests that it can help prevent thrombosis. The herb is popular for treating menopausal upsets and is included in some remedies for premenstrual syndrome, although its main application in over-the-counter products tends to be as a general sedative, particularly suitable for palpitations and other heart complaints. The plant also has some anti-bacterial function, is antispasmodic and also a uterine stimulant.

Remedies and supplements

BioCare PT208; Frank Roberts Alchemilla Compound; Frank Roberts BP Tablets; *Frank Roberts Motherwort Compound Formula; *Gerard House Motherwort Compound; *Lanes Quiet Life Tablets; *Muir's Pick-Me-Up; *Potter's Prementaid; *Potter's Wellwoman Tablets

Simples
Tincture: Neal's Yard Remedies

MUIRA-PUAMA

Dulacia inopiflora

Synonyms: potentwood

Parts used: root

Found in the Amazonian rain forests, muira-puama has a long history of medicinal use in the region although little is known of its active constituents. It is an astringent, spicy herb with a stimulating and aphrodisiac effect and is used for impotence and diarrhoea. It is contained in a few herbal supplements sold as tonics or aphrodisiacs.

Remedies and supplements
Health Aid Herbal Booster; Reevecrest Libidex 5

MULLEIN

Verbascum thapsus

Synonyms: Aaron's rod

Parts used: leaves, flowers

Mullein is a tall biennial with yellow flowers and its leaves covered in thick woolly down. It is expectorant, diuretic and extremely mucilaginous, and is used to produce soothing syrups and oils. It is taken for coughs, influenza, catarrh, bronchitis and is included in a variety of other respiratory remedies. An infused oil made from the flowers is a traditional remedy for earache and may also be applied to sores, boils, chilblains and piles.

Remedies and supplements
Health Aid Herbal Booster; Herbcraft Mullein Formula

Simples
Infused oil: Neal's Yard Remedies
Tincture: Herbcraft; Neal's Yard Remedies

MUSTARD

Brassica nigra

Parts used: seed, oil

Mustard plasters and footbaths may evoke an image of homespun folk medicine but the herb remains extremely effective at stimulating the circulation and digestive system. Mustard poultices were used for rheumatic pain, although the herb can irritate the skin and cause blisters in prolonged contact. It is used in small quantities in warming oils and rubs for muscular stiffness, aches and pains.

Remedies and supplements
External: *Potter's Nine Rubbing Oils

MYRRH

Commiphora myrrh

Synonyms: bola, C. molmol

Parts used: oleo-gum resin

Myrrh resin is obtained from a number of species (including gugulon, *C. mukul*) although the original source is the variety found in the desert scrublands of northern Somalia, Arabia and the Yemen. It is an acrid, bitter tasting herb which is strongly antiseptic and stimulant, anti-inflammatory, antispasmodic and expectorant. It is generally taken internally for indigestion and used as a mouth wash or gargle for tonsillitis, mouth ulcers and gum disease. Externally it can be applied to ulcers, boils and wounds.

Remedies and supplements
*Box's Far Famed Indigestion Tablets; *Culpeper Head Cold and Throat Mixture; *Frank Roberts Nervous Dyspepsia Tablets; *HRI Golden Seal Digestive; *Muir's Catarrh
External: Amber Massage Salve; Dr Shir's Linament; Herbcraft Calendula & Goldenseal Spray; Herbcraft Fresh Breath Cinnamint Spray; Herbcraft Liquorice and Propolis Spray; *Weleda Medicinal Gargle

Simples
Oil: Hartwood Aromatics; Neal's Yard Remedies; Tisserand
Tincture: Neal's Yard Remedies

MYRTLE

Myrtus communis

Parts used: leaves

Myrtle is a urinary antiseptic which will give a characteristic violet-like scent to the urine within 20 minutes of taking the plant internally. It is used for cystitis and urinary infections and may also be helpful for chest infections and congestion. Externally the oil is used for acne, piles and gum diseases.

Remedies and supplements
External: Phytorhuma

NIAOULI

Melaleuca viridiflora

Parts used: essential oil
See Cajuput

NIGHT-BLOOMING CACTUS

Selenicereus grandiflorus

Synonyms: queen of the night, night-blooming cereus

Parts used: stems, flowers

The night-blooming cactus seems almost too beautiful and exotic to be classified as a medicinal herb and many garden writers have regarded it as one of the
world's most exquisite flowers. It contains an alkaloid called cactine which is
similar in action to the digoxin obtained from foxglove and the plant is used for
heart disorders including palpitations and angina pectoris. It also has a diuretic
action.

Remedies and supplements
Blackmores Cactus & Hawthorn

NORWAY SPRUCE

Picea abies

Parts used: needles, bark, oil

Although more familiar to UK householders as a Christmas tree than medicinal
herb, extracts of Norway spruce are traditionally used in pine baths in Germany
as a remedy for rheumatism and muscular aches and pains. Like other varieties of
pine, the plant is also expectorant and demulcent and is occasionally found in
cough remedies.

Remedies and supplements
Bioforce Drosinula; Bioforce Petasan Syrup

NUTMEG

Myristica fragrans

Parts used: seed, oil

Despite its familiarity as a kitchen seasoning, nutmeg is actually quite a
potent hallucinogen and soporific with cases of delirium as the result of over-

consumption reported as early as 1576. The herb is warming, carminative and antispasmodic, and is included in digestive remedies for nausea, abdominal bloating, indigestion and colic. The oil is used externally to relieve muscular aches and pains, and is a traditional childbirth remedy in parts of the Far East where it is massaged into the abdomen during labour to relieve pain. Nutmeg is also helpful for diarrhoea.

• Excess will case headache, dizziness and delirium.

Remedies and supplements
*Potter's Rheumatic Pain Tablets; *Weleda Cough Drops; *Weleda Melissa Comp
External: *Gerard House Dragon Balm Ointment

Simples
Oil: Hartwood Aromatics

OAK

Quercus spp

Parts used: bark

Q. robur, the English or common oak, is used as a highly astringent, antiseptic, anti-inflammatory which can be helpful for many conditions involving bleeding or discharge including diarrhoea, haemorrhage, minor injuries, weeping eczema and vaginal discharges.

Q. alba, the white oak, is a North American plant which the early settlers soon adopted for use in similar ways. It is found in herbal preparations of American origin.

Remedies and supplements
Herbcraft Fresh Breath Cinnamint Spray; *Potter's Peerless Composition Essence

OLIVE

Oleo europaea

Parts used: leaves, oil

Olive is a cooling, astringent, laxative herb which has traditionally been used in folk medicine for lowering fevers and reducing blood pressure. The oil can be massaged into the scalp to improve hair quality and combat dandruff. Olive oil also contains oleic acid (a mono-unsaturated fatty acid) and some *cis*-linoleic acid so is not as valuable as linseed, borage or evening primrose oils. However, according to some theorists, it can be helpful at combating yeast infections and is sometimes advocated as an important component in anti-candida diets. Using the oil in salad dressings would seem as convenient as swallowing capsules.

Remedies and supplements
  BioCare Linseed Oil 500 mg
  External: Health Aid Eczem Oil

Simples
  Capsules: BioCare Omega-Plex Forte; Power Health Olive Oil   (300 mg)

ONION

Allium cepa

Parts used: bulb, fresh juice

Onion is more familiar as an aromatic vegetable than a medicinal herb. Its constituents include a number of sulphur compounds which stimulate the digestive system and also act as antibiotics preventing decay. Onion juice is used to help maintain a healthy gut flora and prevent fermentation; it is also diuretic and expectorant and widely used – mixed with honey or sugar – in traditional household cough remedies. Raw onion also makes a useful standby for treating insect stings.

Recent research suggests that onion can also lower blood sugar levels and it has been used to treat asthma.

Remedies and supplements
  Herbcraft Garlic & Horseradish Winter Formula

Simples
  Juice: Schoenenberger Plant Juice

OREGON GRAPE

Mahonia aquifolia

Synonyms: mountain grape

Parts used: root, root bark

Oregon grape is very similar in actions and chemistry to barberry and is similarly used as a bitter and liver stimulant. It is regarded as a suitably cleansing remedy for skin problems, especially those associated with a sluggish liver condition. It is rather less anti-inflammatory than barberry but seems to have a greater effect on the liver. Creeping Oregon grape (*M. repens*) is very similar and appears in some preparations.

Remedies and supplements
  Herbcraft Dandelion Formula; *Muir's Pick-Me-Up

OSHA

Ligusticum porteri

Synonyms: Porter's lovage, Colorado cough root

Parts used: roots, seed, oil

Osha is regarded by many US herbalists as something of a cure-all; one of the most important herbs from the Rocky Mountains and regarded as sacred by Native Americans who burned it to ward off evil influences. The plant is carminative, diaphoretic, expectorant and stimulating and is largely given for colds, influenza, fevers and coughs. It may also be helpful for rheumatic disorders and indigestion.
• Osha should not be taken in pregnancy.

Remedies and supplements
> Herbcraft Echinacea Formula; Herbcraft Liquorice and Propolis Spray; Herbcraft Mullein Formula

PAEONY

Paeonia officinalis

Synonyms: *Chi Shao Yao, Bai Shao Yao*

Parts used: root

Although various varieties of paeony are used in traditional Chinese medicine, where it is highly regarded for treating liver and blood problems, the native European plant is now rarely found in herbal products. There were once numerous superstitions associating the plant with the moon and it was used for treating convulsions, epilepsy and nervous disorders. It is generally regarded as antispasmodic and tonifying and was also used externally for piles and anal fissures.

Both red (*Chi Shao Yao*) and white (*Bai Shao Yao*) paeony are used in China. The red is regarded as a cooling herb for the blood and is used for treating irritant skin diseases, nosebleeds and to ease the inflammation of sprains and strains, while the white is primarily used as an analgesic, liver tonic and for menstrual and menopausal problems.

Remedies and supplements
> Equillence
> *External:* Golden Yellow Ointment; *Nelsons Haemorrhoid Cream

PALE CATECHU

Uncaria gambier

Synonyms: pale catechu

Parts used: leaves, shoots

Pale catechu is extremely astringent and is thus helpful for chronic diarrhoea, dysentery and chronic catarrh. It can stop excessive mucous discharges and is used topically to stop bleeding.

Remedies and supplements
*Potter's Spanish Tummy Mixture
See Black Catechu

PAPAYA

Carica papaya

Synonyms: pawpaw

Parts used: fruit, seeds, leaves, sap

Papain – an enzyme extracted from the fruit, seeds and leaf – hydrolyses digestive products including amides and polypeptides so improving function. It is also used on wounds and to improve scar tissue. In traditional medicine both the fresh fruit and infusions of the leaves are used for digestive upsets and to counter worm infestations.
See Pineapple

Remedies and supplements
*Gerard House Papaya Plus Tablets; FSC Bromelain Plus; Health Aid Herbal Booster; Lamberts Chewable Bromelain with Papain

PARACRESS

Spilanthes oleracea

Parts used: herb

Paracress is a tropical member of the daisy family which is used as a salad vegetable. It reputedly can also be used externally for fungal infections including thrush, athlete's foot and ringworm. The tincture can be applied neat to affected areas several times a day and it can also be used well diluted as a mouthwash and vaginal douche.

Remedies and supplements
External: Bioforce Seven Herb Cream

Simples
Tincture: Bioforce

PARATUDO

Pfaffia paniculata

Synonyms: suma, Brazilian ginseng

Parts used: root

The name *paratudo* means "for everything" and in the Amazonian rain forests where it grows, *Pfaffia* is regarded as a general cure-all and aphrodisiac. In the West it is used, like ginseng, as a tonic herb, especially helpful in debility and convalescence as well as during the menopause. Like ginseng, too, it is rich in steroidal compounds and saponins, while pfaffic acid derived from the plant has been patented as an anti-tumour drug.

The alternative name "suma" is a recent invention for the US health food market.

Simples

> *Capsules:* Rio Paratudo Pfaffia

PARSLEY

Petroselinum crispum

Parts used: leaves, oil, roots, seed

Familiar as a garnish and in cooking, parsley is also a valuable medicinal herb. Like other plants with a tendency to "rob the soil" it is rich in nutrients and is a valuable source of vitamins and minerals – a useful addition to the diet in anaemia, for example. It is also diuretic, carminative, slightly laxative and antispasmodic. Parsley has some anti-inflammatory action and can be used as a cleansing remedy in rheumatism as well as being included in preparations for "fluid retention" and suggested for premenstrual syndrome. It reputedly reduces the smell of garlic so also finds a place in a number of garlic capsules.

• Parsley should not be used in therapeutic doses in pregnancy; excess oil is toxic.

Remedies and supplements

> BioCare NEF242; Blackmores Odourless Garlic; *Dorwest Mixed Vegetable Tablets; *Gerard House Helonias Compound; Health Aid FemmeVit; Herbcraft Garlic and Horseradish Winter Formula; *Höfels One-a-Day Garlic with Parsley; Kordel's Celery and Juniper; *Lanes Athera; *Lanes Cascade; *Lanes Digest; *Lanes Garlodex; *Lanes Kleer; Professional Herbs Feverfew; Professional Herbs Uva Ursi and Parsley; Solgar Herbal Water Formula Capsules

Simples

> *Juice:* Schoenenberger Plant Juice
> *Oil:* Hartwood Aromatics

PARSLEY PIERT

Aphanes arvensis

Synonyms: *Alchemilla arvensis*, breakstone parsley

Parts used: leaves

Parsley piert is more closely related to the *Alchemilla* family (for example lady's mantle) than to members of the parsley group but takes its name from a superficial resemblance of the leaves. The plant is diuretic, astringent and is primarily used for kidney or bladder stones and other chronic urinary tract disorders. Little is known of its constituents.

Remedies and supplements

*Culpeper Parsley Piert Tablets; *Frank Roberts Buchu Backache Compound Tablets; Frank Roberts Black Willow Compound Tablets; Frank Roberts Parsley Piert Compound Tablets; HRI Water Balance Tablets; *Muir's Water-Ese; *Potter's Diuretabs

PASQUE FLOWER

Pulsatilla vulgaris

Synonyms: meadow anemone

Parts used: flowering plant

Pasque flower is one of our prettiest herbs with attractive red or mauve flowers and feathery leaves. The herb is an important nervine, analgesic and antispasmodic which is included in a number of proprietary remedies for tension and stress. It is helpful for any pain in the reproductive organs and is sometimes used for premenstrual tension. The fresh herb contains an irritant, antibacterial substance, protoanemonin; however, this is destroyed on drying and the plant can then be safely used.

Remedies and supplements

Absorb Plus; *Frank Roberts Calmanite Tablets; Frank Roberts Alchemilla Compound; *Frank Roberts Motherwort Compound Formula; *Frank Roberts Pulsatilla Compound Tablets; *Frank Roberts Valerian Compound; *Potter's Anased Pain Relief Tablets; *Potter's Prementaid; *Weleda Cough Elixir

Simples

Capsules/tablets: Gerard House Pulsatilla
Tincture: Neal's Yard Remedies

PASSION FLOWER

Passiflora incarnata

Synonyms: maypops

Parts used: herb

Passion flower takes its name from the religious symbolism of its flowers rather than any therapeutic effects. It was traditionally used by Native Americans as a tonic and came into the Western herbal repertoire in the nineteenth century, initially as a remedy for epilepsy and later as a cure for insomnia.

Today, it is regarded as an effective, but gentle sedative, antispasmodic and pain killer which will also reduce blood pressure. It is included in a number of day-time mixtures for anxiety and stress but is largely used in insomnia preparations. It is often combined with valerian or hops, although the single herb is also readily available in capsules.

Passion flower may also be helpful for period pain, tension headaches and a number of other nervous conditions such as irritable bowel syndrome and irregular heart beat.

Remedies and supplements

*Bio-Strath Valerian Formula; Bioforce Arterioforce; Bioforce Dormeasan; Blackmores Skullcap & Valerian; Blackmores Valerian Complex; *Cantassium Quiet Nite Sleep; *Cantassium Quiet Tyme; *Frank Roberts Calmanite Tablets; *Frank Roberts Nerfood Tablets; FSC Valerian Formula; *Gerard 99; *Gerard House Motherwort Compound; *Gerard House Valerian Compound Tablets; *Healthcrafts Night Time; *Heath & Heather Becalm; *Heath & Heather Quiet Night; Herbcraft Passiflora and Valerian Formula; HRI Night Tablets; Jay-Vee Tablets; Kordel's Kalm-Ex; Kordel's Quiet Time; *Lanes Quiet Life Tablets; *Muir's Head-Ese; *Muir's Stress-Ese; Neal's Yard Passiflora Tablets; *Potter's Anased Pain Relief Tablets; *Potter's Nodoff Mixture; Professional Herbs Valerian; *Weleda Avena Sativa Comp

Simples

Capsules/tablets: *Arkocaps Phytocalm (230 mg); Culpeper Passiflora Tablets (180 mg); *Gerard House Passiflora; Herbs of Grace Passion Flower; *Lanes Naturest; *Natracalm; Neal's Yard Remedies Passiflora; *Potter's Passiflora; Power Health Passion Flower Oil (250 mg)

Tincture: Bioforce; Neal's Yard Remedies

PATCHOULI

Pogostemon cablin

Synonym: Pogostemon patchouli

Parts used: essential oil

A stimulating and anti-depressant oil, patchouli is a popular ingredient in perfumes and is used in aromatherapy for anxiety and depression. It is also included in skin creams as an astringent and antiseptic.

Simples
> *Oils:* Botanica; Hartwood Aromatics; Neal's Yard Remedies; Tisserand

PAU D'ARCO

Tabebuia impetiginosa

Synonyms: lapacho, ipê-roxa, taheebo

Parts used: wood, inner bark

Like other Amazonian herbs, Western interest in pau d'arco is comparatively recent: it was first investigated in the 1950s when its antibiotic actions were identified and later anti-tumour properties were confirmed. This and other *Tabebuia* spp. have been traditionally used by native tribes for treating cancer and rabies. Various botanical names are found in proprietary products, although the dominant species used in the West as "pau d'arco" is *T. impetiginosa.*

The plant is regarded as an immune stimulant and the tree itself has carnivorous purple flowers which protect it from fungal attack, parasites and pests. It appears in a number of over-the-counter products designed for use in candidiasis but is also generally useful for increasing resistance to infection, countering chronic degenerative diseases and as part of a supportive regime in cancer therapy.

Remedies and supplements
> BioCare Candistatin; Cantassium Didamega

Simples
> *Capsules/tablets:* Full Potency Herbs Pau d'Arco Vegicaps (520 mg); Herbs of Grace Pau d'Arco; Rio Vitalis Lapacho (500 mg)
> *Tea:* Hartwood Aromatics

PEAR

Pyrus communis

Parts used: fruit

Like many fruits, pears are laxative, diuretic and generally cleansing and have been used in rheumatic and tonic remedies for centuries; the juice is also astringent and healing. Hildegard of Bingen recommended a pear and honey combination as a cleansing remedy for toxic problems and migraines.

Remedies and supplements
> BioCare Satasapina Cough Bon-bons; BioCare Satasapina Cough Syrup

PELLITORY-OF-THE-WALL

Parietaria judaica

Parts used: herb

Largely used for urinary tract problems such as cystitis and urinary stones, pellitory-of-the-wall is a cooling diuretic and anti-inflammatory. The plant should not be confused with pellitory (*Anacyclus pyrethrum*) which is a counter-irritant once used for treating toothache.

Remedies and supplements
    *Potter's Watershed Mixture

PEPPER

Piper nigrum

Synonyms: black pepper, white pepper

Parts used: fruits, essential oil

The black and white peppercorns used for seasoning food are simply the dried unripe and ripe berries of the same plant. They are both heating and stimulating for the digestion (hence their popular use in cooking) and they are also expectorant. The oil is sometimes included in warming rubs for arthritis and rheumatism as it is rubefacient – makes the skin red by dilating local blood vessels and increasing blood supply to an area. It is thus warming for cold joints and stiff muscles.

    In Ayurvedic medicine black pepper is mixed with clarified butter (*ghee*) and used in skin inflammations and catarrhal conditions.

Remedies and supplements
    External: Arthur's Formula Bath and Massage Oil; Bee Brand Massage Oil; Neal's Yard Cellulite Oil

Simples
    Oil: Hartwood Aromatics; Tisserand

PEPPERMINT

Mentha × piperita

Synonyms: black mint

Parts used: leaves, essential oils

Members of the mint family readily hybridize and peppermint is generally regarded as a cross between spearmint and water mint (*M. aquatica*). Its characteristic smell is due to a high menthol content and this component can be extracted or synthesized and often appears as an ingredient in herbal remedies.

Numerous varieties have been grown over the years: perhaps the most famous was Mitcham mint, a black peppermint which once formed an important cash crop in what are now London's southern suburbs.

Peppermint is antispasmodic, carminative, diaphoretic and decongestant. The oil is also antiseptic and mildly anaesthetic. It is used in a number of digestive remedies both for its medicinal actions and as a useful flavouring for the more unpleasant tasting herbs. It can help to relieve nausea (including morning sickness) and it is also included in a number of products for catarrh and colds. The oil is used in stimulating rubs for rheumatism as well as soothing creams for skin problems.

Field mint (*M. arvensis*) is rather gentler than peppermint and is similarly used in herbal medicine – especially in Chinese practice. Field mint oil for aromatherapy is available from Nelsons & Russell.

• Peppermint should not be given to babies or toddlers in any form: excess of the oil can irritate the stomach lining and misuse may lead to ulceration. The herb can also cause an allergic reaction in sensitive individuals.

Remedies and supplements

*Bio-Strath Artichoke Formula; *Bio-Strath Valerian Formula; Bioforce Boldocynara; Bioforce IMP (Imperthritica); Blackmores Cape Aloes and Cascara; *Culpeper Elder Flower and Peppermint Mixture; *Frank Roberts Drops of Life Tablets; Gerard House Marshmallow and Peppermint; Gerard House Sooth-a-Tea; *Hactos Cough Mixture; *Heath & Heather Indigestion & Flatulence; Herbcraft Peppermint Formula; Höfels One-a-Day Cardiomax Garlic Pearles; *Lane's Cut-a-Cough; *Lanes Herbelix Specific; *Lanes Honey and Molasses Cough Mixture; *Natraleze; Neal's Yard Anti-Oxidant Herbs Elixir; Neal's Yard Elderflower, Peppermint & Composition Essence; Neal's Yard Eucalyptus & Menthol Lozenges; Neal's Yard Slippery Elm Tablets; *Olbas Pastilles; *Potter's Elderflowers, Peppermint and Composition Essence; *Potter's Life Drops; *Potter's Slippery Elm Stomach Tablets; Pure-fil Romagen Herbal Antioxidant; Reevecrest Gum Thyme; *Revitonil; *Ricola Swiss Herb Lozenges; *Uvacin; *Weleda Clairo Tea; *Weleda Laxadoron Tablets; *Weleda Medicinal Gargle

External: Bioforce Po Ho Oil; Bioforce Po Ho Ointment; Herbcraft Fresh Breath Cinnamint Spray; *Olbas Oil *Potter's Dermacreme Ointment; *Potter's Nine Rubbing Oils; *Weleda Catarrh Cream; *Weleda Oleum Rhinale

Simples

Capsules/tablets: Lamberts Peppermint Oil Capsules (50mg); Obbekjaers Peppermint (200 mg); Power Health Peppermint Oil (250 mg)
Oil: Botanica; Hartwood Aromatics; Neal's Yard Remdies; Tisserand
Tincture: Neal's Yard Remedies

PERSICA

Prunus persica

Synonyms: *Tao Ren*

Parts used: seed

As an expectorant, persica and peach seeds (*P. davidiana*) are both used in China to relieve coughs and asthma, as well as taken for constipation and as a circulatory stimulant. Externally persica and peach are mildly analgesic so figures in rubs for aches and pains.

Remedies and supplements
External: Amber Massage Salve; Dr Shir's Linament; Spring Wind Ointment

PERUVIAN BALSAM

Myroxylon pereirae

Synonyms: balsam of Peru

Parts used: oleo-resin

Like its close relative, tolu, Peruvian balsam is produced by cutting into the tree bark and collecting the resin which oozes out. But while tolu is usually described as cinnamon-flavoured, Peruvian balsam tastes more of vanilla. Like tolu it is antiseptic, stimulant and expectorant but is largely used in external remedies for minor injuries, skin problems, itching skin, sore nipples, wounds and ulcers. It can also be used in creams for nappy rash and ringworm.

Although it can be taken for catarrh and diarrhoea Peruvian balsam seems rarely to be used as such on over-the-counter products.

Remedies and supplements
External: Bioforce Po Ho Ointment; *Gerard House Dragon Balm Ointment; *Weleda Frost Cream

PHELLODENDRON

Phellodendron chinense

Synonyms: *Huang Bai*

Parts used: bark

Regarded in Chinese medicine as bitter and cold, phellodendron bark is used for treating diarrhoea, jaundice, and feverish conditions associated with weak energy states. Externally it is used in ointments, for boils, abscesses and eczema.

Remedies and supplements
External: Golden Yellow Ointment

PILEWORT

Ranunculus ficaria

Synonyms: lesser celandine

Parts used: whole plant

Pilewort is generally regarded as a classic example of the mediaeval Doctrine of Signatures which reasoned that plants indicated their actions by their appearances. The plant's roots are full of tiny nodules which resemble bunches of grapes, or more prosaically, piles. Thus pilewort was recommended as a remedy for haemorrhoids and given its common name. It is used, very effectively, for piles to this day and is highly astringent with saponins which have a specific anti-haemorrhoidal action. It can be used in ointments or taken internally where it is generally combined with laxatives. Like pasque flower, the plant contains protoanemonin which is irritant but destroyed on drying, so fresh pilewort is rarely used.

Remedies and supplements
Culpeper Pilewort Tablets; *Gerard House Pilewort Compound Tablets; *Frank Roberts Pilewort Compound Tablets – Green Label; *Frank Roberts Pilewort Compound Tablets – Orange Label; *Potter's Piletabs
External: *Culpeper Haemorrhoidal Ointment; *Frank Roberts Anti-irritant Ointment; *Frank Roberts Pilewort Ointment; *Potter's Pilewort Ointment

PILL-BEARING SPURGE

Euphorbia hirta

Synonyms: asthma weed, *E. pilulifera*

Parts used: herb

This particular *Euphorbia* species is primarily used as an anti-asthmatic to relieve bronchial spasms and clear phlegm. Other members of the genus are strongly purgative and potentially toxic, but pill-bearing spurge is free of the toxins which cause this effect and is regarded as quite safe to use.

Remedies and supplements
Blackmores Euphorbia Complex; *Culpeper Cough Relief Mixture; *Potter's Antibron Tablets.

PINE

Pinus sylvestris

Synonyms: Scots pine, pumilio pine

Parts used: leaves, young shoots, oil

Pine oil, distilled from the needles, is included in a number of decongestant and expectorant mixtures for coughs and colds. As well as being antiseptic, the plant is topically rubefacient so is used in a variety of external rubs for muscle stiffness and rheumatism. Pine oil makes a useful addition to steam inhalations for colds and catarrh. It is diuretic and is used in aromatherapy as a nerve tonic.

Remedies and supplements

Bioforce Satasapina Cough Syrup; Bioforce Satasapina Bon Bons; Bioforce Usnean Cough Lozenges; *Lane's Sage and Garlic Catarrh Remedy; Pycnogenol
External: Bee Brand Massage Oil; *Culpeper Healing Ointment; *Gerard House Dragon Balm Ointment

Simples

Oil: Hartwood Aromatics; Neal's Yard Remedies; Tisserand

PINEAPPLE

Ananas sativa

Synonyms: Ananas comosus

Parts used: stem

Few people would immediately classify pineapple as a medicinal herb; most regard it as a refreshing fruit. It is, however, rich in an enzyme called bromelain, which is very similar to the papain found in the papaya fruit. Both papaya and pineapple have traditionally been regarded as digestive stimulants and researchers believe that these protolytic enzymes are the reason.

Both have a local action on the digestive tract but are not significantly absorbed into the system so they do not affect the liver. Both papaya and pineapple are used in over-the-counter remedies, notably in mainland Europe, where they are generally suggested for indigestion and gastritis. Papain has also been used to treat threadworm and roundworm infestations. Both fruits can also be used on ulcers and slowly healing wounds.

As a digestive stimulant, pineapple is sometimes suggested as a slimming aid while the juice has been used topically in France to tonify the skin.

Remedies and supplements

BioCare Buccalzyme; FSC Bromelain Plus; Lamberts Chewable Bromelain with Papain; Solgar Bromelain Tablets
External: *Weleda Larch Resin Lotion
Simple: Capsules: Arkocaps Phytoshape (325 mg)

PLEURISY ROOT

Asclepias tuberosa

Synonyms: butterfly weed

Parts used: root

Pleurisy root originates from the USA where it grows in dry, grassy places in the south and east. The plant was used by Native Americans as a remedy for chest conditions. It was introduced into Europe during the eighteenth century and became a favourite with the physiomedicalists in the nineteenth. As such, its use remains more common in the UK, where North American herbal traditions are strongest, than in mainland Europe. The plant has a nutty, bitter taste and is used as an expectorant, tonic, antispasmodic and diaphoretic. As the name implies, its main use was in treating pleurisy although it also features in a number of bronchitis and general cough remedies as well.

Remedies and supplements

*Culpeper Influenza Mixture; *Culpeper Cough Relief Mixture; Herbcraft Mullein Formula; Neal's Yard Horehound & Aniseed Linctus; *Potter's Antibron Tablets; *Potter's Chest Mixture; *Potter's Horehound and Aniseed Cough Mixture; *Potter's Vegetable Cough Remover

POISON IVY

Rhus toxicodendron

Synonyms: poison oak, *R. radicans*

Parts used: bark

Poison oak or ivy is a North American shrub famed for its ability to cause severe contact dermatitis. The plant is not used in conventional herbal therapy but is a favourite in homoeopathy where it is used in ointments for sprains (ideally where the joint is hot and inflamed) and also to relieve the irritation of chicken pox.

Remedies and supplements

Neal's Yard Rhus Tox and Ruta Ointment; *Nelsons Rhus Tox Cream; *Weleda Rhus Tox Ointment

POKEROOT

Phytolacca americana

Synonyms: pokeweed, red ink plant, *Phytolacca decandra*

Parts used: berries, root

Pokeroot is a traditional Native American healing herb used as an anti-rheumatic, emetic and pain killer by a number of tribes. It was included in the US Pharmacopoeia until 1916 and is still widely used in American folk medicine. It appeared in Europe in the nineteenth century and was once very popular with British herbalists, although there have been concerns over its toxicity and excess will cause vomiting and diarrhoea. As well as its use for rheumatism, the plant is anti-inflammatory, anti-catarrhal, purgative and mildly analgesic.

Recent work has focused on its immune-stimulant action in AIDS therapy. As a stimulant and cleanser for the lymphatic system it can also be useful for glandular fever and tonsillitis.

Externally, pokeroot is included in ointments for joint inflammations, skin problems and piles.

Remedies and supplements
*Frank Roberts Catarrh Tablets; Frank Roberts Golden Seal Compound Tablets
External: Frank Roberts Phytolacca Cream; *Potter's Parasolv Ointment

Simples
Tincture: Neal's Yard Remedies

POLYPODY

Polypodium vulgare

Parts used: rhizomes, flowers

Polypody rhizomes are used as an expectorant and diuretic which also stimulate the liver and gall bladder, and improve digestion. The plant is little used today but was once popular for dry coughs, chest infections, indigestion and arthritic problems. Like other ferns, polypody is also used to expel worms (including tape worms). Anthroposophical medicine uses the flowers, which are gentler, as a digestive remedy.

Remedies and supplements
*Weleda Digestodoran Tablets

POPLAR

Populus spp

Synonyms: abele, white poplar, black poplar

Parts used: bark

The white poplar and its close relatives *P. nigra* (black poplar) and aspen (*P. tremula*) are used medicinally in very similar ways. The bark of these trees is astringent, diuretic, anti-inflammatory and analgesic and can be used as a cleansing remedy for arthritic disorders, rheumatism and general debility. It is added to cystitis preparations and has also been used for liver problems. The main constituents are salicylates (also found in willow) which account for the anti-inflammatory action, and it can also be helpful for reducing fevers. Externally poplar bark can be used for chilblains, piles and sprains although it is rarely used in this way in proprietary preparations.

Remedies and supplements

Bioforce Cystaforce; Bioforce Prostasan; *Frank Roberts Cold Tablets; *Frank Roberts Prickly Ash Compound Tablets; *Gerard House Ligvites; *Potter's Peerless Composition Essence; *Potter's Tabritis

POTATO

Solanum tuberosum

Parts used: tuber

As well as being an important source of minerals and vitamins, the juice of the humble potato can be helpful for relieving excessive stomach acid. It is mildly laxative.

Simple:

Juice: Schoenenberger Plant Juice

PRICKLY ASH

Zanthoxylum americanum

Synonyms: toothache tree, yellow wood

Parts used: bark

Prickly ash is primarily used as a circulatory stimulant and anti-rheumatic. It is a warming, spicy herb that can also help to relieve pain and stimulate the digestion. As its common name implies it is a traditional treatment for toothache helping to encourage saliva flow; prickly ash is also used to reduce fevers, and can be included in internal skin remedies where poor circulation is a contributory factor.

Remedies and supplements

*Frank Roberts Avexan Tablets; *Frank Roberts Prickly Ash Compound Tablets; *Muir's Rheumatic Pain; *Potter's Peerless Composition Essence; *Potter's Tabritis; *Rheumasol

Simples

Capsules/tablets: Gerard House Prickly Ash Tablets
Tincture: Neal's Yard Remedies

PUMPKIN

Cucurbita maxima

Synonyms: winter squash

Parts used: seed, seed oil, juice

In the past, one of the main uses of pumpkin seed was to kill tapeworms, when a dose of the herb was combined with saline purgatives.

Today we're more likely to sprinkle the seeds on salads or chew them as a healthy snack. The seeds are rich in zinc, which is a helpful supplement for both the immune system and prostate gland – hence the herb's inclusion in male-oriented remedies. The seed oil is also a good source of *cis*-linoleic acid and other essential fatty acids.

Pumpkin flesh and juice is mildly laxative and diuretic and can be used as a gentle digestive stimulant.

Remedies and supplements
    Super Garlic Perles for Men

Simples
    Capsules: Power Health Pumpkin Seed Oil (250 mg)
    Juice: Schoenenberger Plant Juice

PURPLE LOOSESTRIFE

Lythrum salicaria

Parts used: flowering plant

Purple loosestrife is used in parts of France, Germany and Switzerland to treat diarrhoea and digestive upsets. It is mildly anti-bacterial and astringent and may also be helpful for heavy periods, haemorrhage and vaginal discharges. Externally it can be used for sores, skin infections and eczema.

Remedies and supplements
    Bioforce Tormentavena

PYRETHRUM

Tanacetum cinerariifolium

Synonyms: Dalmatian pellitory

Parts used: flowers

The dried flowers of pyrethrum are useful as an insecticide and can be made into household and greenhouse sprays. The plant is quite safe to use and is sometimes included in insect repellents and remedies for insect bites.

Remedies and supplements
    External: *Nelsons Pyrethrum Spray

QUASSIA

Picrasma excelsa

Synonyms: bitter ash

Parts used: wood chips

A bitter appetite stimulant that is also insecticide and a digestive tonic. The herb is mainly used for indigestion and for liver disorders, although a wash can also be used externally for parasitic infestations including scabies and lice while an enema is given for threadworms.

Remedies and supplements
    *Lanes Herbelix Specific

QUEEN'S DELIGHT

Stillingia sylvatica

Synonyms: yaw root

Parts used: root

Originating in North America, queen's delight is considered to be a "blood puri-fier" useful for skin complaints and digestive problems; it is also laxative and diuretic. The herb contains potentially irritant compounds which, however, tend to be unstable and break down on drying and when processed in extracts.

Remedies and supplements
    Blackmores Sarsparilla Complex

RAMSONS

Allium ursinum

Synonyms: bear's garlic, wild garlic

Parts used: herb, juice

Ramsons grow wild throughout Europe adding a wonderful garlicky scent to spring woodlands. The plant has been used in folk medicine since Greek times – much as cultivated garlic has been – as a remedy for infections, chest complaints and digestive disorders. It is traditionally regarded as a blood purifier and spring tonic. Like garlic, ramsons also help to reduce blood cholesterol levels and have been used to treat high blood pressure associated with arteriosclerosis as well as yeast-related infections where it can help to normalise the gut flora.

Ramsons are rather milder in flavour than ordinary garlic and may be better tolerated by those with sensitive stomachs.

Remedies and supplements
Bioforce Arterioforce

Simples
Juice: Schoenenberger Plant Juice
Tincture: Bioforce

RASPBERRY

Rubus idaeus

Parts used: leaves, fruit

Raspberry leaf is best known for its tonifying effect on the uterus and its use as a preparative for childbirth. It is generally taken for eight weeks before the confinement and the tea may also be sipped during labour to help strengthen the womb for the exertions in store. As a uterine relaxant and tonic, raspberry leaf has been recommended for period pain, although a number of other herbs can be more effective at easing spasmodic cramps. The herb is also astringent so is used in gargles for sore throats and may be taken for diarrhoea.

Remedies and supplements
*Gerard House Helonias Compound; Gerard House Vig-a-Tea; Herbcraft Echinacea, Eyebright and Bilberry Formula; Kordel's Women's Multi

Simples
Capsules/tablets: Blackmores Raspberry Leaf; Frank Roberts Raspberry Leaf Tablets (500 mg); Gerard House Raspberry Leaf; Heath & Heather Raspberry Leaf; Herbs of Grace Red Raspberry; Neal's Yard Raspberry Leaf Capsules; *Potter's Raspberry Leaf
Tincture: Neal's Yard Remedies

RED BEET

Beta conditiva alef

Parts used: root, juice

Beetroot juice has been used since medieval times as an easily digested and nutritious food in illness. It helps to regulate the digestive system and is believed to stimulate the lymphatics to improve resistance to infection and generally help the immune system. In recent years beetroot juice has been included in a number of dietary regimes for cancer treatment with significant results.

In general therapy, red beet is used much as it was in the middle ages – as a nourishing food for sensitive stomachs and a kidney stimulant.

Simples
> *Capsules:* BioCare Beetroot Extract
> *Juice:* Schoenenberger Plant Juice

RED CLOVER

Trifolium pratense

Parts used: flowers

Red clover is mainly used by herbalists as a cleansing remedy for skin problems such as psoriasis and eczema. It is a useful expectorant and diuretic, helpful for both dry coughs and gout. The herb was used in the 1930s in cancer therapy and still finds a role in the treatment of breast and skin cancers.

Remedies and supplements
> Absorb Plus; Blackmores Echinacea Complex; Colon Cleanse; Honeyrose Herbal Cigarettes; Natural Flow Colonite

Simples
> *Capsules:* Herbs of Grace Red Clover
> *Tincture:* Neal's Yard Remedies

REISHI

Ganoderma lucidem

Synonyms: *Ling Zhi,* lacquered bracket fungus

Parts used: fruiting body

The reishi mushroom was highly regarded by the ancient Taoists as a spiritual tonic and one which could enhance longevity. The herb is now known to stimulate the immune system and is also sedative and expectorant. It will lower blood sugar and cholesterol levels and generally has a tonic effect on the system.

Remedies and supplements
> Herbcraft Reishi Shiitake; Mycoherb Myco Forte; Mycoherb Rei Shi Gen; Mycoherb Tri Myco Gen

Simples
> *Tincture:* Mycoherb Rei-Gen (East-West Herbs)

RESTHARROW

Ononis spinosa

Synonyms: cammock, spiny rest harrow

Parts used: root

Although restharrow has a long tradition of use as a diuretic, it has not always seemed particularly effective. It would appear that the plant is very sensitive to growing conditions – if it produces saponins then it will have diuretic properties; if the soil is not ideal to create these chemicals, then the plant can prove quite ineffective.

Restharrow is rather more popular in mainland Europe than in the UK and there, unusually, the root is used as an infusion rather than a decoction as its active constituents are easily destroyed in steam. Saponin-rich restharrow can increase urinary output by 20%, although the effect is reduced in time so short treatments with the herb are preferable.

Remedies and supplements
    Bioforce Nephrosolid

RHATANY

Krameria triandra

Parts used: roots

An astringent, largely used for diarrhoea and haemorrhage, rhatany is included in ointments for piles and chilblains as well as given internally for excessive menstrual bleeding. It can be used as a gargle for sore throats, gum disease and pharyngitis.

Remedies and supplements
    *Weleda Medicinal Gargle

RHUBARB

Rheum palmatum

Synonyms: Chinese rhubarb, Turkey rhubarb, Indian rhubarb, *Da Huang*

Parts used: rhizome

Rhubarb originally came from China and was imported into Europe along the spice trade route through India and Turkey – hence its various geographic names. The medicinal plant is quite different from the familiar edible variety, which was developed through hybridization in the nineteenth century. Rhubarb root is a strong laxative, astringent and digestive tonic. It is mainly used for chronic constipation and in liver and gall bladder remedies. The Chinese also believe it will cool the blood and prescribe it for various menstrual problems, nose bleeds and skin eruptions. As with other herbal laxatives it contains anthraquinones and works by irritating the gut lining.
• Rhubarb root should not be taken in pregnancy or lactation.

Remedies and supplements

BioCare Phytosterol Complex; Colon Cleanse; *Dorwest Digestive Tablets; Frank Roberts Acidosis Tablets; *Frank Roberts B & L Tablets; *HRI Golden Seal Digestive; *Lanes Herbelix Specific; Ortis Fruit & Fibres; *Potter's Acidosis; *Potter's Indian Brandee; *Potter's Stomach Mixture; Professional Herbs Cascara and Rhubarb
External: Dr Shir's Liniment; Golden Yellow Ointment

Simples

Tincture: Neal's Yard Remedies

RIBWORT PLANTAIN

Plantago lanceolata

Parts used: leaves

Ribwort plantain has long pointed leaves and will grow to around 30–40 cm/12–16 in in height – quite unlike its familiar relative common plantain which nestles comfortably in lawns and paving cracks. It is astringent, anti-inflammatory and a potent anti-catarrhal largely used for colds, hay fever and allergic rhinitis. The plant also obtains minerals and trace elements from the soil: it is particularly rich in zinc, potassium and silica and also contains aucubin – an antibiotic glycoside – all of which helps to make the plant very healing and supportive for the immune system.

Remedies and supplements

Bioforce Usneasan Cough Lozenges; *Ricola Swiss Herb Lozenges

Simples

Juice: Schoenenberger Plant Juice
Tincture: Bioforce, Neal's Yard Remedies

ROSE

Rosa spp

Parts used: petals, hips, oil

The rose is probably one of the West's most neglected medicinal herbs – although certainly until the 1930s rose tincture was the pharmacist's standby for sore throats and diarrhoea. Rosehips are still used in a number of preparations as an important source of vitamin C and rose oil can generally be obtained (at a price) for use in skin problems, as a nerve tonic, anti-depressant and aphrodisiac. Several varieties of rose are used in Chinese medicine as tonics, liver restoratives, and menstrual remedies but sadly rose petals – useful though they can be – are rarely included in over-the-counter products as anything more than a flavouring.

Remedies and supplements

Rose: Honeyrose Herbal Cigarettes

Rosehips: American Nutrition Acerola Plus and Super Acerola Plus; Blackmores Rosehips; Gerard House Eez-a-Tea

Simples

Capsules: Frank Roberts Rosehip Tablets
Oil: Hartwood Aromatics; Neal's Yard Remedies; Tisserand

ROSE GERANIUM

Pelargonium graveolens

Synonyms: geranium Bourbon

Parts used: essential oil

Rose geranium oil was originally produced at Grasse in France, but as labour costs increased, production migrated first to Algeria and later to the island of Réunion in the Indian Ocean. The island was once known as île Bourbon and the oil thus became Bourbon oil or geranium Bourbon. Enthusiasts for the oil claim that the Réunion oil is still the best, although it is now also sourced in China and Egypt. The Bourbon oil is particularly rich in citronellol and has a powerful fragrance.

The oil is used in aromatherapy for premenstrual and kidney problems and can also be used for acne, eczema and fungal infections. The high citronellol content also makes it a useful component of insect repellents.

Remedies and supplements

External: *Potter's Medicated Extract of Rosemary

Simples

Oil: Hartwood Aromatics; Neal's Yard Remedies; Nelson & Russell; Tissersand

ROSEMARY

Rosmarinus officinalis

Parts used: leaves, oil

Rosemary is a valuable tonic herb, stimulating thanks to the presence of a substance called borneol, and very warming. It is useful for temporary fatigue and over-work and makes a pleasant tea. The herb is also astringent, antiseptic, carminative, diuretic, anti-spasmodic and will stimulate the circulation. It can be used to relieve headaches, migraines, indigestion and the cold feelings that come with poor circulation. The oil is also a valuable remedy for arthritis, rheumatism, muscular aches and pains.

Rosemary is widely used in hair treatments: it is reputed to darken greying hair, makes a good rinse for auburn, and will also help to clear dandruff. Like thyme and marjoram, rosemary has also recently been investigated as an anti-oxidant which can prevent premature ageing of cells.

Remedies and supplements

BioCare Oxydent; *Frank Roberts Supa-Tonic Tablets; Gerard House Vig-a-Tea; Neal's Yard Anti-Oxidant Herbs Elixir; Pure-fil Romagen Herbal Antioxidant
External: Neal's Yard Ginger and Juniper Warming Oil; Neal's Yard Sports Salve; *Potter's Adiantine; *Potter's Medicated Extract of Rosemary; *Rickard's Woodsap Ointment; *Weleda Frost Cream; *Weleda Rhus Tox Ointment

Simples

Juice: Schoenenberger Plant Juice
Oil: Botanica; Hartwood Aromatics; Neal's Yard Remedies; Nelson & Russell; Tissersand
Tincture: Neal's Yard Remedies

ROSEWOOD

Aniba roseaodora

Synonyms: pau rosa, cara-cara

Parts used: essential oil

Used as a stimulating oil in aromatherapy, rosewood is anti-depressant and uplifting. It can also help to strengthen the immune system and has analgesic properties. Aromatherapists sometimes use it for headaches and to aid concentration.

Simples

Oil: Botanica; Nelson & Russell; Tisserand

RUE

Ruta graveolens

Synonyms: herb of grace

Parts used: leaves

An extremely bitter herb, rue was once thought to give protection from the plague and was an ingredient in the "four thieves vinegar" which was taken as a prophylactic by those who stole from the bodies of plague victims. The herb was long associated with eye complaints and was a favourite with the itinerant eye-doctors of the Middle Ages. It is a warming, diaphoretic, uterine stimulant, that also acts on the digestion and – thanks to the high rutin content – will strengthen the blood vessels.

In homoeopathy, rue is a specific for injuries to the shinbone and also for strains and bruising. It is often recommended as a follow-up treatment to arnica in easing traumatic injuries and severe bruising.

Remedies and supplements
> Neal's Yard Rhus Tox and Ruta Ointment; *Nelsons Strains Ointment; *Weleda Ruta Ointment

SAFFLOWER

Carthamus tinctorius

Synonyms: saffron thistle, false saffron, dyer's saffron

Parts used: flowers, seed oil

Safflower has traditionally been used as a diuretic and laxative. It is a bitter aromatic herb once used to reduce fevers and treat cuts and grazes. Extracts from the flowers are also believed to act as a heart stimulant and are used in China to treat menstrual irregularities and blood clotting disorders. The oil contains essential fatty acids – mainly *cis*-linoleic and oleic acids – and makes a useful dietary supplement.

Remedies and supplements
> Efamol Evening Primrose Oil with Linseed and Safflower; FSC Siberian Ginseng
> *External:* Amber Massage Salve; Dr Shir's Linament; Spring Wind Ointment

Simples
> *Capsules:* Power Health Safflower Oil Capsules (250 mg); Solgar Safflower Oil

SAGE

Salvia officinalis

Parts used: leaves, oil

Regular drinking of sage tea was once regarded as a guarantee of longevity, and country rhymes reminded all that "he who drinks sage in May, shall live for aye". We now know that the plant's reputation may have something to do with its high oestrogen content so it could almost be regarded as an early, and very gentle, form of hormone replacement therapy. As well as this hormonal aspect the plant also dries up body fluids so the two activities combined make it an ideal choice both for relieving night sweats at the menopause and for drying up milk in lactating mothers when it is time for weaning.

Sage also has an affinity with the throat and makes an excellent gargle and mouth wash for minor infections and inflammations. It is astringent. antiseptic, anti-inflammatory, antispasmodic, anti-depressant and a digestive stimulant.

The purple variety (*S. officinalis purpura*) is often preferred by herbalists although all members of the group display similar properties. Sage ointment is popular in parts of Europe as a household standby for minor cuts and insect bites.

Remedies and supplements
> *Bio-Strath Chamomile Formula; *Cantassium Hay Fever; *Lane's Sage and Garlic Catarrh Remedy; Neal's Yard Anti-Oxidant Herbs Elixir; Neal's Yard Lemon &

Honey Lozenges; Pure-fil Romagen Herbal Antioxidant; *Ricola Swiss Herb Lozenges; *Weleda Fragador Tablets
External: Bioforce Seven Herb Cream; Neal's Yard Ginger and Juniper Warming Oil; *Weleda Medicinal Gargle

Simples
Capsules: Arkocaps Phytomenopause (220 mg)
Juice: Schoenenberger Plant Juice
Oil: Hartwood Aromatics; Neal's Yard Remedies
Tincture: Bioforce Menosan; Neal's Yard Remedies

SANDALWOOD

Santalum album

Parts used: essential oil

Sandalwood is important in Ayurvedic medicine as a cooling, anti-spasmodic herb that stimulates the mind and improves digestive energy. In aromatherapy the oil is regarded as generally relaxing, anti-depressant, carminative, diuretic and antispasmodic. It is used for urinary problems, nervous disorders and chest complaints and can be added to bathwater to encourage restful sleep.

Simples
Oil: Botanica; Hartwood Aromatics; Neal's Yard Remedies; Nelson & Russell; Tisserand

SANICLE

Sanicula europaea

Parts used: herb

Although rarely used in herbal medicine today, sanicle was once listed in several European pharmacopoeia as a wound herb and gargle for sore throats. It contains tannins and saponins and is an effective astringent. It is still used in European folk medicine for haemorrhages.

Remedies and supplements
External: Bioforce Seven Herb Cream

SARSPARILLA

Smilax aristolochiaefolia

Synonyms: Mexican sarsparilla

Parts used: roots, rhizome

A number of *Smilax* spp. originating in Central and South America are used medicinally and they include *S. regelii* (Honduran sarsparilla) and *S. febrifuga* (Ecuadorian sarparilla), as well as the Mexican variety. The plant is largely used as a cleansing remedy, anti-inflammatory and antiseptic that can be helpful for irritant and chronic skin problems including psoriasis. The Chinese use similar *Smilax* spp. for treating venereal disease, dysentery and rheumatism, although Western use is largely confined to skin preparations.

Remedies and supplements

Absorb Plus; BioCare PT208; Blackmores Echinacea Complex; Blackmores Sarsparilla Complex; *Gerard House Blue Flag Root; *Gerard House Ligvites; Gerard House Seaweed and Sarsparilla Tablets; Herbcraft Burdock & Nettle Formula; *HRI Clear Complexion Tablets; *Potter's Skin Eruptions Mixture

Simples

Tincture: Neal's Yard Remedies
Capsules: Full Potency Herbs Sarsparilla Root Vegicaps (520 mg); *Potter's Jamaican Sarsparilla

SASSAFRAS

Sassafras albidum

Parts used: root bark, root

The volatile oil obtained from sassafras contains safrole, which is now believed to be carcinogenic so use of the plant is restricted in some areas. It was once a popular carminative, diaphoretic, diuretic and anti-rheumatic used for digestive upsets, rheumatism and skin complaints. The plant was introduced into Europe in the sixteenth century by the Spanish who used it as a remedy for venereal disease (similarly introduced at about the same time). Only small quantities of the herb should be used, not only because of the toxicity of safrole but because excess can cause vomiting and liver damage.

Remedies and supplements

Blackmores Sarsparilla Complex

SAW PALMETTO

Serenoa repens

Synonyms: *Sabul serrulata*

Parts used: fruits

Saw palmetto berries originate in the south-eastern states of the USA and were a popular food among Native Americans and early settlers. They were highly valued for their tonic effect, as a strengthening remedy in debility and convalescence and the herb was traditionally used for cystitis and prostate problems.

In recent years researchers have demonstrated that saw palmetto prevents the conversion of the male hormone testosterone into dihydrotestosterone which is believed to be the substance responsible for benign prostate enlargement. The herb further encourages breakdown of any DHT that may have formed, thus preventing and helping to cure the problem, rather than simply relieving it superficially. Saw palmetto is included in a number of general tonic preparations, usually targeted at older men, as well as in specifics for urinary and prostate disorders.

Remedies and supplements

Bioforce Prostasan; *Dorwest Damiana and Kola Tablets; *Frank Roberts Strength Tablets; *Frank Roberts Supa-Tonic Tablets; La Gelee Royale; Nature's Plus Prost-Actin; *Potter's Antiglan Tablets; *Potter's Elixir of Damiana and Saw Palmetto; *Potter's Strength Tablets; Prostex; Serenoa-C

Simples

Capsules: Full Potency Herbs Saw Palmetto Berries Vegicaps (520 mg); *Sabalin (95 mg)
Tincture: Herbcraft; Neal's Yard Remedies

SCHISANDRA

Schisandra chinensis

Synonyms: *We Wei Zi*

Parts used: berries

The Chinese call schisandra berries " *Wu Wei Zi*" or five taste fruit suggesting an all-round medicine that can influence many parts of the body. The berries are highly regarded in the East as an aphrodisiac and tonic, and have a tradition of enhancing female beauty. They are also useful for certain types of allergic skin problems and are particularly good as a kidney tonic.

Simples

Capsules: Arkocaps Phytosuperior (300 mg)
Tincture: Neal's Yard Remedies

SEAWEED

See Kelp

SENEGA

Polygala senega

Synonyms: rattlesnake root

Parts used: root

Senega is rich in saponins making it a potent expectorant and emetic. It is primarily used for bronchitis, catarrh and asthma. Traditionally it was used by Native American for treating snake bites – hence the common name.

Remedies and supplements

Blackmores Euphorbia Complex; Blackmores Liquorice Complex; *Potter's Antibron Tablets; *Potter's Chest Mixture

SENNA

Senna alexandrina

Synonyms: *Cassia angustifolia*, Alexandrian senna, Tinnevally senna

Parts used: leaves, pods

Senna pods and leaves have been used as laxatives for at least 2,000 years and probably longer. The plant contains anthraquinone glycosides which irritate the gut lining and thus stimulate peristalsis. It is generally combined with carminatives, such as fennel or aniseed, to prevent excessive griping, but is used in a considerable number of over-the-counter remedies for constipation and piles.

Excessive use of senna can lead to nausea, vomiting and deterioration in bowel function with the risk of diverticulitis. It should not be taken in pregnancy or by those suffering from colitis or irritable bowel syndrome.

Remedies and supplements

Bioforce Linoforce; Blackmores Cape Aloes and Cascara; *Dorwest Natural Herb Tablets; Frank Roberts Constipation Tablets; *Frank Roberts Pilewort Compound Tablets – Green Label; *Frank Roberts Pilewort Compound Tablets – Orange Label; Frank Roberts Uva-Ursi Compound Tablets; *Gerard House Pilewort Compound; Health Aid Liver Guard Forte; *Lanes Athera; *Lanes Dual-Lax Extra Strong; *Lusty's Herbalene; Neal's Yard Cascara Compound; Ortisan Liquid; Ortilax; Ortisan; *Potter's Cleansing Herb; *Potter's Kas-Bah Herb; *Potter's Out of Sorts Tablets; *Potter's Senna Tablets; *Weleda Clairo Tea; *Weleda Laxadoron Tablets

Simples

Capsules: Arkocaps Phytosenalax (300 mg)
Tincture: Neal's Yard Remedies

SESAME

Sesamum indicum

Synonyms: benne, gingili

Parts used: seeds, seed oil

The pungent, nutty flavour of sesame oil is well known from Chinese, Middle Eastern and Indian cookery. Extracts, known as tahini, are an important flavouring in many traditions, while the seeds themselves are a good source of calcium. Sesame is regarded as an important tonic herb in Ayurvedic tradition and both the seeds and oil are widely used for chronic coughs, constipation and period problems, or externally for burns and ulcers. The oil is also a good source of linolenic and linoleic acids.

Remedies and supplements
External: Amber Massage Salve

SHEPHERD'S PURSE

Capsella bursa-pastoris

Synonyms: mother's hearts

Parts used: herb

Shepherd's purse is a common and persistent garden weed. It takes its name from the heart shaped seed-pods and is used in both Western and Chinese herbal traditions to stop haemorrhage.

Shepherd's purse is astringent and a urinary antiseptic so is ideal for severe cystitis which may involve blood in the urine and chronic colitis; it is also used for treating heavy periods for which there is no clear pathological cause. It has a role in over-the-counter remedies for cystitis.

Remedies and supplements
Frank Roberts Uva-Ursi Compound Tablets; *Muir's Sciatica; *Potter's Antitis Tablets; *Potter's Sciargo; *Potter's Sciargo Herb

Simples
Tincture: Bioforce, Neal's Yard Remedies

SHIITAKE

Lentinus edodes

Synonyms: *Xiang Gu*, snake butter

Parts used: fruiting body

Shiitake mushrooms are now a familiar item on Western supermarket produce shelves, but the plant has been valued as a medicine in Japan and China for more than 2,000 years. It is immune-enhancing, anti-viral and will also act as a tonic and restorative for the liver. It has been used in AIDS therapy, candidiasis, colds, influenza and as a supportive remedy in cancer. The plant will also reduce high cholesterol levels and can be helpful in urine incontinence in the elderly.

Remedies and supplements
Herbcraft Reishi Shiitake; Mycoherb Myco Forte; Mycoherb Rei Shi Gen; Mycoherb Tri Myco Gen

Simples
Tinctures: Mycoherb Shi-Gen (East-West Herbs)

SIBERIAN GINSENG

Eleutherococcus senticosus

Parts used: root

Although various varieties of *Eleutherococcus* have been used in traditional Chinese medicine for some 2,000 years, it is a comparative newcomer to the West, its
properties "rediscovered" in the 1950s and the herb then extensively used by
Soviet athletes to increase stamina and enhance performance. The herb stimulates the immune and circulatory systems and also helps to regulate blood pressure and lower blood sugar levels. Its main application is, however, as a tonic,
helping the body to cope with increased stress levels and to provide extra energy.

It is useful to take Siberian ginseng before a particularly stressful period –
such as in the weeks before exams or an arduous business trip – rather than in the
heat of a crisis. It is usually regarded as gentler in action than Korean ginseng and
may be a preferred choice for women.

Remedies and supplements
BioCare AD206; BioCare Oxy-B15; FSC Siberian Ginseng; HealthAid Ginseng;
Health Aid Herbal Booster; Health Aid Liquid Herbal Booster; Healthcrafts GEB6
Combination; Healthcrafts Korean and Siberian Ginseng; Imuno-Strength; Lady-
Care: For Women going through the Menopause; Natural Flow Triple Ginseng;
Reevecrest Libidex 5; Super Gre-Caps

Simples
Capsules: Arkocaps Phytoforce (250 mg); Full Potency Herbs Ginseng (Siberian)
Vegicaps (250 mg); Full Potency Herbs Siberian Ginseng Vegicaps (520 mg);
Health Aid Siberian Ginseng (250 mg); Health Aid Sibergin Siberian Ginseng
(2500mg); Healthcrafts Siberian Ginseng (600 mg); Herbs of Grace Siberian
Ginseng; Power Health Siberian Ginseng
Tinctures: Bioforce

SILVER BIRCH

Betula pendula

Synonyms: *B. alba*, *B. verrucosa*, white birch

Parts used: leaves, bark, oil, sap

Birch is a bitter and astringent herb that is also diuretic and mildly laxative. An oil distilled from the bark is known as birch tar oil and has been used to treat psoriasis and eczema. Internally the plant is generally used as a cleansing remedy for rheumatism, arthritis and for urinary tract disorders including cystitis and kidney stones.

Remedies and supplements

Bioforce Golden Grass Tea; Bioforce Imperthritica; Bioforce Nephrosolid; Gerard House Sleek-a-Tea; Reevecrest Gum Thyme; Weleda Birch Elixir

Simples

Juice: Schoenenberger Plant Juice
Tincture: Neal's Yard Remedies

SILVERWEED

Potentilla anserina

Synonyms: cramp weed

Parts used: herb

Silverweed is a decorative, low growing plant commonly cultivated as a garden flower. Like its relative tormentil, it is highly astringent, but is generally regarded as an anti-catarrhal rather than a remedy for diarrhoea. The juice is rich in minerals and also contains an anti-spasmodic constituent which accounts for its traditional role in treating cramps and spasmodic pain. Silverweed can be used internally for colic (and, of course, diarrhoea) or externally on sores and weeping eczema.

Remedies and supplements

Bioforce Imperthritica; Bioforce Nephrosolid; Herbcraft Fresh Breath Cinnamint Spray

Simples

Juice: Schoenenberger Plant Juice
Tincture: Bioforce.

SKULLCAP

Scutellaria lateriflora

Synonyms: mad dog herb

Parts used: herb

The variety of skullcap most widely used in medicine today originates from Virginia and was introduced into Europe in the eighteenth century as a treatment for rabies – hence the alternative name. It was used by the Cherokee for menstrual problems but is widely regarded now as an extremely effective sedative and nervine. It is cooling, anti-bacterial, styptic, reduces fevers, lowers blood pressure and cholesterol levels, calms the foetus in pregnant women and acts as a stimulant for the digestion.

Although skullcap can thus be used internally for diarrhoea, jaundice, urinary tract infections, haemorrhage and threatened miscarriage it tends to be confined to over-the-counter products for anxiety, tension and insomnia. The European variety of skullcap (*S. galericulata*) has similar properties.

Remedies and supplements

Blackmores Skullcap & Valerian; Blackmores Valerian Complex; *Cantassium Quiet Days; *Cantassium Quiet Tyme; *Culpeper Head Cold and Throat Mixture; *Dorwest Scullcap and Gentian Tablets; *Gerard House Biophylin; *HRI Calm Life Tablets; Kordel's Quiet Time; *Muir's Pick-Me-Up; Neal's Yard Scullcap Compound Capsules; *Potter's Newrelax; *Potter's Nodoff Mixture; *Potter's Vegetable Cough Remover; *Potter's Wellwoman Herbs; *Potter's Wellwoman Tablets; Professional Herbs Valerian

Simples

Capsules: Full Potency Herbs Scutellariae Vegicaps; Herbs of Grace Scullcap
Tincture: Neal's Yard Remedies

SKUNK CABBAGE

Symplocarpus foetidus

Synonyms: skunkweed, polecat weed

Parts used: rhizome and root

Like other traditional North American healing herbs, there has been little research into the pharmacology of skunk cabbage and its actions are not well understood. The Winnebago and Dakota Indians used it as an expectorant in asthma, while the MicMac treated headaches by tying the herb in bundles and smelling it – hardly a pleasant experience: the settlers gave the plant the name polecat weed because of it particularly foul smell.

The roots are known to contain 5-hydroxytryptamine (serotonin) which acts as a neurotransmitter in the human body.

It is used by Western herbalists primarily as an expectorant, sedative and antispasmodic given for bronchitis, asthma, whooping cough and catarrh.

Remedies and supplements

*Culpeper Head Cold and Throat Mixture; Neal's Yard Horehound and Aniseed Linctus; *Potter's Horehound and Aniseed Cough Mixture

SLIPPERY ELM

Ulmus rubra

Synonyms: *U. fulva*, red elm

Parts used: inner bark

Slippery elm is a highly mucilaginous herb mainly used to coat the stomach and provide protection in cases of gastritis, heartburn and ulceration. It is also a valuable nutrient which can be made into a gruel and flavoured with honey and spices for convalescents or the seriously debilitated. Externally it makes an effective drawing ointment for splinters and boils and can also soothe wounds and burns.

Remedies & supplements
BioCare Buccalzyme; BioCare Gastroplex; Blackmores Liquorice Complex; *Frank Roberts Althaea Compound Tablets; *Frank Roberts Cranesbill Compound Tablets; *Gerard House Fenulin; *Gerard House Papaya Plus Tablets; *Lanes Biobalm; *Lanes Pileabs; *Natraleze; Natural Flow Regular Ten Powder; Neal's Yard Slippery Elm Tablets; *Potter's Slippery Elm Stomach Tablets
External: *Rickard's Woodsap Ointment

Simples
Capsules/tablets: Blackmores Slippery Elm; *Gerard House Slippery Elm Tablets; Herbs of Grace Slippery Elm

SNAKEGOURD

Trichosanthes kirilowii

Synonyms: *Tian Hua Fen*

Parts used: root

An anti-bacterial root that is used in traditional Chinese medicine externally as an anti-inflammatory and for clearing boils and abscesses. Internally it is given for coughs and is also hypoglycaemic. The peel and seeds of the gourd are also used medicinally, largely as expectorants.

Remedies and supplements
External: Golden Yellow Ointment

SNOW FUNGUS

Tremella fuciformis

Synonyms: *Bai Mu Er*

Parts used: fruiting body

The snow fungus is common on deciduous trees in China and the southern states of the USA. Traditionally it was used as an energy tonic in China to strengthen the circulation and heart and invigorate the brain. Recent scientific studies have demonstrated that the plant also reduces cholesterol levels, countering arteriosclerosis, and confirmed its supportive action on the heart. It can also help strengthen the immune system and has an antioxidant effect on cells.

Remedies and supplements
  Mycoherb Myco Forte

Simples
  Tincture: Mycoherb Baimu-Gen (East-West Herbs)

SOUTHERNWOOD

Artemisia abrotanum

Synonyms: old man, lad's love

Parts used: leaves

Several members of the *Artemisia* genus have well-established medicinal properties, but they only rarely feature in over-the-counter herbal remedies and supplements. All the family are strongly aromatic bitters which stimulate the digestion; most are also anthelmintic destroying a range of intestinal worms. Southernwood is generally believed to stimulate hair growth, although there is no real evidence that this is more than a folkloric tradition. Its country name "lad's love" is said to derive either from attempts to use it to stimulate beard growth or from its other folk use as an abortifacient.
• No *Artemisia* spp should be given to pregnant women.

Remedies and supplements
  St Hildegard-Posch Ebberautem Elixir
  External: *Potter's Adiantine; St Hildegard-Posch Eberrautem Cream; *Weleda Frost Cream

SPATHOLOBUS

Spatholobus suberectus

Synonyms: *Ji Zue Teng*

Parts used: stems

In Chinese traditional medicine the stems of this relative of the bean family are considered as a warming remedy for liver and spleen to encourage circulation and act as a general cleansing remedy. The herb is included in various menstrual and menopausal preparations as well as being used in arthritic problems and lumbago.

Remedies and supplements
    Equillence

SPEARMINT

Mentha spicata

Synonyms: garden mint

Parts used: leaves, oil

The familiar garden mint which so often accompanies roast lamb is usually a variety of spearmint. It acts as a carminative and antispasmodic, but is much gentler than peppermint and is mainly used for minor problems such as wind, indigestion and also in children's fevers and stomach upsets.

Remedies and supplements
    *Frank Roberts Nervous Dyspepsia Tablets

SPEEDWELL

Veronica officinalis

Synonyms: heath speedwell, fluellen

Parts used: herb

Although little used medicinally today, speedwell makes a pleasant-tasting addition to herbal tea mixtures. In the past it was used for stomach upsets, chesty coughs and rheumatic problems and is regarded as weakly diuretic and expectorant.

Remedies and supplements
    *Ricola Swiss Herb Lozenges

SQUILL

Drimia maritima

Synonyms: Indian squill, sea onion

Parts used: bulb

Squill vinegar and syrup of squills have long been listed in the British Pharmacopoeia and have been widely used in cough mixtures for generations. Indeed, Dioscorides gives a recipe for making squill vinegar dating from around AD 60 that is much the same as the method used today. Like many expectorants, squill acts by irritating the digestive tract (which by reflex action then irritates the lungs) so it tends to cause nausea and vomiting in excess. The herb is also diuretic and a heart tonic, and as such was once used for dropsy. Squill has also been used in the past as a hair tonic and dandruff remedy.

Remedies and supplements

*Culpeper Balm of Gilead Cough Mixture; *Gerard House Lobelia Compound; *Heath & Heather Balm of Gilead Cough Mixture; *Heath & Heather Balm of Gilead Cough Pastilles; *Heath & Heather Catarrh; *Lane's Cut-a-Cough; *Lanes Honey and Molasses Cough Mixture; Neal's Yard Balm of Gilead; *Potter's Balm of Gilead; *Potter's Chest Mixture

ST JOHN'S WORT

Hypericum perforatum

Parts used: herb

St John's wort is usually held as an excellent example of the Doctrine of Signatures: a mediaeval theory that by their appearance plants would suggest their beneficial properties. It yields a red oil when infused and the leaves appear to have tiny holes in them (in fact these are translucent oil sacs) so St John's wort was deemed a wound herb good for inflammations and burns. It is still used in that way and is locally antiseptic and anti-inflammatory.

Taken internally, the herb is a good sedative and anti-inflammatory. It can be useful for depression, nervous tension and for emotional upsets associated with the menopause. Its anti-depressant action is said to be due to its ability to inhibit the enzyme monoamine oxidase (MAO) which itself inhibits neurotransmitters involved in stimulating the brain. MAO inhibitors are widely used in orthodox medicine and some researchers suggest that St John's wort has similar action but without the usual side-effects of orthodox drugs. The herb is also used for premenstrual syndrome and can ease some period pains.

Recent interest has focused on chemicals known as hypericins, found in St John's wort, which have an affect on the immune system and have been trialled in AIDS therapy.

• Prolonged use can increase the photosensitivity of the skin.

Remedies and supplements

Bioforce Cystaforce; Bioforce Hyperiforce; Bioforce Hyperisan; Herbcraft Echinacea Formula; Kordel's Women's Multi

External: Bioforce Po Ho Ointment; Bioforce Seven Herb Cream; Neal's Yard Hypericum and Urtica Ointment; Neal's Yard Hypercal Ointment; *Nelsons Burns Ointment; *Nelsons Hypercal Cream; *Nelsons Hypercal Tincture; *Nelsons Pyrethrum Spray; *Weleda Hypericum/Calendula Ointment

Simples

Capsules/tablets: Blackmores Hypericum (500 mg); Gerard House St John's Wort; Kira; Power Health Pure St John's Wort (200 mg)

Juice: Schoenenberger Plant Juice

Infused oil: Bioforce, Neal's Yard Remedies

Tincture: Bioforce; Herbcraft; Neal's Yard Remedies

STINGING NETTLES

Urtica dioica

Parts used: herb

Nettles sting thanks to the hairs on their stems and leaves which contain histamine and thus act as a potent irritant. The plant is an astringent diuretic that will also stop bleeding. It is a useful tonic thanks to its ability to "rob the soil" of relevant nutrient and thus concentrate minerals and vitamins in its leaves. Nettle makes an ideal "spring tonic" to cleanse the system, using either the juice or a soup made from the young shoots, to clear out the stagnations of winter. Nettle is used externally in creams for irritant skin rashes and rheumatic pain, and it can also be taken internally for similar complaints as well as heavy periods, gout and anaemia.

The Romans reputedly planted the related Roman nettle (*U. pilulifera*) along British roadsides as they believed the climate would be so cold they would need to beat themselves with nettles to irritate and encourage blood flow to the skin to keep warm. The treatment remained a folk therapy for rheumatism until comparatively recently.

Remedies and supplements

Bioforce Alfavena; Bioforce Tormentavena; Bioforce Urticalan; Blackmores Celery Complex; Blackmores Sarsparilla Complex; *Frank Roberts Kelp and Nettle Compound; Herbcraft Burdock & Nettle Formula; *Lanes Kleer; *Weleda Fragador Tablets

External: Neal's Yard Hypericum and Urtica Ointment; St Hildegard-Posch Stinging Nettle Oil

Simples

Capsules: Arkocaps Phytofluid (210 mg); Power Health Pure Nettle Leaf (200 mg)
Juice: Schoenenberger Plant Juice
Tincture: Herbcraft; Neal's Yard Remedies

STONE ROOT

Collinsonia canadensis

Synonyms: horse balm, rich weed

Parts used: rhizome

As with other North American herbs introduced into Europe in the eighteenth and nineteenth centuries, stone root has been little researched and its constituents are largely unknown. It is unusual in that while the root is readily tolerated, small amounts of the leaves will cause nausea and vomiting. It is generally considered as a diuretic and digestive remedy, mainly used for treating kidney stones as the name implies. Stone root is also astringent and has a tonic effect on the capillaries.

Remedies and supplements
　　Culpeper Pilewort Tablets; *Potter's Piletabs

SUK GOK

Dendrobium nobile

Synonyms: *Shi Hu*

Parts used: stems

Suk gok – the usual commercial name for this herb – is Korean. The Chinese call it *Shi Hu* and have regarded it as a tonic remedy for at least 2,000 years. It was believed to bring longevity and strengthen kidney energy, making it an important remedy for the reproductive organs. Suk gok is mildly analgesic and will also reduce fevers.

Remedies and supplements
　　East West Shi Hu and Gan Cao Tea

SUNDEW

Drosera rotundifolia

Synonyms: dew plant

Parts used: herb

The sundew is a carnivorous plant capturing small insects on its sticky leaves and sucking the nutrients from them. It grows in peat bogs throughout Europe and is a useful anti-tussive herb particularly indicated for whooping cough and asthma. It is a relaxing antispasmodic, ideal for asthmatic coughs, and also shows some anti-microbial activity. It is soothing and mucilaginous and has been used for various gastric complaints.

Remedies and supplements
　　Bioforce Drosinula Cough Syrup; *Weleda Cough Elixir

SWEET ANNIE

Artemisia annua

Synonyms: sweet wormwood, *Qing Hao*

Parts used: whole plant

Sweet Annie has hit the headlines in recent years as an effective remedy for drug-resistant strains of malaria. The plant is used in Chinese medicine for feverish colds and heat stroke. It is anti-bacterial, will also stop bleeding, and is markedly less bitter than other members of the *Artemisia* family.

Remedies and supplements
    BioCare Artemisia Complex; BioCare Eradicidin Forte

SWEET SUMACH

Rhus aromatica

Synonyms: fragrant sumach

Parts used: root bark, berries

Sweet sumach is a traditional remedy for childhood bedwetting. The plant is a North American shrub and is given in drop doses of the tincture or fluid extract before bed. Scientific evidence for its efficacy is scant and some herbalists regard it as a panacea, especially, perhaps, since sweet sumach is known to have diuretic properties as well.

Remedies and supplements
    Bioforce Cystaforce

SWEET VIOLET

Viola odorata

Synonyms: blue violet

Parts used: herb

Sweet violets are rich in saponins and mucilage and have been used as a soothing expectorant for bronchitis and other respiratory problems. The herb has long been used in cancer treatment, notably for breast and skin cancers and is also found in general skin creams, notably in Germany and Austria.

Remedies and supplements
    External: St Hildegard-Posch Violet Salve

TAMARIND

Tamarindus indica

Synonyms: Indian date

Parts used: fruit

Used for fevers and jaundice in traditional medicine, tamarind occurs in proprietary remedies for constipation as a means of keeping the intestine moist and lubricating the stool. It is astringent and stimulating and is also mildly antiseptic. Externally it is used for sore eyes and rheumatism.

Remedies and supplements

Ortisan; Ortis Fruit & Fibres; Ortisan Liquid

TANGERINE

Citrus reticulata

Synonyms: *Chen Pi, Qing Pi*

Parts used: peel, essential oil

The Chinese use tangerine peel as a carminative and expectorant for coughs. It is a warming herb that is also anti-inflammatory to reduce swellings. The oil is considered by aromatherapists as uplifting and relaxing.

Remedies and supplements

External: Golden Yellow Ointment

Simples

Oil: Botanica; Nelson & Russell

TEA

Camellia sinensis

Parts used: leaf buds

Tea has been drunk in China since around 3000 BC and is regarded as a good digestive stimulant, an astringent for clearing phlegm and a digestive remedy. Indeed, when it was first introduced into Europe it was considered very much as a medicinal herb and seventeenth century advertisements extol its virtues as a digestive remedy and cure for over-indulgence.

The black tea, most widely drunk in Britain, is a fermented form of the leaf, while green tea is made from leaves that have been pan-fried and then dried. Oolong tea comes in between as a partly fermented variation.

Green tea is believed to improve resistance to stomach and skin cancers and stimulate the immune system while oolong tea is generally regarded as a digestive remedy. Black tea is highly astringent and useful for treating diarrhoea.

Simples

Capsules: Arkocaps Phytotrim (300 mg); Full Potency Herbs Green Tea Vegicaps (520 mg)

TEA TREE

Melaleuca alternifolia

Synonyms: ti tree

Parts used: essential oil

Interest in tea tree oil dates back to the 1920s when its strong antibacterial action was first investigated in France. The tree comes from Australia, where it was used in traditional Aboriginal medicine, and by the Second World War it was a regular component in field dressing kits among Australian troops.

In the past few years a thriving tea tree industry has grown up which has led to a number of highly adulterated oils appearing on the market. True tea tree oil is one of the few oils which does not irritate mucous membranes and it can be used neat on the skin or a few drops added to tampons can be used for topical treatment of vaginal thrush.

As well as its antibacterial action, tea tree oil is anti-fungal and anti-viral; it stimulates the immune system and if taken internally (not recommended without professional guidance) acts as an expectorant and diaphoretic. It is available in a wide range of creams which can be used in antiseptic dressings for cuts and grazes, on acne and other skin infections, applied to all sorts of fungal infections (including thrush and athlete's foot) and is also effective on cold sores, warts, verrucas and insect bites. The oil, used neat on a comb, or added to shampoos is a good way to treat head lice. Tea tree oil is also used (generally in combination with other herbs) for sore throats.

Remedies and supplements
Herbcraft Fresh Breath Cinnamint Spray; Thursday Plantation Throat Lozenges
External: BioCare Dermasorb; *Lanes Kleer Ti-Tree and Witch Hazel Cream; *Lane's Number 44 Skin Ointment; Nelsons Tea Tree Cream; *Potter's Skin Clear Ointment; Thursday Plantation Antiseptic Cream; Thursday Plantation Walkabout

Simples
Oil: Botanica; Hartwood Aromatics; Neal's Yard Remedies; Nelson & Russell; Tisserand

THYME

Thymus vulgaris

Parts used: herb, essential oil

Widely used in cooking, thyme – like many culinary herbs – is a carminative helping to ease the digestion as it copes with rich foods. The plant (particularly the oil) is also extremely antiseptic, and it is a good expectorant both to clear phlegm and, thanks to its antibacterial action, combats chest infections. Thyme is included in a number of cough remedies and digestive stimulants. The oil is also stimulating and tonic and can usefully be added to baths to combat exhaustion and added to rubs for muscular aches, pains and stiffness.

Remedies and supplements

*Bio-Strath Thyme Formula; BioCare Oxydent; Bioforce Bronchosan; Efalex; Gerard House Eez-a-Tea; Neal's Yard Anti-Oxidant Herbs; Neal's Yard Horehound & Honey Lozenges; Pure-fil Romagen Herbal Antioxidant; Reevecrest Gum Thyme; *Ricola Swiss Herb Lozenges; *Weleda Cough Elixir; *Weleda Herb and Honey Cough Elixir

External: Chirali Old Remedy Strain & Sprain Cream; *Potter's Nine Rubbing Oils; *Weleda Catarrh Cream

Simples

Capsules/Tablets: Arkocaps Phytocoff (250 mg)
Juice: Schoenenberger Plant Juice
Oil: Hartwood Aromatics
Tincture: Neal's Yard Remedies

TOLU

Myroxylon balsamum

Synonyms: tolu balsam

Parts used: oleo-resin

The South American Incas used tolu balsam, which was collected by cutting into the bark of this tropical tree and then collecting the sap which congeals into a thick resin, for flavouring. It was brought back to Europe by the *conquistadores* for use in perfumes. Tolu is antiseptic, expectorant and stimulating, and is largely used as a pleasant tasting ingredient for cough and throat remedies. It is also included in friar's balsam – a remedy still listed in the official British Pharmacopoeia – for use in steam inhalants for catarrh and colds.

Remedies and supplements

*Lanes Herbelix Specific; *Lanes Honey and Molasses Cough Mixture

TORMENTIL

Potentilla erecta

Synonyms: *Potentilla tormentilla*, blood root, tormentilla

Parts used: root

Tormentil is a bitter astringent herb which has mainly been used for diarrhoea and colitis. It contains a high proportion of tanins and can be used externally for wounds and sores. Some immune-stimulating action has been identified and it also has mild anti-allergic properties.

Remedies and supplements
    Bioforce DBT (Diabetisan); Bioforce Tormentavena

Simple
    Tincture: Bioforce

TUCKAHOE

Wolfiporia cocos

Synonyms: *Fu Ling, Fu Shen, Poria cocos*, Indian bread

Parts used: whole plant

Tuckahoe grows on the roots of various conifers and hardwoods and has long been used in China as a sedative and diuretic. In Chinese medicine nervous agitation is seen as a sign of disturbed heart energy and tuckahoe is believed to be suitably calming in such cases. It is also considered to be cooling and thus effective for fevers. The central part of the fungus, known as *Fu Shen*, is largely used as a sedative, while the exterior (*Fu Ling*) is generally preferred as a diuretic. Modern research has highlighted immune-stimulating properties and the herb has also been used to treat viral hepatitis. The plant is mainly valued as a diuretic and tonic and is used in menopausal remedies.

Remedies and supplements
    Equillence

Simples
    Tincture: Mycoherb Fu-Gen (East-West Herbs)

TURMERIC

Curcuma longa

Parts used: rhizome

Turmeric is an important ingredient of curries and curry powder and has a distinctive smell and bitter taste. It is not widely used in Western herbal medicine, although in Ayurvedic tradition it is considered as a natural antibiotic that will strengthen the digestion and improve the gut flora. It is also a circulatory stimulant, carminative and wound herb and is included in external creams and ointments for sprains, bruises and itching skin. Recent research has suggested that turmeric can help to cleanse and restore the liver and it also shows some anti-inflammatory activity.

Remedies and supplements
    BioCare Boswellic Acid Complex; BioCare Silymarin Complex; FSC Ginger and Turmeric; Healthcrafts Kelp
    External: Bee Brand Massage Oil; Dr Shir's Linament; Golden Yellow Ointment

USNEA

Usnea spp

Parts used: lichen

Several hanging lichens of the *Usnea* genus are used medicinally. Their action is similar to Iceland moss – expectorant and soothing for the mucous membranes.

Remedies and supplements

Bioforce Usneasan Cough Lozenges; Herbcraft Echinacea, Eyebright and Bilberry Formula

External: Herbcraft Liquorice and Propolis Spray

VALERIAN

Valeriana officinalis

Parts used: root

Valerian certainly ranks as one of the most widely used over-the-counter herbal sedatives, featuring in around 50 products. It reduces high blood pressure and is sometimes included in remedies for hypertension and heart conditions.

Valerian is a non-addictive tranquillizer and can be used for both day time stresses, anxiety and insomnia. It is popular in remedies targeted at menopausal women and also for anxiety associated with premenstrual syndrome and period pain. It has been extensively researched and its actions are believed to be due to a combination of valerianic acids (also found in other sedative herbs) and valepotriates, which are a complex group of chemicals that also show anti-tumour activity. Extracts are sometimes used in skin creams for eczema.

Remedies and supplements

*Bio-Strath Valerian Formula; BioCare Artemisia Complex; Bioforce Dormeasan; Blackmores Skullcap & Valerian; Blackmores Valerian Complex; *Cantassium Quiet Days; *Cantassium Quiet Nite Sleep; *Cantassium Quiet Tyme; *Dorwest Digestive Tablets; *Dorwest Natural Herb Tablets; *Dorwest Scullcap and Gentian Tablets; Frank Roberts Alchemilla Compound; Frank Roberts BP Tablets; Frank Roberts Constipation Tablets; *Frank Roberts Calmanite Tablets; *Frank Roberts Motherwort Compound Formula; *Frank Roberts Nerfood Tablets; *Frank Roberts Pulsatilla Compound Tablets; *Frank Roberts Valerian Compound; FSC Valerian Formula; *Gerard 99; *Gerard House Biophylin; *Gerard House Gladlax; *Gerard House Valerian Compound Tablets; Health Aid FemmeVit; *Healthcrafts Night Time; *Heath & Heather Becalm; *Heath & Heather Quiet Night; Herbcraft Passiflora and Valerian Formula; *HRI Calm Life Tablets; *HRI Golden Seal Digestive; HRI Night Tablets; Jay-Vee Tablets; Kordel's Kalm-Ex; Kordel's Quiet Time; *Lanes Kalms; *Lanes Quiet Life Tablets;*Muir's Stress-Ese;*Muir's Head-Ese; *Muir's Pick-Me-Up;

*Natrasleep; Neal's Yard Scullcap Compound Capsules; *Potter's Newrelax; *Potter's Nodoff Mixture; *Potter's Prementaid; *Potter's Wellwoman Tablets; Professional Herbs Valerian; *Valerina – Day-Time; *Valerina – Night -Time; *Weleda Avena Sativa Comp.

Simples

Capsules/tablets: Bare Foot ValerianTablets; Culpeper Valerian Tablets (150 mg); Full Potency Herbs Valerian Root Vegicaps (520 mg); Herbs of Grace Valerian; Power Health Pure Valerian (270 mg)
Juice: Schoenenberger Plant Juice
Tincture: Bioforce; Herbcraft; Neal's Yard Remedies

VERVAIN

Verbena officinalis

Parts used: herb

The Romans held vervain sacred to Jove and used it to anoint altars and provide a protective talisman for emissaries. The plant was also sacred to the Druids and was associated with fortune-telling until well into the seventeenth century. Today it is regarded as a useful nervine and liver tonic. It is bitter and stimulating for the digestion and is ideal as a tonic in convalescence and debility. Vervain is sedating and features in a number of over-the-counter remedies for anxiety and stress and it can also be helpful for neuralgia and migraine. As a liver tonic it is used for jaundice and gall bladder problems.
• Vervain should be avoided in pregnancy but can be taken in labour to stimulate contractions.

Remedies and supplements

*Cantassium Hay Fever; *Dorwest Scullcap and Gentian Tablets; Frank Roberts Alchemilla Compound; HRI Night Tablets; *Lanes Athera; *Muir's Head-Ese; *Muir's Stress-Ese; Neal's Yard Scullcap Compound Capsules; *Potter's Newrelax; *Potter's Prementaid

Simples

Tincture: Neal's Yard Remedies

VINE

Vitis vinifera

Parts used: leaves

Although little used in modern herbal medicine, the vine is astringent, diuretic and anti-inflammatory: it improves the circulation and can help to control bleeding. Vine extract can be used both internally and externally for varicose veins, and can be made into gargles for sore throats and inflamed gums. Wine – made, of course, from the fruit of the vine – has numerous therapeutic properties: it can help reduce cholesterol levels and provide some protection from heart disease – in moderation, of course. Hildegard of Bingen suggests vine ash as a remedy for dental problems and gum disease and various products based on this are marketed in Germany and Austria.

Remedies and supplements
External: Phytovarix

WAHOO

Euonymus atropurpreus

Synonyms: burning bush, spindle tree

Parts used: bark

Wahoo was a Native American remedy used by nineteenth century settlers as a diuretic and heart remedy. Today it is mainly regarded as a liver herb stimulating bile flow, with a laxative as well as diuretic action. It is a mild heart tonic and circulatory stimulant and is generally used in gall bladder and liver preparations. The European variety, *Euonymus europaeus*, also known as spindle tree, is similarly used.

Remedies and supplements
*Frank Roberts Black Root Compound Tablets; *Potter's GB Tablets; *Potter's Indigestion Mixture

WALNUT

Juglans regia

Parts used: leaves, bark, fruit, oil

Walnut leaves and bark have traditionally been used in Europe as a remedy for constipation and skin problems while the Chinese regarded the nuts as a tonic for the kidneys. In recent years walnut oil pressed from the seeds, has been found to contain essential fatty acids (*cis*-linoleic and *alpha*-linolenic acids) which like the more widely promoted *gamma*-linolenic acid from evening primrose oil, is vital for normal bodily function. A recent US study suggests that regular consumption of walnuts can also reduce cholesterol levels and lower the risk of heart attacks.

Remedies and supplements
Absorb Plus; Bioforce DBT (Diabetisan); Colon Cleanse

WATERCRESS

Nasturtium officinale

Parts used: leaves

Familiar in salads and soups, watercress is also a medicinal plant that will stimulate the digestion, liver function and kidney metabolism and act as a valuable cleansing remedy for skin problems. Combined with nettle juice it makes a good "spring cleaning" potion used as a restorative after the winter. It is also diuretic and, as such, is included in blood pressure remedies.

Remedies and supplements
> Blackmores Cactus & Hawthorn; *Dorwest Mixed Vegetable Tablets

Simples
> *Tincture:* Bioforce

WEST INDIAN BAY

Pimenta racemosa

Synonyms: bayberry tree, wild clove

Parts used: oil

Bay rum, which consists largely of the distilled leaves of the West Indian bay tree, was once a favourite hair treatment used to bring gloss and lustre. The oil is now synthesized for the commercial cosmetics market, but the herb is still used by Potter's in some of its dandruff preparations.

Remedies and supplements
> *External:* *Potter's Adiantine; *Potter's Medicated Extract of Rosemary

Simples
> *Oil:* Hartwood Aromatics

WHITE HOREHOUND

Marrubium vulgare

Synonyms: hoarhound

Parts used: herb

White horehound has long been a favourite for cough lozenges and throat sweets and "horehound candy" was once widely available from confectioners and chemists. The herb is expectorant, antiseptic and bitter and is used for bronchitis, coughs, colds and catarrh. As a bitter tonic it also has a stimulant effect on the digestive system particularly the liver. It can be used externally for grazes and skin rashes although is more often regarded as an internal remedy. It is used in a number of herbal remedies and supplements for respiratory problems including candies and throat lozenges.

Remedies and supplements

Bioforce Bronchosan; *Cantassium Hay Fever; *CatarrhEeze; *CoughEeze; *Culpeper Influenza Mixture; *Frank Roberts Rod-Bron Tablets; *Heath & Heather Catarrh; *Lanes Honey and Molasses Cough Mixture; Neal's Yard Horehound & Honey Lozenges; Neal's Yard Horehound & Aniseed Linctus; *Potter's Chest Mixture; *Potter's Horehound and Aniseed Cough Mixture; *Potter's Vegetable Cough Remover;*Ricola Swiss Herb Lozenges; Thursday Plantation Throat Lozenges; *Weleda Cough Elixir; *Weleda Herb and Honey Cough Elixir

Simples

Tincture: Neal's Yard Remedies

WHITE WILLOW

Salix alba

Parts used: leaves, bark

The *Salix* genus gives its name to "salicylates": the group of anti-inflammatory and analgesic compounds familiar in aspirin and present in significant amounts in the bark and leaves of the white willow. The plant, like aspirin, is used for relieving pain and reducing fevers and is helpful for rheumatism, gout, arthritis, feverish chills and headaches. It is included in several over-the-counter products for arthritic conditions and is also sometimes used for digestive disorders. The North American black willow (*S. nigra*) is used in the same way as the European species.

Remedies and supplements

Arthur's Formula; *Bio-Strath Willow Formula; BioCare Salicidin; Frank Roberts Black Willow Compound Tablets; *Gerard House Ligvites; Herbcraft Passiflora and Valerian Formula; Kordel's Celery 3000 Plus; Kordel's Feverfew and Willow; *Weleda Digestodoran Tablets

Simples

Capsules: Power Health Pure White Willow (200 mg)
Tincture: Neal's Yard Remedies

WILD CARROT

Daucus carota

Synonyms: Queen Anne's lace, bee's nest plant

Parts used: herb, seeds, oil

Wild carrot acts as a diuretic and carminative: the whole plant is preferred for urinary stones, cystitis and gout, while the seeds are taken for indigestion and wind. They will also promote menstrual flow. The oil is used in skin cream, as a reputed anti-wrinkle remedy, and to treat eczema and dermatitis.

Wild carrot root is white and inedible, and the familiar orange vegetable comes from the cultivated variety – *D. carota* subsp. *sativa*. This is rich in *beta*-carotene which is a precursor of vitamin A, and carrot extracts are used for strengthening night vision and also for skin conditions. Carrots are also a good source of vitamins B and C and are regarded as an important addition to anti-cancer diets. Carrot juice has been used as a remedy for intestinal worms and is used for diarrhoea and indigestion. *Beta*-carotene is also said to provide some protection from the sun's ultra-violet rays and is suggested by beauticians as a useful supplement before sun-tanning.

• Vitamin A is one of the few vitamins that can be extremely toxic in large doses affecting the liver and turning the skin a yellow colour. However, *beta*-carotene is believed to be rather safer as any surplus is simply excreted.

Remedies and supplements

*Muir's Sciatica; *Potter's Sciargo; *Potter's Sciargo Herb; *Potter's Watershed Mixture

Simples

Capsules/tablets: Arkocaps Phytobronz (370 mg root); Power Health Carrot Oil (250 mg)
Juice: Schoenenberger Plant Juice
Infused oil: Neal's Yard Remedies
Oil: Hartwood Aromatics; Tisserand

WILD CHERRY

Prunus serotina

Synonyms: black cherry, wild rum cherry

Parts used: bark, fruit

Wild cherry bark is generally used as a cough suppressant and sedative although the Cherokee in North America also recommended it to relieve labour pains. The bark is astringent and has been given for diarrhoea. It is a bitter tasting herb so will stimulate the digestion and some anti-viral activity has been recorded. Extracts containing cherry fruit and juice are reputedly anti-oxidant.

Remedies and supplements

BioCare Procydin; Neal's Yard Horehound & Aniseed Linctus; *Potter's Horehound & Aniseed Linctus; Thursday Plantation Throat Lozenges

Simples

Tincture: Herbcraft; Neal's Yard Remedies

WILD LETTUCE

Lactuca verosa

Synonyms: lettuce opium

Parts used: leaves, dried juice

Until the 1930s, the dried white juice or latex from lettuce was widely sold as "lettuce opium", used as a sedative, pain killer and to counter insomnia. The herb is still used in this way and is included in a number of over-the-counter remedies for sleeplessness, anxiety and nervous tension. It can also be helpful for irritable and nervous coughs and has been used to ease rheumatic pain and also to calm hyperactive children.

Remedies and supplements

*Cantassium Quiet Nite Sleep; *Frank Roberts Calmanite Tablets; FSC Valerian Formula; *Gerard House Valerian Compound Tablets; Herbcraft Passiflora and Valerian Formula HRI Night Tablets; Ladies Meno-Life Formula; *Lanes Quiet Life Tablets; *Muir's Head-Ese; *Muir's Stress-Ese; *Potter's Anased Pain Relief Tablets; *Potter's Antibron Tablets

WILD OATS

Avena sativa

Synonyms: groats

Parts used: seeds, whole unripe plant

Oats form one of the world's most important cereal crops used as a staple food in northern Europe for centuries. Medicinally, the plant is anti-depressant, tonic and regarded as emotionally uplifting. More recently it has been shown to reduce blood cholesterol levels. Externally oats, generally in the form of oatmeal, are included in products for eczema and dry skin, while internally it is given for depression, nervous exhaustion, emotional upsets associated with the menopause, or debility following illness. Oat straw was a mediaeval remedy for rheumatism.

The whole plant, pressed while still green, gives a rich juice which is used much like the seeds as a nerve tonic.

Several herbal remedies combine oats with ginseng in a tonic mix and it is also contained in a number of general purpose remedies for anxiety and stress as well as those aimed at menopausal women.

Remedies and supplements

Bioforce Alfavena; Bioforce Cystaforce; Bioforce Dormeasan; Bioforce Ginsavena; Bioforce Ginsavita; Bioforce Neuroforce; Bioforce Tormentavena; *Culpeper Herbal Tonic for Digestive Disorders; *Frank Roberts Avexan Tablets; *Frank Roberts Nerfood Tablets; Herbatone; Herbcraft Burdock & Nettle Formula; Kordel's Kalm-Ex; *Muir's Head-Ese; *Muir's Stress-Ese; *Weleda Avena Sativa Comp

Simples
>   *Juice:* Schoenenberger Plant Juice
>   *Tincture:* Bioforce; Herbcraft; Neal's Yard Remedies

WILD ROSEMARY

Ledum palustre

Synonyms: marsh tea, march cistus

Parts used: leaves

A reputed narcotic, said to cause delirium, the *Ledum* spp. are members of the heather family and are similarly diuretic and astringent. Externally the plant acts as an insecticide and was once sprinkled among clothes and in grain stores to deter vermin. It can be used internally for diarrhoea or externally for scabies, parasites and skin irritation.

Remedies and supplements
>   *External:* *Nelsons Pyrethrum Spray

WILD STRAWBERRY

Fragaria vesca

Parts used: leaves, fruits

Strawberry leaves are mildly astringent and diuretic and are often added to herbal tea blends. They can be used for diarrhoea and digestive upsets while the fruits are sometimes used in skin lotions for sunburn. Anthroposophical theory regards the leaves as cooling and calming.

Remedies and supplements
>   *Weleda Fragador Tablets

WILD YAM

Dioscorea villosa

Synonyms: colic root, Mexican wild yam

Parts used: rhizome, root

Wild yam's main claim to fame is as the original source of the oral contraceptive pill. It is rich in steroidal saponins which provided the diosgenin that was converted into oestrogen- and progesterone-like substances until the pharmaceutical industry found a way to synthesize these hormones. Wild yam is also antispasmodic, anti-inflammatory, mildly diaphoretic and stimulates bile flow. It is largely used for colic and rheumatism but may also be included in products for period pain, cramps, asthma, gastritis and gall bladder problems.

Remedies and supplements
BioCare AD206; Herbcraft Fresh Breath Cinnamint Spray

Simples
Tincture: Herbcraft; Neal's Yard Remedies
Capsules/Tablets: Gerard House Wild Yam; Herbs of Grace Wild Yam

WINTERGREEN

Gaultheria procumbens

Synonyms: checkerberry, teaberry

Parts used: leaves, oil

Wintergreen oil with its characteristic smell was once a familiar standby in a wide range of ointments for rheumatism and muscular aches and pains. Infusions of the leaves were occasionally used internally, but the plant was mainly valued for its oil. This is very rich in methyl salicylate which is anti-inflammatory, anti-rheumatic and diuretic. Today, synthetically produced methyl salicylate has largely replaced wintergreen in many over-the-counter products, although a few do still claim to contain the genuine article.

• Wintergreen oil is toxic in excess and should also be avoided by those sensitive to aspirin.

Remedies and supplements
*Olbas Pastilles
External: Arthur's Formula Cream; Chirali Old Remedy Strain & Sprain Cream; *Olbas Oil; *Potter's Dermacreme Ointment

WITCH HAZEL

Hamamelis virginiana

Parts used: leaves, branches, bark

Distilled witch hazel is a familiar first aid remedy for bruises, sprains, cuts and grazes. It is astringent and stops bleeding and commonly used to ease varicose veins and piles, on spots and blemishes, and for all sorts of minor household injuries. The solution is available as a generic from chemists and is also used in a number of cosmetic preparations, often combined with rosewater.

The tincture, well diluted, can be used much as generic distilled witch hazel and a number of proprietary creams and ointments are available. Witch hazel is used internally as a potent astringent for diarrhoea, colitis, excessive menstruation and haemorrhage.

Remedies and supplements

    External: Bioforce Po Ho Ointment; Bioforce Seven Herb Cream; Frank Roberts Cade Oil Ointment; Gerard House Witch Hazel Ointment; *Lanes Heemex; *Lanes Kleer Ti-Tree and Witch Hazel Cream; *Nelsons Haemorrhoid Cream; Phytovarix; *Potter's Adiantine; *Potter's Varicose Ointment

Simples

    Capsules: Arkocaps Phytovarix (220 mg)
    Tincture: Bioforce; Neal's Yard Remedies

WORMWOOD

Artemisia absinthum

Parts used: leaves, juice

Like southernwood, wormwood is a bitter, anthelmintic used to stimulate the digestion. It contains thujone which is a highly toxic and addictive hallucinogen and the herb should only be used for short periods. It once formed the key flavouring in the alcoholic drink, absinthe, which although very popular in the nineteenth century was later banned because of its toxicity. However, thujone is only significantly soluble in alcohol so fresh pressed juices and infusions are quite safe to use. As a strong digestive bitter, wormwood can help to stimulate gastric function, improve appetite and ease flatulence and stomach upsets.

Remedies and supplements

    BioCare Candicidin

Simples

    Juice: Schoenenberger Plant Juice
    Tincture: Neal's Yard Remedies

YARROW

Achillea millefolium

Synonyms: soldier's woundwort, nosebleed, milfoil

Parts used: herb, oil

A common meadow herb, yarrow is astringent and bitter used as an anti-inflammatory, diaphoretic, diuretic, or wound herb. It relaxes the peripheral blood vessels so can help to reduce high blood pressure and it is also cooling in fevers. Like chamomile flowers, yarrow flowers also contain anti-allergenic compounds which are activated by hot water and are thus found in infusions and the distilled essential oil.

    The herb is used in over-the-counter remedies for colds, hay fever and catarrh which focus on its astringent and fever reducing properties. As a diuretic it also occurs in urinary remedies and those designed to counter fluid retention or reduce blood pressure.

The oil is sometimes found commercially and is both anti-inflammatory and anti-allergenic. It can be used in steam inhalations for hay fever or in chest rubs for colds and catarrh.

• Yarrow should be avoided in pregnancy as it is a uterine stimulant. The fresh herb can sometimes cause contact dermatitis and in rare cases, prolonged use may increase the skin's photosensitivity.

Remedies and supplements

Bioforce Cystaforce; Bioforce Gastrosan; Bioforce Hyperisan; Bioforce Imperthritica; *Cantassium Hay Fever; *CatarrhEeze; Frank Roberts BP Tablets; *Frank Roberts Cold Tablets; *Frank Roberts Drops of Life Tablets; Gerard House Fem-a-Tea; Health Aid Liver Guard; *Potter's Rheumatic Pain Tablets; *Potter's Tabritis; *Potter's Wellwoman Tablets; *Potter's Wellwoman Herbs; *Ricola Swiss Herb Lozenges; *Weleda Carminative Tea; *Weleda Laxadoron Tablets

Simples

Juice: Schoenenberger Plant Juice
Oil: Tisserand
Tincture: Bioforce, Neal's Yard Remedies

YELLOW DOCK

Rumex crispus

Synonyms: curled dock

Parts used: root

Yellow dock is regarded as a cleansing herb suitable for chronic skin problems and arthritic complaints. It is also laxative and stimulates bowel flow so may be found in remedies for constipation and liver problems.

Remedies and supplements

Blackmores Echinacea Complex; Blackmores Sarsparilla Complex; Discovery Coliclens; Health Aid Herbal Booster; Herbcraft Burdock & Nettle Formula; *Muir's Rheumatic Pain; Natural Flow Colonite; *Potter's Skin Eruptions Mixture
External: *Nelsons Pyrethrum Spray

Simples

Capsules: Herbs of Grace Yellow Dock
Tincture: Neal's Yard Remedies

YELLOW GENTIAN

Gentiana lutea

Parts used: roots, rhizomes

Gentian is one of the most popular bitter digestive stimulants in Europe. It is widely used to improve appetite and digestive function and to treat a range of gastrointestinal problems including nausea, diarrhoea, indigestion, gastritis and heartburn. The herb has a tonic effect and, like all bitters, can be helpful in fever management. It has an extremely bitter taste and is generally used in quite small quantities.

• Gentian should not be taken by those suffering from gastric or duodenal ulcers.

Remedies and supplements

*Bio-Strath Liquorice Formula; Bioforce Gastrosan; Blackmores Dandelion Complex; Blackmores Skullcap & Valerian; *Box's Far Famed Indigestion Tablets; *Culpeper Herbal Tonic for Digestive Disorders; *Dorwest Scullcap and Gentian Tablets; FSC Valerian Formula; Herbcraft Peppermint Formula; Herbatone; Kordel's Quiet Time; *Lanes Herbelix Specific; *Lanes Kalms; *Potter's Appetiser Mixture; *Potter's Indigestion Mixture; *Potter's Stomach Mixture; Professional Herbs Cayenne & Ginger; St Hildegard-Posch Enzian Wine

Simples

Tincture: Bioforce; Neal's Yard Remedies

YLANG YLANG

Cananga odorata

Parts used: essential oil

Ylang ylang oil comes from a tall tree grown in the East Indies. It is anti-depressant and sedative and is popularly used in aromatherapy for impotence and frigidity. It can be useful for nervous tension and to ease palpitations.

Simples

Oil: Botanica; Hartwood Aromatics; Neal's Yard Remedies; Nelson & Russell; Tisserand

YUCCA

Yucca elata

Parts used: root

Although the yucca is mentioned in John Gerard's herbal of 1597 as a "hot and dry" plant, and he was clearly impressed by its novelty, he does not have any suggestions as to its use. Roots of some varieties have been used as detergents, due to the high saponin content in the root, and others have a reputation as a strong purgative. Some reports suggest that the plant can have an action on the gut flora helping to absorb bacterial toxins and improve function and it is also reputedly anti-inflammatory and analgesic.

Recent research in Dublin highlighted the fact that yuccas also extract nitrogen containing compounds from the air as a source of nutrients. Kept in a lavatory the plants will thus absorb urine smells.

Remedies and supplements
Kordel's Celery 3000 Plus

Simples
Capsules: Full Potency Herbs Yucca Vegicaps (520 mg)
Tincture: Herbcraft

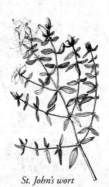

St. John's wort

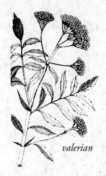

valerian

A–Z of Herbal Remedies and Supplements

This section lists around 900 over-the-counter herbal preparations available in the UK. Those which have a product licence and are of proven efficacy and safety are marked with an asterisk (*), others are sold as food supplements or may be single herbs which are exempt from licensing under the 1968 Medicines Act and The Medicines (Retail Sale and Supply of Herbal Remedies) Order 1977. Many suppliers of supplements are currently obtaining product licences for these lines so many more of the items featured may become licensed in the near future. Medicinal claims can be made for licensed products and these are indicated. For supplements a brief description is given of the main attributes of the herbs they contain while for single herb products refer to notes given in the A–Z of Herbs. Cautions given by the relevant suppliers are included in each entry but also check in the A–Z of Herbs for any additional warnings, and see Pregnancy and Childbirth in the A–Z of Common Complaints for herbs to be avoided in pregnancy. Technically, unlicensed products cannot give a recommended "dosage" only a suggested intake – however, for simplicity the word "dosage" is used throughout, although not all suppliers are willing to make such recommendations.

ABSORB PLUS

Sold as a supplement, this product is promoted as a digestive cleansing mixture largely containing fibre (beet fibre and oat bran), the sorts of "friendly" bacteria which comprise the gut flora, and a mixture of herbs. These are walnut, which is a laxative, cornsilk (a diuretic), chaparral and agrimony (both used to treat diarrhoea amongst other things) and fennel (a carminative). Perhaps less relevant for digestive problems are sarsparilla largely regarded as a skin remedy and anti-inflammatory although Chinese species have been used for dysentery; red clover – primarily a skin remedy and expectorant; and pasque flower which is largely used as a sedative and to ease pain in the reproductive organs.

HEALTH PLUS

*AGNOLYT

This is essentially a 1:5 tincture of chastetree berry which is licensed for occasional bloatedness and sold as "a gentle non-diuretic, non-hormonal, herbal medicine" for women aged 18–45.
• Not recommended in pregnancy, breast feeding or if taking hormonal preparations.

Dosage: 40 drops in a little fluid on an empty stomach each morning. Continue for up to three months.

MADAUS (UK DISTRIBUTOR NATURAL TOUCH)

AMBER MASSAGE SALVE

This is a Chinese product containing a mixture of essential oils and traditional Chinese remedies which can be used for aching and stiff muscles, joints, tendons and bruises. Active herbal ingredients are *Dang Gui*, peach seeds, lithospermum, safflower and myrrh, as well as the resinous extract from a type of oriental rattan known as dragon's blood. The mixture also contains amber resin which the Chinese used to reduce swellings and improve circulation, as well as mastic which is a gum from the *Pistacia lentiscus* tree more often used in making varnish, in a base of sesame oil and beeswax. The potion can be massaged into affected areas two or three times a day but should not be used on open wounds.
• External use only.

SPRING WIND HERBS (EAST WEST HERBS IN THE UK)

AMERICAN NUTRITION ACEROLA PLUS AND SUPER ACEROLA PLUS

Acerola is a very rich natural source of vitamin C. The "Acerola Plus" supplement provides 100 mg of the vitamin and Super Acerola Plus has 500 mg. The tablets also contain blackcurrant and rosehip powders in a lactose base. Depending on individual requirements 1000 mg or more of vitamin C can be taken daily.

FERROSAN HEALTHCARE

*AQUALETTE

Licensed for fluid retention and maintaining a normal water balance, Aqualette contains two diuretic herbs – horsetail and dandelion. In this product dandelion root is used which is also a liver stimulant. The tablet base is lactose. It is not recommended for children under 16.

Dosage: 2–3 tablets three times a day.

MEDIC HERB

ARKOCAPS

Arkopharma produces a number of herbal capsules each containing a single herb. Most are sold as supplements but generally try to convey in their names general areas of applications. Details of the plants involved are included in the A–Z of herbs but the following table summarizes contents and dosages. More of these products may become licensed in future.

ARKOPHARMA

Table 4: Arkocaps single herb capsules (supplements)

Product	Content	Dosage
Arkocaps Alfalfa	310 mg alfalfa	2 capsules morning and evening
Arkocaps Dandelion	250 mg dandelion root	1–2 capsules, three times a day
Phytobronz	370 mg carrots	2 capsules morning and evening
Phytochol	340 mg gugulon	2 capsules in the morning and evening
Phytoclense	230 mg alder buckthorn	2 capsules three times a day before meals
Phytocoff	250 mg thyme	2 capsules three times a day
Phytodesensatine	200 mg common plantain	2 capsules three times a day
Phytoderma	270 mg burdock root	2 capsules morning and evening
Phytodigest	150 mg globe artichoke	3 capsules twice a day before main meals
Phytodreams	240 mg Californian poppy	Adults: 2 tablets at midday and 3 in the evening Children age 6 and over: 1

continued

Product	Content	Dosage
		capsule one hour before bed
Phytoenergyze	340 mg guarana seeds	2 capsules morning and lunchtime at the start of meals
Phytoexcel	240 mg gotu kola	1 capsule three times a day
Phytofeverfew	200 mg feverfew	2–3 capsules morning and evening; maintenance dose 1 capsule a day for 3 months once symptoms are relieved
Phytofibre	350 mg isphaghula husks	Adults: 2–3 capsules a day with each of the two main meals. Children: 1 capsule with each of the two main meals
Phytofluid	210 mg stinging nettles	2 capsules morning and evening during meals
Phytoforce	250 mg Siberian ginseng	3 capsules morning and at mid-day
Phytoimune	330 mg garlic	2 capsules three times a day
Phytokold	250 mg *Echinacea purpurea*	2 capsules morning and evening
Phytomemo	180 mg ginkgo	2 capsules morning and evening
Phytomenopause	220 mg sage	2 capsules morning and evening
Phytophrodisiac	250 mg damiana	2 capsules morning and evening
Phytopremenstrual	150 mg hops	2 capsules, three times a day before meals
Phytorhuma	330 mg devil's claw	During the painful phase take 2 capsules morning, mid-day and evening; as a maintenance dose take 2 capsules in the morning and evening
Phytosenalax	300 mg senna leaf	3 capsules morning and evening

continued

Product	Content	Dosage
Phytoseptik	230 mg eucalyptus leaves	2 capsules three times a day
Phytoshape	325 mg pineapple stems	2–3 capsules morning and evening
Phytosilica	270 mg bamboo gum	2 capsules morning and evening
Phytosistitus	270 mg cherry stalks	2 capsules three times a day
Phytoslim	200 mg bean husks	2 capsules morning, lunchtime and evening
Phytosuperior	300 mg shisandra fruits	1 capsule three times a day
Phytotravel	280 mg ginger	2 capsules morning and evening
Phytotrim	300 mg green tea	2 capsules morning and evening
Phytovainetone	230 mg bilberry leaves	2 capsules morning and evening
Phytovarix	220 mg of witch hazel leaf	3 capsules morning and evening

*ARKOCAPS PHYTOCALM

A licensed product for nervousness and insomnia, Phytocalm capsules contain 230 mg of passion flower.

Dosage: adults – for insomnia take 2 tablets at night before dinner and 3 before bed; for nervousness take 2 tablets morning and evening with meals; children age 6 and over – 2 capsules in the evening one hour before bed

ARKOPHARMA

ARKOFLUID MEGA GLA

Capsules containing borage oil which offer 24% GLA.

Dosage: 2–3 capsules daily.   ARKOPHARMA

ARKOFLUIDS EPO

Capsules containing evening primrose oil.
Dosage: 2–3 capsules daily.

ARKOPHARMA

ARTHUR'S FORMULA

These tablets combine devil's claw and white willow – both herbs widely used for rheumatism and arthritis – with garlic and calcium.

Dosage: 1 tablet three times a day increasing to 2 tablets three times a day if required.

POWER HEALTH

ARTHUR'S FORMULA CREAM

This is an unlicensed cream containing wintergreen oil which is rich in methyl salicylate and has been used for arthritic conditions, and lavender oil which can be helpful for muscular aches and pains. Other ingredients are marigold oil – generally considered useful for wounds and varicose veins; marjoram oil, antispasmodic and helpful for insomnia; evening primrose oil and kava kava extract which is mainly regarded as a diuretic but has been used for rheumatism and gout. The mixture is in a groundnut oil base and should be massaged daily into joints.

• External use only.

POWER HEALTH

ARTHUR'S FORMULA BATH AND MASSAGE OIL

An unlicensed oil mixture sold as a massage treatment and bath additive that may be suitable for arthritis and rheumatism. The mixture contains four essential oils: juniper, lavender, pepper and benzoin, all of which are regarded by aromatherapists as useful for easing muscular aches and stiffness. The oil also contains vitamin E which helps to act as a preservative and generally protects cells from oxidation. The oils should be used as a massage twice a week.

• External use only.

POWER HEALTH

BACH FLOWER REMEDIES

The Bach Flower Remedies were discovered by Dr Edward Bach in the 1930s and are essentially the "dew" collected from certain flowers preserved in brandy. This basic essence (almost homoeopathic by definition) is believed to incorporate some unseen energy from the flower which imbues the remedy with some sort of healing properties that act on the human psyche. Sceptics say any action the remedies achieve is actually just the preserving brandy, but they do seem to help many people and are widely used. Details of Dr Bach's 38 healing remedies are listed in Table 5 below; more detailed guidelines for each remedy's action are available in a number of specialist books some of which are listed in the Glossary.

Dr Bach's Rescue Remedy – a combination of Cherry Plum, Impatiens, Rock Rose and Star of Bethlehem – can be used as an all-purpose first aid treatment for shock, trauma and the sort of nervousness that accompanies exams or visits to the dentist.

Dosage: Having chosen a suitable selection of remedies four drops of each should be put into a 10 ml dropper bottle and this then filled with spring water. Drop doses of the remedy can then be taken on the tongue as required.

A NELSON & CO

Table 5: The Bach Flower Remedies

Remedy	*Dr Bach's suggested use*
Agrimony	For those who suffer mental torture behind a "brave face"
Aspen	For vague fears of an unknown origin
Beech	For critical intolerance of others
Centaury	For the weak-willed
Cerato	For those who doubt their own judgement and seek advice of others
Cherry Plum	For fears of mental collapse
Chestnut Bud	For a refusal to learn from past mistakes
Chicory	For possessiveness and selfishness
Clematis	For the inattentive and dreamy escapist
Crab Apple	A cleansing remedy for those who feel unclean or ashamed
Elm	For those temporarily overcome by feelings on inadequacy
Gentian	For the despondent and easily discouraged
Gorse	For hopelessness and despair
Heather	For the self-centred obsessed with their own troubles
Holly	For those who are jealous, angry or feel hatred for others
Honeysuckle	For home sickness and nostalgia
Hornbeam	For "Monday morning feelings" and procrastination
Impatiens	For the impatient
Larch	For those who lack confidence
Mimulus	For fear of known things
Mustard	For deep gloom and severe depression

continued

Remedy	*Dr Bach's suggested use*
Oak	For those who struggle on against adversity
Olive	For complete exhaustion
Pine	For guilt feelings and self-blame
Red Chestnut	For excessive fear for others, especially loved ones
Rock Rose	For extreme terror
Rock Water	For the self-repressed who overwork and deny themselves any relaxation
Scleranthus	For uncertainty and indecision
Star of Bethlehem	For shock
Sweet Chestnut	For extreme anguish; the limit of endurance
Vervain	For tenseness, over-enthusiasm and over-effort
Vine	For the dominating and inflexible
Walnut	For protection at times of change such as the menopause or during other major lifestage transitions
Water Violet	For the proud and reserved
White Chestnut	For mental anguish and persistent nagging worries
Wild Oat	For uncertainty about which path to take; an aid to decision taking
Wild Rose	For the apathetic who lack ambition
Willow	For the resentful and bitter who are fond of saying "not fair"

BARE FOOT FEVERFEW TABLETS

Unlicensed simple feverfew tablets.

POTTER'S

BARE FOOT VALERIAN TABLETS

Unlicensed simple valerian tablets.

POTTER'S

BEE BRAND MASSAGE OIL

Based on an Indonesian recipe, this massage oil contains a combination of warming herbs which would have a rubefacient effect on the skin, warming and stim-

ulating blood flow. It contains essential oils of cajuput, clove, pine and lemon-grass with extracts of pepper leaves, ginger, turmeric, garlic and galangal all in a coconut oil base. In the East the mix is widely recommended for arthritis, rheumatism, muscular aches and pains, colds, chills and dry irritant skin. It can be massaged into affected areas once or twice a day or added to bath water.
• External use only.

EAST-WEST HERBS

*BIO-STRATH ARTICHOKE FORMULA

This is based on Bio-Strath Elixir (see below) with additional extracts of arti-choke leaves, milk thistle seeds and peppermint leaves. Both artichoke and milk thistle are good liver stimulants and tonics. It is licensed as a remedy for indiges-tion caused by eating fatty foods which may be related to gall-bladder problems.
• Not recommended for children under 12.

Dosage: 20 drops in water three times a day.

CEDAR HEALTH

*BIO-STRATH CHAMOMILE FORMULA

This is based on Bio-Strath Elixir (see below) with additional extracts of sage and chamomile: herbs which are antiseptic and anti-inflammatory. It is licensed for minor acute painful conditions of the mouth and throat including mouth ulcers and gum disorders.
• Not recommended for children under 12.

Dosage: 20 drops in water three times a day which can be used as a mouth wash.

CEDAR HEALTH

*BIO-STRATH ELIXIR

The basic Bio-Strath Elixir is derived from the *Saccharamyces cerevisiae* yeast. The product originates from Switzerland and extensive research there and in Ger-many has suggested that the mixture can improve mental performance in both young and old. The Elixir is the base for a number of other herbal products and is licensed as a tonic for use during convalescence, to help symptoms of fatigue and tiredness, and to improve appetite.
• Not recommended for children under the age of 12.

Dosage: 5 ml three times daily.

CEDAR HEALTH

*BIO-STRATH LIQUORICE FORMULA

This is based on Bio-Strath Elixir (see above) with additional extracts of liquorice, chamomile and yellow gentian extracts. Liquorice has a laxative action, chamomile is carminative and gentian is a bitter digestive stimulant. It is licensed as an aid to digestion.
• Not recommended for children.

Dosage: 20 drops in water three times a day.

CEDAR HEALTH

*BIO-STRATH THYME FORMULA

This is based on Bio-Strath Elixir (see above) with additional extracts of thyme leaves and cowslip roots. Both these herbs are strongly expectorant and the mixture is licensed to provide symptomatic relief from coughs.
• Not recommended for children.

Dosage: 20 drops in water three times a day.

CEDAR HEALTH

*BIO-STRATH VALERIAN FORMULA

This is based on Bio-Strath Elixir (see above) with additional extracts of valerian, passion flower and peppermint. Both valerian and passion flower are good herbal sedatives; peppermint is more stimulating but no doubt improves the flavour. The mixture is licensed to provide symptomatic relief from tension, irritability, stress and insomnia.
• Not recommended for children.

Dosage: 20 drops in water three times a day.

CEDAR HEALTH

*BIO-STRATH WILLOW FORMULA

This is based on Bio-Strath Elixir (see above) with additional extracts of willow bark and cowslip root extracts. Willow is a good anti-inflammatory widely used for arthritic and rheumatic disorders; cowslip root does have antispasmodic action although is generally valued as an expectorant. The product is licensed for the symptomatic relief of backache, lumbago, sciatica, fibrositis and muscular pain.
• Not recommended for children under 12.

Dosage: 50 drops in water three times a day.

CEDAR HEALTH

BIOCARE AD206

This is a food supplement combining tonic herbs and a mixture of vitamins and minerals. It contains Siberian ginseng, gotu kola, wild yam and liquorice as well as pantothenic acid, niacin, vitamins B_6 and C, magnesium, chromium and zinc salts, and small amounts of the enzymes protease, cellulase, lipase, and amylase. The product is suggested as a tonic for the adrenal cortex.
• Not for use in pregnancy or if pregnancy is planned.

Dosage: 1 capsule, twice a day.

BIOCARE

BIOCARE ARTEMISIA COMPLEX

This food supplement contains a number of herbs to stimulate the digestive system – anise, golden seal, hyssop and liquorice – with echinacea which is a good anti-bacterial and valerian (a sedative). The main herb is, however, sweet Annie which has some anti-bacterial action but is significantly less bitter than other members of the *Artemisia* family.
• Do not use in pregnancy or Crohn's disease

Dosage: 1 capsule three times a day.

BIOCARE

BIOCARE BEETROOT EXTRACT

A food supplement containing beetroot extract and promoted as a natural mineral and vitamin source.

Dosage: 1 capsule three times a day.

BIOCARE

BIOCARE BIOCIDIN/BIOCIDIN FORTE

This food supplement is one of a number targeted at those suffering from candidiasis and is designed to support the intestinal flora. It contains grapefruit seeds which are reputedly antiparasitic and anti-fungal. Two versions are available: Biocidin with 75 mg of grapefruit seed and Biocidin Forte with 150 mg. BioCare also produces a liquid version (see p. 262).
• Do not use in colitis or ulcerative conditions of the colon

Dosage: 1 capsule, three times a day.

BIOCARE

BIOCARE BOSWELLIC ACID COMPLEX

Sold as a food supplement, this mixture contains ginger as a carminative, turmeric extract as a liver stimulant, bilberry flavonoids which, like similar extracts (such as rutin), can improve blood vessels and boswellic acid extracted from trees similar to those which produce frankincense. The mixture may be supportive for digestive function.

Dosage: 1 capsule three times a day.

BIOCARE

BIOCARE BUCCALZYME

This supplement contains immune stimulating herbs along with a reasonably large amount of vitamin C so may be helpful in cases of recurrent infections. Herbal ingredients are astragalus, echinacea, liquorice and marigold, with slippery elm which will ease digestion. It also contains zinc salts, vitamin A and bromelain extracted from pineapple – another digestive remedy.

Dosage: 1 capsule twice a day.

BIOCARE

BIOCARE CANDICIDIN

A food supplement intended as part of a yeast-free diet, it contains extracts of oregano, clove, wormwood and ginger which all act on the digestive tract, along with borage oil as a rich source of *gamma*-linolenic acid. The mixture is in a base of grapeseed oil and lauric acid – a coconut extract which also supports the gut flora.
• Not to use in pregnancy or if pregnancy is planned; not to use in cases of intestinal ulceration and gastritis.

Dosage: 1 capsule twice a day.

BIOCARE

BIOCARE CANDISTATIN

A combination of anti-fungal and digestive stimulant herbs to improve the general quality of the gut flora. The supplement is used in anti-candida treatments and contains pau d'arco, garlic, barberry, golden seal and milk thistle.
• Not for use in pregnancy or if pregnancy is planned.

Dosage: 1 capsule three times a day.

BIOCARE

BIOCARE CELERY SEED

Unlicensed simple celery seed capsules; each contains extracts equivalent to 2.5 g.

Dosage: 1 capsule twice a day.

BIOCARE

BIOCARE CITRIMAX FORTE

Like other products containing extracts of Malabar tamarind, this is targeted at those trying to lose weight. The capsules also contain pantothenic acid, vitamin C, manganese and chromium salts.
• Not recommended for those with a history of migraine or citrus allergy

Dosage: 1 tablet three times a day, 30–60 minutes before meals.

BIOCARE

BIOCARE COLON CARE

As its name suggests this supplement is sold as part of a colon improving regime suitable for those with problems of constipation or generally sluggish digestion. Capsules contain isphaghula, golden seal and cascara sagrada so will have a significant laxative effect. They also contain 50 mg of pepsin, a digestive enzyme.
• Do not use in intestinal obstruction.

Dosage: 1 capsule three times a day taken with half a glass of water.

BIOCARE

BIOCARE COQ10 PLUS

A dietary supplement containing 800 mg of linseed oil as a rich source of essential fatty acids. Capsules also contain coenzyme Q10, lecithin and vitamin E.
• Not to be used with anticoagulant drugs, warfarin, heparin, coumarin.

Dosage: 1 capsule daily.

BIOCARE

BIOCARE CP227

Cranberry extract has been shown to ease symptoms of cystitis and in this supplement it is combined with vitamin C and *Lactobacillus acidophilus* which will help to combat infections and improve the natural gut flora.

Dosage: 1 level teaspoon mixed with water, twice a day.

BIOCARE

BIOCARE DERMASORB

An unlicensed cream combining tea tree with *Lactobacillus acidophilus* – the friendly bacteria found in our guts – that could help to discourage opportunist skin infection by yeasts.
• External use only.

BIOCARE

BIOCARE EFA COMPLEX

A combination of essential fatty acids derived from linseed oil with *gamma*-linolenic acid from an unnamed source. The capsules also contain lecithin and vitamin E.
• Not to be used with anticoagulant drugs, warfarin, heparin, coumarin or in epilepsy.

Dosage: 1 capsule twice a day.

BIOCARE

BIOCARE EPO

Capsules containing 250 mg of evening primrose oil providing 20 mg of *gamma*-linolenic acid.

Dosage: 1 capsule daily.

BIOCARE

BIOCARE ERADICIDIN FORTE

This supplement contains sweet Annie which has some anti-bacterial action along with barberry – a bitter digestive stimulant – and grapefruit seeds which are anti-fungal. It comes from a range of products aimed at supporting the gut flora.

Dosage: 1 capsule, three times a day.

BIOCARE

BIOCARE GARLICIN

An unlicensed simple garlic supplement with 400 g of freeze-dried garlic concentrate which is said to be rich in allicin and alliin.
• BioCare's Garlicin Plus also contains 200µg of biotin which is anti-fungal.

Dosage: 1 capsule daily with the evening meal.

BIOCARE

BIOCARE GASTROPLEX

Primarily aimed at easing indigestion this product contains slippery elm and marshmallow. Capsules also include a substance called *gamma*-oryzanol which stimulates the digestive enzymes.

Dosage: 1 capsule three times a day.

BIOCARE

BIOCARE GINKGO PLUS

Unlicensed supplement containing ginkgo and bilberry flavonoids which could help the circulation. It also includes vitamin C and potassium.

Dosage: 1 capsule, three times a day.

BIOCARE

BIOCARE LINSEED OIL 1000 MG

A supplement containing 1 g of linseed oil as a source of essential fatty acids, as well as lecithin and vitamin E.
• Not to be used with anticoagulant drugs, warfarin, heparin, coumarin.

Dosage: 1 capsule twice daily.

BIOCARE

BIOCARE LINSEED OIL 500 MG

A supplement containing 500 mg of linseed oil as a source of essential fatty acids, as well as lecithin, vitamin E and a little olive oil.
• Not to be used with anticoagulant drugs, warfarin, heparin, coumarin.

Dosage: 1 capsule, twice daily.

BIOCARE

BIOCARE LIV243

A digestive stimulant combining a mixture of enzymes and primarily liver herbs, this supplement contains extracts of greater celandine, fringe tree, dandelion and globe artichoke, all of which have a good cleansing and stimulating effect on the liver and gall bladder. The capsules also contain amylase, lipase, protease and cellulase.

Dosage: 1 capsule three times a day.

BIOCARE

BIOCARE NEF242

This supplement combines the digestive enzymes amylase, lipase, protease and cellulase, with a selection of diuretic and nutritional herbs that could act as a general tonic for the kidney. These are alfalfa, parsley, horsetail, celery seed and acerola.

Dosage: 1 capsule three times a day between meals.

BIOCARE

BIOCARE OMEGA-PLEX FORTE

This is essentially cold-pressed olive oil with the addition of *gamma*-linolenic acid from an unnamed source, and vitamins A, D and E sold as a general dietary supplement.

Dosage: 1×5 ml teaspoonful mixed into food or used as a salad dressing, daily.

BIOCARE

BIOCARE OXY-B15

A general tonic offering based on Siberian ginseng with the addition of vitamins B_{15} (pangamic acid), C, E and co-enzyme Q10.

Dosage: 1 capsule daily.

BIOCARE

BIOCARE OXYDENT

Both rosemary and thyme oil, contained in this supplement, have been shown to act as strong anti-oxidants clearing free radicals and helping to prevent the ageing of cells. Capsules also contain selenium, vitamin E, a vitamin A analogue and grapeseed oil.

Dosage: 1 capsule daily.

BIOCARE

BIOCARE PARACIDIN

Liquid version of BioCare's Biocidin products (see p. 257) based on grapefruit seed extract.
• Do not use in colitis or ulcerative conditions of the colon.

Dosage: 2 drops twice a day diluted in half a glass of water; it can also be used as a gargle or vaginal douche.

BIOCARE

BIOCARE PHYTOSTEROL COMPLEX

The herbs in this supplement all may have some sort of hormonal action due to the high proportion of plant steroids they contain. These are: hops, celery seed, alfalfa, liquorice and rhubarb. The capsules also contain 5 mg of silica which generally helps to heal and strengthen human tissues.
• Do not use in pregnancy, malignant disease or with high blood pressure.

Dosage: 1 capsule three times a day.

BIOCARE

BIOCARE PROCYDIN

A combination of fruit extracts which are all rich in vitamins, flavonoids and anti-oxidant compounds and could be useful as a dietary supplement. Capsules contain extracts of black cherry, blackberry and bilberry.
• Not suitable for hyperactive children.

Dosage: 1 capsule three times a day.

BIOCARE

BIOCARE PT208

This supplement contains chastetree and motherwort extracts which generally have a hormonal action and may be helpful for menstrual irregularities. It also contains sarsparilla which is primarily an anti-inflammatory, and a mixture of mineral salts, rutin, digestive enzymes, vitamins B, E, and sugars.
• Do not use in pregnancy or hormone related malignancies.

Dosage: 1 capsule twice a day.

BIOCARE

BIOCARE SALICIDIN

This blend of digestive and anti-bacterial herbs could be helpful for a range of digestive upsets including irritable bowel syndrome. The mixture includes white willow, liquorice, golden seal and echinacea along with anti-fungal grapefruit seeds.
• The suppliers recommend that it should not to be used by asthmatics or by individuals allergic to aspirin.

Dosage: 1 capsule three times a day.

BIOCARE

BIOCARE SILYMARIN COMPLEX

This supplement contains a mixture of herbs that have a stimulating and cleansing effect on the liver: milk thistle, turmeric, artichoke and black radish, so it could be a useful supplement in cases of liver sluggishness.
• Not to be used in hepatitis or cancerous conditions of the liver.

Dosage: 1 capsule three times a day.   BIOCARE

BIOCARE UR 228

This product is very similar to BioCare's CP227 product and combines cranberry extract with vitamin C and *Lactobacillus acidophilus* in a capsule rather than powder format.

Dosage: 1 capsule with half a glass of water each morning.

BIOCARE

BIOCOSMETICS STARFLOWER OIL

Capsules containing borage oil (offering 23% *gamma*-linolenic acid) with vitamin E.

Dosage: 2 capsules daily for adults; 1 capsule daily for children.

POWER HEALTH

BIOFORCE ALFAVENA

A combination of herbs rich in minerals and vitamins which could provide a useful source of iron in some types of anaemia. The supplement contains alfalfa, stinging nettle and wild oats.

Dosage: 2–5 tablets daily for adults and 1 or 2 tablets for children.

BIOFORCE

BIOFORCE ARTERIOFORCE

Most Bioforce products are based on fresh herbal tinctures produced in Switzerland. This one is sold in both capsule and liquid format and contains herbs which generally have a beneficial effect on the circulatory system. These are garlic, ramsons, hawthorn and arnica. The mix also includes passion flower which is a sedative and vitamin E which is regarded as beneficial in heart problems.

Dosage: 5–15 drops in water three times a day. Capsules are also available.

BIOFORCE

BIOFORCE BOLDOCYNARA

This mixture contains herbs that are primarily liver and gall bladder stimulants and tonics – globe artichoke, milk thistle, dandelion and boldo – with the addition of a little peppermint which will improve the flavour and act as a carminative for the digestion.

Dosage: 10–15 drops in water three times a day which should be reduced to 5–8 drops if the response is too drastic.

BIOFORCE

BIOFORCE BRONCHOSAN

Another of the Bioforce tincture range, this is a combination of expectorant herbs which would be useful for a wide range of coughs. It includes thyme, white horehound, liquorice, anise and eucalyptus. Less familiar in the UK is the use of ivy and burnet which are continental favourites for coughs and catarrh. Ivy forms a significant proportion of this product and is potentially toxic but the recommended dosage clearly takes this into consideration and should not be exceeded.

Dosage: 10 drops in water three times a day.

BIOFORCE

BIOFORCE CARDIAFORCE

This supplement combines hawthorn and lemon balm as a tonic wine. Hawthorn has a recognised beneficial effect on the heart, helping to regulate function, while lemon balm is largely sedating.

Dosage: 1 tablespoon four times a day in water sweetened with honey or grape sugar.

BIOFORCE

BIOFORCE COMFREY CREAM

An unlicensed cream containing comfrey.
• External use only.

BIOFORCE

BIOFORCE CYSTAFORCE

A combination of Bioforce's fresh Swiss tinctures containing a mixture of diuretics and antispasmodics for the urinary system that could be helpful in conditions like cystitis. The mixture includes the diuretics aspen, bearberry and yarrow, with sweet sumach and St John's wort which are sometimes used for bed wetting problems in children, along with echinacea which is an anti-bacterial, lemon balm (largely calming and sedative), a small amount of deadly nightshade which is a powerful anti-spasmodic, and wild oats – a restoring nervine. Bearberry and echinacea account for some 50% of the combination.

Dosage: 15 drops in water at night.

BIOFORCE

BIOFORCE DBT (DIABETISAN)

This combination of herbal tinctures includes a number of plants with a hypoglycaemic action which could act as a dietary supplement in late-onset diabetes. These are: bilberry, kidney beans, walnut and alfalfa. The mix also contains tormentil which is astringent and immune-stimulant, and bitter cress which is little used by UK herbalists but generally considered a good source of vitamin C so is presumably also supportive of the immune system.

Dosage: 5–10 drops in water three times a day.

BIOFORCE

BIOFORCE DORMEASAN

This supplement contains the classic combination of sedating herbs used in many of the over-the-counter products listed here for anxiety, tension and insomnia: passion flower, hops, and valerian. It also contains wild oats (a good nerve tonic) and lemon balm – sedating and anti-depressant.

Dosage: 10–20 drops in water, three times a day for general use, or 20–30 drops sweetened with honey or sugar at night.

BIOFORCE

BIOFORCE DROSINULA COUGH SYRUP

Sundew is one of the herbalist's most effective expectorants and this product also contains extracts of elecampane and ipecacuanha which are popular herbs for all sorts of coughs and bronchitis. Less familiar is extract of Norway spruce which, like other conifers, has some expectorant properties and ivy which is a strong purgative but is used in parts of Europe in homoeopathic doses for coughs and catarrh.

Dosage: one or two teaspoons every 2–3 hours; 1 teaspoon every 2–3 hours for children aged 6–12.

BIOFORCE

BIOFORCE ECHINACEA CREAM

An unlicensed cream containing echinacea.
• External use only

BIOFORCE

BIOFORCE ECHINAFORCE

Essentially a simple echinacea tincture using *E. purpurea*. The same extract is produced in tablet form.

BIOFORCE

BIOFORCE GARLIC CAPSULES

Unlicensed garlic capsules containing 270 mg of extract.

Dosage: 1–3 capsules, three times a day before meals.

BIOFORCE

BIOFORCE GASTROSAN

A combination in tincture format of largely liver-stimulating herbs that may be helpful for a sluggish digestion and gastric upsets. The mixture contains dandelion, yellow gentian, holy thistle, angelica and centaury which are all bitter digestive stimulants. It also contains lemon balm which has a carminative effect and yarrow, a digestive tonic useful for settling digestion and in gastritis.

Dosage: 20–30 drops in water three times a day before meals.

BIOFORCE

BIOFORCE GINSAVENA

A tincture combining wild oats and ginseng as a generally tonic mixture to combat stress.

Dosage: 10–20 drops in water three times a day.

BIOFORCE

BIOFORCE GINSAVITA

Similar to Bioforce Ginsavena (wild oats and ginseng) only in a tablet form.

Dosage: 2 tablets three times a day.

BIOFORCE

BIOFORCE GOLDEN GRASS TEA

This tea contains silver birch, golden rod and horsetail which are extensively used as diuretics and urinary antiseptics in treating cystitis. Less familiar in the UK is knotweed which is an astringent also used in parts of Europe as a diuretic, and heartsease, largely used in cough and skin remedies but also a cleansing herb with some diuretic action.

Dosage: 1 tablespoon of tea to 500 ml of boiling water. Infuse for 10–20 minutes and drink a little at a time through the day.

BIOFORCE

BIOFORCE HYPERIFORCE

This tincture contains a combination of sedative and anti-depressant herbs: St John's wort, lemon balm and hops and is suggested to "help maintain mood stability". UK herbalists however, generally recommend that hops should be avoided in depression.

Dosage: 30 drops in water three to five times a day.

BIOFORCE

BIOFORCE HYPERISAN

This tincture contains horse chestnut which is generally regarded as a useful tonic for blood vessels and venous circulation; arnica which is rarely used internally in the UK but can be helpful for tissue repair; as well as yarrow and St John's wort which are both anti-inflammatory wound herbs.

Dosage: 10–20 drops in a little water three times a day.

BIOFORCE

BIOFORCE IMP (IMPERTHRITICA)

This tincture is designed to ease arthritis and rheumatism although the combination of herbs it uses derives from central European rather than UK tradition. It uses knotweed, golden rod, yarrow, horsetail and silver birch which are all diuretic, along with butterbur which is an antispasmodic useful in pain relief, and silverweed another antispasmodic used for treating cramping pain. Also in the mixture is homoeopathic extract of autumn crocus which can also ease pain, and mistletoe which may be there to improve the circulation. The tincture includes a small amount of peppermint – probably to improve the flavour.

Bioforce suggests combining this mixture with potato juice to improve efficacy.

Dosage: 5–10 drops in water three times a day, one hour before meals.

BIOFORCE

BIOFORCE KELPASAN

Unlicensed simple kelp tablets derived from the seaweed *Macrocysris pyrfera*.

Dosage: 1 tablet morning and noon before meals.

BIOFORCE

BIOFORCE LINOFORCE

A mixture of laxatives combining bulking herbs like linseed with more irritant ones containing anthraquinones (senna and alder buckthorn). The mix also contains ginger as a carminative to counter griping and it is flavoured with sugar (which also has a laxative effect) and vanilla.

Dosage: 1 teaspoon morning and evening in 500 ml of water.

BIOFORCE

BIOFORCE MENOSAN

Sage tincture as a simple.

Dosage: 15–20 drops in water three times a day.

BIOFORCE

BIOFORCE NEPHROSOLID

This tincture contains a combination of diuretic and urinary antiseptic herbs: golden rod, silver birch, restharrow, horsetail, juniper and knotweed as well as silverweed which is antispasmodic, to relieve cramping, and heartsease which is largely used in cough and skin remedies but is also cleansing with some diuretic action.
• The mixture contains juniper which can irritate the kidneys in prolonged use so should only be taken for short periods.

Dosage: 10–15 drops three times a day in a little water or combined with Bioforce Golden Grass Tea.

BIOFORCE

BIOFORCE NEUROFORCE

This is a similar combination to the same company's Ginsavena product combining wild oats and ginseng as a generally tonic supplement. Tablets also contain calcium and sodium salts, glutamic acid and lecithin as additional nutrients.

Dosage: one or two tablets, three times a day after meals.

BIOFORCE

BIOFORCE PETAFORCE

Unlicensed capsules containing butterbur as a simple.

Dosage: 1 or 2 capsules three times a day.

BIOFORCE

BIOFORCE PETASAN

A tincture combining mistletoe and butterbur which has been used in parts of Europe in cancer therapy and convalescence.

Dosage: 5–10 drops three times a day, half an hour before meals.

BIOFORCE

BIOFORCE PETASAN SYRUP

A traditional European combination for coughs containing butterbur and Norway spruce extracts.

Dosage: 1 or 2 teaspoons three times a day, or as required.

BIOFORCE

BIOFORCE PO HO OIL

A combination of essential oils of peppermint, eucalyptus, juniper, caraway and fennel which have some immune stimulant and anti-catarrhal actions for colds and catarrh. Although essential oils are rarely used internally in the UK, practice is quite different elsewhere in Europe.
• The mixture contains juniper so should be avoided in pregnancy and by those with kidney disease.

Dosage: Bioforce suggests 3–5 drops of the oil in a herb tea as an internal remedy repeated several times a day or in water as a gargle and mouth wash.

BIOFORCE

BIOFORCE PO HO OINTMENT

This is an external version of the Po Ho Oil designed as a chest rub or for topical application for bruises and abrasions. It contains St John's wort, Peruvian balsam and marigold which are antiseptic and healing; witch hazel, also healing and astringent; peppermint which has a stimulating and warming effect on the skin; and citron oil which is an uncommon member of the *Citrus* genus but is similar in action to lemon – useful for countering infections and easing sore throats.
• External use only

BIOFORCE

BIOFORCE PROSTASAN

This tincture contains around 93% of saw palmetto, a herb widely used for treating prostate problems. The herb mix also includes echinacea to counter infection, golden rod (a diuretic) and a small amount of aspen which is diuretic, anti-inflammatory and analgesic.

Dosage: 10–20 drops in water three times a day.

BIOFORCE

BIOFORCE SATASAPINA COUGH BON BONS

A similar mixture to the Satasapina Cough Syrup with the addition of a little peppermint oil as flavouring, honey and pine buds.

Dosage: The bon bons are suitable for adults and children and can be sucked as required.

BIOFORCE

BIOFORCE SATASAPINA COUGH SYRUP

This gentle mixture contains pine extract in a base of pear juice and honey to soothe coughs and sore throats. It is quite safe for children.

Dosage: adults – 1 or 2 teaspoons several times a day; children – half the adult dose.

BIOFORCE

BIOFORCE SEVEN HERB CREAM

An unlicensed general purpose healing cream which may be suitable for a wide range of minor sores and abrasions. It contains extracts of familiar wound herbs like St John's wort, chamomile, marigold, arnica, witch hazel and sage as well as the less common sanicle and paracress derived from central European tradition. The herbs are in a base of lanolin with sunflower and avocado oils.
• External use only.

BIOFORCE

BIOFORCE TORMENTAVENA

This combination of tinctures includes astringent, anti-bacterial and relaxing herbs which are generally used for diarrhoea, gastric upsets and spasmodic cramps. The main ingredient is tormentil (68%) with purple loosestrife, hemp nettle, knotweed and butterbur. A small amount of wild oats extract is also included which may have an uplifting, tonic effect.

Dosage: 20–30 drops in water three to five times a day.

BIOFORCE

BIOFORCE URTICALAN

Basically a homoeopathic calcium supplement using stinging nettles as a mineral source along with various silica, calcium and sodium salts.

Dosage: 2 tablets, three times a day.

BIOFORCE

BIOFORCE USNEASAN COUGH LOZENGES

A combination of expectorant and anti-bacterial herbs for throat infections and coughs. The lozenges are based on liquorice juice with the addition of ribwort plantain, blue flag, Iceland moss, pine, larch and the *Usnea* spp. lichens which give the lozenges their name.

Dosage: 1 lozenge every 1–2 hours.

BIOFORCE

BLACKMORES ALFALFA TABLETS

Unlicensed simple containing 380 mg of alfalfa.

BLACKMORES

BLACKMORES CACTUS & HAWTHORN

These tablets contain extracts of night-blooming cactus and hawthorn which are both effective heart tonics. Watercress and bearberry are included as diuretics, which can be helpful for high blood pressure, and the mixture also includes cola which is rich in caffeine and so has a stimulating effect on the heart.

BLACKMORES

BLACKMORES CAPE ALOES AND CASCARA

As the name implies, this is largely a combination of laxative herbs: aloes, senna and cascara sagrada, with the addition of ginger, cardamom and peppermint which are all carminatives to counter griping.

BLACKMORES

BLACKMORES CELERY COMPLEX

The herbs in this product are traditional cleansing remedies used in preparations for arthritis: celery seed, guaiacum, burdock and stinging nettle. The product also contains echinacea which is sometimes included in arthritis remedies to counter any possible infection that may be contributing to the condition.

BLACKMORES

BLACKMORES CORNSILK COMPLEX

This is a combination of urinary antiseptics and diuretic herbs which would be relevant for treating such problems as cystitis. The mixture includes buchu, bearberry and couch grass.

BLACKMORES

BLACKMORES DANDELION COMPLEX

The herbs in this mixture all have an effect on the liver as cleansing remedies and tonics. It includes dandelion, barberry, yellow gentian, boldo and centaury which produce a bitter and stimulating mix.

BLACKMORES

BLACKMORES ECHINACEA COMPLEX

As well as echinacea this combination includes herbs that are generally regarded as cleansing and helpful for skin problems: red clover, sarsparilla, burdock and yellow dock.

BLACKMORES

BLACKMORES EUPHORBIA COMPLEX

Pill-bearing spurge (*Euphorbia* spp.) is generally regarded as an effective expectorant for asthma and bronchitis. In this product it is combined with gumplant, senega and liquorice to make a powerful combination for stubborn coughs. The mixture also includes ginger, which can combat nausea and is a warming herb for lung problems.

BLACKMORES

BLACKMORES GARLIX

This is a strong garlic product with the equivalent of 2 g of freeze-dried garlic per tablet. This is not deodorized in any way but is in an enteric coating which will help to reduce initial garlic smells.

BLACKMORES

BLACKMORES GINGER TABLETS (TRAVEL CALM)

Unlicensed simple containing 400 mg of ginger per capsule. It is said to be suitable for both children and adults.

BLACKMORES

BLACKMORES HYPERICUM

Unlicensed simple containing 400 mg of St John's wort per capsule.

BLACKMORES

BLACKMORES LIQUORICE COMPLEX

This is a combination of potent expectorants – senega, gumplant and liquorice – with soothing demulcents (marshmallow and slippery elm) that could be helpful to loosen tight coughs.

BLACKMORES

BLACKMORES ODOURLESS GARLIC

A garlic product that becomes "odourless" thanks to the addition of parsley (20 mg to 10 mg of garlic extract) rather than by a reduction in beneficial sulphur compounds. It is said to be suitable for both children and adults.

BLACKMORES

BLACKMORES RASPBERRY LEAF

Unlicensed simple containing 300 mg raspberry leaf. Dolomite is also included largely to bind the tablet.
• Raspberry leaf should not be taken during pregnancy until the last weeks.

BLACKMORES

BLACKMORES ROSEHIPS

A vitamin C supplement combining 450 mg of rosehips with fruit sugar and dolomite to bind the tablet. It is said to be suitable for both adults and children.

BLACKMORES

BLACKMORES SARSPARILLA COMPLEX

The herbs in this mixture are largely cleansing remedies used for skin problems: they include sarsparilla, yellow dock, stinging nettle and queen's delight. Such disorders often respond to liver-stimulating remedies and the mixture includes greater celandine which is often used in this way. The product also contains sassafras which is rarely used these days because of concerns over its toxicity.

BLACKMORES

BLACKMORES SKULLCAP & VALERIAN

Both skullcap and valerian are, of course, excellent sedatives to counter tension and anxiety. The product also includes passion flower and hops (also effective sedatives) and includes yellow gentian and cayenne which would have a more stimulating, warming effect. The formula is marketed as "Nervaids" in Australia.

BLACKMORES

BLACKMORES SLIPPERY ELM

Unlicensed simple containing 350 mg of slippery elm. Tablets also include 125 mg of dolomite as a binding agent.

Dosage: 1 or 2 tablets before meals with 1–2 glasses for water as slippery elm absorbs intestinal fluids.

BLACKMORES

BLACKMORES VALERIAN COMPLEX

A traditional combination of relaxing and sedative herbs which could be used to counter tensions and stress. It includes valerian, passion flower, hops and skullcap as well as black haw which is generally used for relaxing sore muscles and relieving pain but (like its relative cramp bark) also has a calming effect on the nerves.

BLACKMORES

*BOX'S FAR FAMED INDIGESTION TABLETS

A licensed product for the symptomatic relief of indigestion this contains a combination of carminatives, digestive stimulants and laxatives. It is largely made up of ginger, cayenne and aloes, as well as yellow gentian, myrrh – both extremely bitter and thus stimulating for the digestion – and cajuput oil which is an antispasmodic used in aromatherapy for gastric upsets.

• Not recommended in pregnancy and when breast feeding.

Dosage: 1 or 2 tablets night and morning, after meals.

RICKARD LANE'S & W H BOX

BUMBLES PROPOLIS, ANISEED & LIQUORICE LOZENGES

An unlicensed combination of liquorice and aniseed with propolis. Liquorice is expectorant, soothing and demulcent for sore throats and coughs while aniseed is also an expectorant and is often used as a flavouring.

Dosage: adults and children over five years – 1 lozenge as required.

POWER HEALTH

BUMBLES PROPOLIS, MENTHOL & EUCALYPTUS LOZENGES

An unlicensed combination of menthol and eucalyptus with propolis. Eucalyptus can be helpful for catarrh and sore throats while menthol is one of the active constituents of peppermint and is potentially irritant for the gastric lining so should not be given to small children.

Dosage: adults – not more than 6 in 24 hours; children over 12 years – not more than 3 in 24 hours.

POWER HEALTH

CANTASSIUM AGNUS CASTUS

Unlicensed simple containing 500 mg of chastetree per capsule.

LARKHALL GREEN FARM

*CANTASSIUM BOLDO AID

A licensed remedy for the treatment of occasional water retention. This product largely comprises diuretics – boldo, clivers, dandelion and bearberry – with the addition of bladderwrack which is a metabolic stimulant.
• Not recommended in pregnancy or for children. Overdose may cause nausea and vomiting.

Dosage: 1 or 2 tablets, three times a day with water.

LARKHALL GREEN FARM

CANTASSIUM CONCENTRATED CRANBERRY

Unlicensed tablets containing 400 mg of cranberry concentrate with an additional 20 mg of vitamin C.

Dosage: 1 tablet, morning and evening.

LARKHALL GREEN FARM

CANTASSIUM DIDAMEGA

A mixture of largely anti-fungal and anti-bacterial herbs combined with caprylic acid, vitamins, minerals, amino acids and friendly gut bacteria that could be used as a nutritional supplement for those on a yeast-free diet. Herbs used are: garlic, pau d'arco, echinacea and feverfew.

Dosage: 1 to 3 tablets daily.

LARKHALL GREEN FARM

CANTASSIUM ECHINACEA 500

Unlicensed simple containing 200 mg of echinacea powder and extracts.

Dosage: 1 to 3 tablets daily.

LARKHALL GREEN FARM

CANTASSIUM EVENING GOLD

Evening primrose oil sold in 15 ml phials which can be used directly on the skin or taken internally (one drop is equivalent to 50 mg of oil).

LARKHALL GREEN FARM

CANTASSIUM GARLIC OIL CAPSULES

Unlicensed simple containing the equivalent of 660 mg of fresh garlic per capsule.

LARKHALL GREEN FARM

CANTASSIUM GARLIMEGA 2000

Unlicensed simple containing the equivalent of 2 g of fresh garlic per capsule.

Dosage: 1 capsule per day.

LARKHALL GREEN FARM

CANTASSIUM GINKGO 2000

Unlicensed simple containing the equivalent of 2 g of ginkgo leaf per capsule.

Dosage: 1 or 2 tablets daily

LARKHALL GREEN FARM

*CANTASSIUM HAY FEVER

A licensed product for the symptomatic relief of hayfever and summer catarrh. It contains a combination of anti-catarrhal, anti-inflammatory and antispasmodic herbs – sage, white horehound, yarrow, indian tobacco, and boneset – with the addition of some warming cayenne and vervain which, amongst other things, is a liver tonic. Liver remedies are often included in hay fever treatments to help strengthen and cleanse the system.

Dosage: adults – 1 or 2 tablets, three times a day; children – 1 tablet three times a day.

LARKHALL GREEN FARM

CANTASSIUM MICRO GARLIC

Unlicensed garlic tablets in a mini-size format for children and those who find it difficult to swallow pills.

LARKHALL GREEN FARM

*CANTASSIUM QUIET DAYS

Licensed product for the symptomatic relief of mild anxiety – although it is currently sold only as a food supplement. The tablets contain a popular combination of sedative herbs: valerian, skullcap and hops.

Dosage: 1 or 2 tablets per day.

LARKHALL GREEN FARM

*CANTASSIUM QUIET NITE SLEEP

A licensed product for the treatment of occasional insomnia. Tablets contain some of the most widely used sedative herbs – valerian, hops, chamomile and passion flower – with the addition of wild lettuce which is a good soporific.

Dosage: 2 or 3 tablets at night.

LARKHALL GREEN FARM

*CANTASSIUM QUIET TYME

Licensed product for the symptomatic relief of mild anxiety which contains the popular combination of valerian, skullcap, hops and passion flower.
• Not recommended for children.

Dosage: 2 tablets, three times a day.

LARKHALL GREEN FARM

CANTASSIUM RED GINSENG 600

Unlicensed simple containing the equivalent of 500 mg of ginseng.

Dosage: 1 or 2 tablets per day.

LARKHALL GREEN FARM

CANTASSIUM RED PANAX GINSENG

Unlicensed simple containing the equivalent of 500 mg of ginseng.

Dosage: 1 or 2 tablets per day.

LARKHALL GREEN FARM

*CANTASSIUM RHEUMATIC PAIN

A licensed product for the symptomatic relief of pain in musculo-skeletal disorders. It includes herbs regularly used for treating rheumatism and arthritis – guaiacum, celery and bogbean – with the addition of dandelion as a cleansing diuretic.
• Not recommended for children.

Dosage: 1 or 2 tablets after each meal.

LARKHALL GREEN FARM

CANTASSIUM TONG KWAI

Unlicensed simple containing the equivalent of 600 mg of *Dang Gui.*

Dosage: 3 tablets daily.

LARKHALL GREEN FARM

*CANTASSIUM TRAVEL SICKNESS

Licensed product for the relief of travel sickness and nausea. Each capsule contains 250 mg ginger.

Dosage: adults – 3 tablets; children aged six to 12 years – 1 or 2 tablets all to be taken half an hour before travelling.

LARKHALL GREEN FARM

*CATARRHEEZE

A licensed product for the relief of nasal congestion containing white horehound, elecampane and yarrow. Both white horehound and elecampane are also expectorants used in cough remedies.

Dosage: adults – 2 tablets three times a day; children aged five to 12 years – 1 tablet three times a day.

ENGLISH GRAINS HEALTHCARE

CHIRALI OLD REMEDY STRAIN & SPRAIN CREAM

An unlicensed cream containing oils traditionally used for muscular aches and pains, and rheumatism. It includes wintergreen, thyme and eucalyptus essential oils with bay, which is less commonly used but was once popular for sprains and bruises, and evening primrose oil which provides important nutrients.

EAST WEST HERBS

CITRI-TRIM

An unlicensed slimming product based on the Malabar taramind.

HEALTH PLUS

*COLDEEZE

This product contains two very common herbal ingredients – garlic and echinacea – and is licensed for the symptomatic relief of bronchial cough, respiratory catarrh, rhinitis, colds and influenza. The same herbs are included in similar products licensed for skin problems.

Dosage: 2 tablets three times a day.

ENGLISH GRAINS HEALTHCARE

COLON CLEANSE

A combination of fruit fibre extracts (apple and beetroot) plus herbs and *Lactobacillus acidophilus* bacteria suggested as a cleansing remedy for the digestive system. Although the herbal mix includes rhubarb, it is not a strongly laxative combination, focusing more on general liver and digestive tonics and carminatives. Other herbs in the mixture are walnut, red clover, chamomile, dandelion, agrimony, fennel and milk thistle.

Dosage: 1 or 2 capsules daily after meals; up to three times a day.

LAMBERTS HEALTHCARE

*COUGHEEZE

A licensed remedy for the relief of chesty, productive coughs, this product contains a combination of expectorants: ipecacuanha, white horehound and elecampane.

Dosage: adults – 2 tablets three times a day; children aged eight to 12 years – 1 tablet three times a day.

ENGLISH GRAINS HEALTHCARE

*CULPEPER BALM OF GILEAD COUGH MIXTURE

A licensed remedy for the symptomatic relief of coughs, this contains balm of gilead which is a pleasant tasting herb often included in cough products for children. It also includes squill vinegar which is a rather more potent expectorant, lungwort and Indian tobacco (an antispasmodic and expectorant).

Dosage: adults – 2 × 5 ml teaspoons three or four times a day; children over 5 years –1 × 5 ml teaspoon every three hours.

CULPEPER

*CULPEPER COMFREY OINTMENT

This particular comfrey ointment is licensed so can claim effectiveness for the relief of bruises, sprains and strains. It should be applied to affected areas two or three times a day.

• External use only.

CULPEPER

*CULPEPER COUGH RELIEF MIXTURE

A licensed remedy for coughs, this mixture contains expectorants – pill-bearing purge and gumplant – often used by herbalists to treat asthma and bronchitis. It also contains lungwort, liquorice and pleurisy root which are all also highly expectorant and soothing, and aniseed oil which will improve the flavour and provide additional expectorant action.

Dosage: adults 1 or 2 × 5 ml teaspoons three times a day; children over 5 years – 1 × 5 ml teaspoon three times a day.

CULPEPER

*CULPEPER ELDER FLOWER AND PEPPERMINT MIXTURE

A licensed combination for the symptomatic relief of colds, chills and influenza. As well as elder and peppermint the mixture includes warming herbs like bayberry, hemlock spruce, cayenne, cassia oil and ginger which is very similar to the equivalent Potter's product. It also includes pimento oil *(Pimenta dioica)* which is from the same plant that produces allspice used in cooking. This herb is largely used for indigestion but is also warming and stimulating and is sometimes included in external chest rubs for coughs and colds.

Dosage: adults and children over eight years – 2 × 5 ml teaspoons in a third of a cup of warm water, three times a day.

CULPEPER

CULPEPER EVENING PRIMROSE CAPSULES

Unlicensed capsules containing evening primrose oil.

CULPEPER

CULPEPER FEVERFEW TABLETS

Unlicensed simple containing 200 mg of feverfew per tablet.

CULPEPER

CULPEPER GARLIC CAPSULES

Unlicensed simple capsules containing garlic extract.

Dosage: 3 capsules per day.

CULPEPER

CULPEPER GINGER ROOT CAPSULES

Unlicensed simple containing 300 mg of ginger per capsule.

Dosage: 3 capsules half an hour before a journey; repeat after two or three hours if necessary.

CULPEPER

CULPEPER GINSENG CAPSULES

Unlicensed simple containing 460 mg of ginseng per capsule.

Dosage: 1 capsule each morning, taken for a month at a time.

*CULPEPER HAEMORRHOIDAL OINTMENT

A licensed ointment for the symptomatic relief of piles, this contains pilewort as a simple. It should be applied to the affected area two or three times a day.
• External use only.

*CULPEPER HEAD COLD AND THROAT MIXTURE

A licensed remedy for the symptomatic relief of head colds, sore throats and associated headaches, this contains a warming combination of herbs which are largely antispasmodic and anti-bacterial including cayenne, Indian tobacco, myrrh and camphor. It also contains skunk cabbage which is an expectorant, and skullcap: although this herb is largely regarded as a sedative it is also cooling and has a traditional role in the treatment of fevers. American valerian is largely a sedative and antispasmodic but because of increasing concerns of its rarity this plant is little used these days.

Dosage: adults – 1 × 5 ml teaspoon every three hours; children over eight years – 1 × 5 ml teaspoon, once a day.

*CULPEPER HEALING OINTMENT

A licensed ointment containing eucalyptus and camphor as a warming rub for the relief of muscular stiffness, sprains, strains and muscular aches and pains. The product also contains colophony resin extracted from long leaf pine *(Pinus palustris)* which is distilled to produce turpentine. Like other pine oils, this extract can be helpful for muscular aches and pains.

*CULPEPER HERBAL MIXTURE FOR ACIDITY, INDIGESTION AND FLATULENCE

A licensed remedy for the symptomatic relief of acidity, indigestion and flatulence which contains herbs also regularly used for treating stomach upsets and gastritis. These include marshmallow, meadowsweet, dandelion, liquorice and aniseed oil.

Dosage: 1 × 5 ml teaspoonful every three hours.

*CULPEPER HERBAL TONIC FOR DIGESTIVE DISORDERS

Described as "a licensed remedy for the symptomatic relief of stomach discomfort dues to the stresses and strains of everyday life" this is a mixture of wild oats, yellow gentian and cola. Wild oats are largely considered as a good anti-depressant and tonic for the nervous system while yellow gentian and cola are both digestive stimulants.

Dosage: 1 × 5 ml teaspoon every three hours.

CULPEPER

*CULPEPER INFLUENZA MIXTURE

A licensed remedy for influenza and the common cold this is a combination of warming herbs, anti-catarrhals and expectorants providing a broad spectrum of symptomatic relief. It contains: bayberry, boneset, white horehound, hemlock spruce, pleurisy root, clove oil, cassia oil, cayenne and ginger.

Dosage: adults and children over eight years – 1 × 5 ml teaspoonful in water every four hours.

CULPEPER

*CULPEPER PARSLEY PIERT TABLETS

A licensed product for urinary problems that includes parsley piert, buchu, bearberry and dandelion, herbs used in treating infections and inflammations (such as cystitis) and urinary stones.

Dosage: adults – 1 or 2 tablets, three times a day; elderly – 1 tablet three times a day.

CULPEPER

CULPEPER PASSIFLORA TABLETS

Unlicensed simple containing the equivalent of 180 mg of passion flower.

Dosage: 2 tablets three times a day for daytime use; 2 tablets at tea-time and 2 at bedtime for night time use.

CULPEPER

CULPEPER PILEWORT TABLETS

This product contains pilewort and agrimony which are both astringent and used in treating piles along with stone root and cascara sagrada which are laxatives used in constipation.

Dosage: 2 tablets three times a day for a minimum of 10 days.

CULPEPER

*CULPEPER RHEUMATIC TABLETS

A licensed remedy to relieve rheumatism which contains agrimony, guaiacum and garlic. This is an unusual combination but contains herbs that are diuretic and cleansing to help clear toxins which may be contributing to the problem.

Dosage: 1 tablet three times a day.

CULPEPER

CULPEPER SEAWEED TABLETS

Unlicensed combination of kelp and bladderwrack.

Dosage: 1 table three times a day.

CULPEPER

CULPEPER VALERIAN TABLETS

Unlicensed simple tablets each containing 150 mg of valerian.

Dosage: 1 or 2 tablets, three times a day for daytime use; 2–4 tablets at bedtime if required.

CULPEPER

DISCOVERY COLICLENS

A cleansing mixture for the digestive system containing the bulking laxative isphaghula, blessed thistle (largely used as a liver and digestive stimulant) and yellow dock which is laxative along with potassium bicarbonate, vitamin C and assorted minerals from Dead Sea extracts.

FINDERS INTERNATIONAL

*DORWEST DAMIANA AND KOLA TABLETS

A licensed remedy for the symptomatic relief of fatigue, this product contains cola which is rich in caffeine and thus very stimulating, along with the tonic herbs damiana and saw palmetto which are also often used in aphrodisiac preparations.

Dosage: 2–3 tablets as required.

DORWEST HERBS

*DORWEST DIGESTIVE TABLETS

A licensed remedy for indigestion, heartburn, hyperacidity and nausea this product contains golden seal which will stimulate the liver and tonify the digestion, rhubarb (a laxative), carminative ginger and valerian which is generally regarded as a tranquilliser but is also carminative and antispasmodic for digestive problems.

Dosage: 1 tablet after meals.

DORWEST HERBS

*DORWEST GARLIC AND FENUGREEK TABLETS

A licensed remedy for the common cold, coughs and catarrh, containing garlic and fenugreek. Garlic is highly anti-bacterial while fenugreek is warming and expectorant.

Dosage: 3 tablets at night.

DORWEST HERBS

*DORWEST KELP SEAWEED

A licensed remedy for rheumatic pain and to regulate weight containing 170 mg of bladderwrack.

Dosage: 2 tablets twice a day.

DORWEST HERBS

*DORWEST MIXED VEGETABLE TABLETS

A licensed remedy for "rheumatic pain and to improve urinary function" containing a combination of diuretics – watercress, celery and parsley – with horseradish which is warming, stimulating and also diuretic.

Dosage: 2 tablets twice a day.

DORWEST HERBS

*DORWEST NATURAL HERB TABLETS

A combination of mainly laxative herbs licensed as a remedy for constipation and including senna, aloes, cascara sagrada and dandelion root. The mix also contains valerian which is generally regarded as a tranquilliser but is also carminative and helpful to ease intestinal cramps.

Dosage: 2 tablets at night.

DORWEST HERBS

*DORWEST SCULLCAP AND GENTIAN TABLETS

This remedy contains the sedative herbs valerian, vervain, and skullcap, and is licensed to relieve irritability and insomnia. It also contains yellow gentian which is a digestive stimulant and tonic.

Dosage: 3 tablets three times a day.

DORWEST HERBS

DR SHIR'S LINIMENT

An unlicensed liniment containing a mixture of herbs traditionally used in Chinese medicine to relieve sprains, strains and arthritic pains. These are: rhubarb, safflower, myrrh, arisaema, persica, *Dang Gui,* turmeric, and camphor as well as dragon's bone and mastic (see Amber Massage Salve). It should be massaged gently into affected areas daily for 20–30 minutes
• Not to be used on open lesions; external use only.

SPRING WIND HERBS (EAST WEST HERBS IN THE UK)

EAST WEST AMACHAZURU TEA

A tea containing dried amachazuru as a simple.

EAST-WEST HERBS

EAST WEST JU HUA TEA

A tea containing dried chrysanthemum flowers as a simple.

EAST–WEST HERBS

EAST WEST SHI HU AND GAN CAO TEA

A tea containing a combination of suk gok and liquorice.

EAST-WEST HERBS

ECHINEX

Echinacea as a 10:1 simple tincture.

Dosage: 20 drops three times a day, neat or diluted in water.

ORTIS

EFACAL

A combination targeted at the menopausal market containing 400 mg of evening primrose oil, 100 mg of calcium and 44 mg of fish oil per capsule.

Dosage: 4 capsules each evening for 12 weeks followed by 2 capsules each evening.

EFAMOL

EFALEX

This is an interesting combination of evening primrose oil, thyme oil and fish oils which has been tested as a supplement for children suffering from dyslexia and an inability to concentrate. Recent research suggests that these problems could be associated with an imbalance of lipids (fatty substances) within the body, which early work suggests can be improved by the oils used in this product. Reports of the results have been impressive.

Dosage: 8 capsules a day for up to three months, then 4 capsules a day.

EFAMOL

EFAMOL MARINE

A supplement containing 430 mg of evening primrose oil with 107 mg of fish oil per capsule. A "high strength" version containing twice as much oil per capsule is also available.

Dosage: 8 capsules a day for up to 12 weeks followed by 2 capsules a day.

EFAMOL

EFAMOL ORIGINAL

Efamol produces evening primrose oil in a variety of formats, generally with the addition of vitamins C and E which act as anti-oxidants and preservatives. The oil is available in dropper bottles as well as 500 mg and 1000 mg capsules.

Dosage: Oil – half a teaspoonful daily for 12 weeks then reduced to a quarter of a teaspoonful; topical application as required.
Capsules: 3 capsules per day for 12 weeks then reduced to 1 capsule per day.

EFAMOL

EFAMOL ORIGINAL HIGH STRENGTH PRE-MENSTRUAL PACK

This product combines Efamol Original evening primrose oil (1000 mg) with Efavite tablets containing vitamins C and B_6, niacin and zinc in a ten-day course to be taken each month before menstruation.

EFAMOL

EFAMOL PLUS

A dietary supplement in two versions containing evening primrose oil combined with either multivitamins and minerals, or fish oil and co-enzyme Q10.

Dosage: 1 capsule daily

EFAMOL

EFAMOL WITH SAFFLOWER AND LINSEED OILS

While evening primrose is a good source of *gamma*-linolenic acid, nutritionists also point to the body's need for *alpha*-linolenic and *cis*-linoleic acids. This multi-oil product combines all three with the addition of vitamin E as an anti-oxidant.

Dosage: 4 capsules daily for the first 12 weeks, followed by 2 capsules daily.

EFAMOL

EQUILLENCE

A combination of royal jelly and eight Chinese herbs frequently used for menopausal and menstrual irregularities: Chinese foxglove *(Sheng Di Huang),* *Dang Gui,* chrysanthemum, paeony (white), tuckahoe *(Fu Shen),* glossy privet, Chinese dates and spatholobus. The product is designed to be taken by menopausal women.

REGINA

*FO TI TIENG

A licensed product, based on a traditional combination, for use as a general tonic and pick-me-up. It contains cola, meadowsweet and gotu kola.

Dosage: adults – 1 capsule three times a day; children over 12 years – 1 capsule daily

JESSOP MARKETING

FRANK ROBERTS ACIDOSIS TABLETS

A combination of carminatives and soothing gastric herbs that could be useful for indigestion. The mixture includes meadowsweet, cinnamon, cardamom, caraway and aniseed with rhubarb (a laxative) and charcoal which is sometimes included in herbal stomach mixtures to absorb excessive acid.

Dosage: 2 or 3 tablets three times a day.

FRANK ROBERTS HERBAL DISPENSARIES

FRANK ROBERTS AGNUS CASTUS TABLETS

An unlicensed simple containing chastetree.

Dosage: 2 tablets three times a day.

FRANK ROBERTS HERBAL DISPENSARIES

FRANK ROBERTS ALCHEMILLA COMPOUND

The herbs in this unlicensed mixture are traditionally used to relieve menstrual disorders – lady's mantle, motherwort, helonias and pulsatilla – with the addition of valerian and vervain which are calming and sedative.
• Not to be taken in pregnancy.

Dosage: 2 tablets three times a day.

FRANK ROBERTS HERBAL DISPENSARIES

*FRANK ROBERTS ALTHAEA COMPOUND TABLETS

A licensed remedy for use in gastritis and irritable bowel syndrome. It contains meadowsweet, liquorice, slippery elm and marshmallow: herbs that are soothing for the gastric mucosa and are also antacid and anti-inflammatory.

Dosage: 2 tablets three times a day.

FRANK ROBERTS HERBAL DISPENSARIES

*FRANK ROBERTS ANTI-IRRITANT OINTMENT

A licensed ointment containing pilewort, zinc oxide, sulphur and menthol (a peppermint extract) intended for use on irritating piles.
• External use only.

FRANK ROBERTS HERBAL DISPENSARIES

*FRANK ROBERTS AVEXAN TABLETS

A licensed mixture of wild oats (a nerve tonic and anti-depressant) with prickly ash bark which is generally warming and stimulant. The mixture is recommended to counter mental fatigue and overwork.

Dosage: 1 tablet four times a day.

FRANK ROBERTS HERBAL DISPENSARIES

*FRANK ROBERTS B & L TABLETS

This product is now licensed as a laxative for constipation although in the past it has been promoted as a more specific remedy for the liver and gall bladder. The herbs it contains include black root, a liver stimulant and purgative, as well as the laxatives aloes, rhubarb and cascara sagrada. Cayenne is included as a warming stimulant with ginger as a carminative in order to counter griping.

Dosage: 1 tablet twice a day.

FRANK ROBERTS HERBAL DISPENSARIES

*FRANK ROBERTS BLACK ROOT COMPOUND TABLETS

This is a licensed product containing herbs that are stimulating for the liver and gall bladder – black root, fringe tree bark and wahoo – along with cayenne and ginger which are both warming and stimulating. The mixture is now recommended for the relief of "indigestion, nausea and colic associated with fatty meals".

Dosage: 2 tablets three times a day.

FRANK ROBERTS HERBAL DISPENSARIES

FRANK ROBERTS BLACK WILLOW COMPOUND TABLETS

This unlicensed mixture contains corn silk, buchu and parsley piert which are largely diuretic for use in a number of urinary problems. The mix also includes black willow which, like white willow, is considered as an analgesic and anti-inflammatory, golden seal (also anti-inflammatory) and helonias which is usually considered as a remedy for menstrual disorders but was used in traditional Native American medicine for urinary problems as well.

Dosage: 2 tablets, three times a day.

FRANK ROBERTS HERBAL DISPENSARIES

FRANK ROBERTS BP TABLETS

An unlicensed combination of herbs that can be used in treating high blood pressure and related disorders: yarrow, lime flowers, valerian and motherwort.

Dosage: Dosage: 2 tablets, three times a day.

FRANK ROBERTS HERBAL DISPENSARIES

*FRANK ROBERTS BUCHU BACKACHE COMPOUND TABLETS

A licensed product for treating backache which is associated with urinary dysfunction. It contains the diuretics and urinary antiseptics buchu, bearberry and parsley piert.

Dosage: 2 tablets three times a day.

FRANK ROBERTS HERBAL DISPENSARIES

FRANK ROBERTS CADE OIL OINTMENT

An unlicensed ointment containing cade oil (an extract made from juniper twigs traditionally used for psoriasis), witch hazel and zinc oxide.
• External use only.

FRANK ROBERTS HERBAL DISPENSARIES

FRANK ROBERTS CAJUPUT RUB

An unlicensed rub containing cajuput, cayenne and camphor – all traditionally used for rheumatism and muscular aches and pains – as well as methyl salicylate which is often used as a substitute for wintergreen.
• External use only.

FRANK ROBERTS HERBAL DISPENSARIES

*FRANK ROBERTS CALMANITE TABLETS

A licensed combination to treat sleeplessness associated with tension and stress. It contains a popular combination of herbs – hops, passion flower, pasque flower, wild lettuce and valerian – which are found in a number of similar products.

Dosage: 2 or 3 tablets 30 minutes before bedtime.

FRANK ROBERTS HERBAL DISPENSARIES

*FRANK ROBERTS CATARRH TABLETS

A licensed remedy for catarrh containing Indian tobacco, pokeroot and echinacea. Echinacea is, of course, anti-bacterial while Indian tobacco is largely regarded as antispasmodic and can relieve coughing. Pokeroot is anti-catarrhal.

Dosage: 1 or 2 tablets three times a day.

FRANK ROBERTS HERBAL DISPENSARIES

*FRANK ROBERTS COLD TABLETS

One of Frank Roberts' traditional remedies dating back around 50 years, this licensed product contains a warming combination of anti-catarrhals and expectorants for treating colds and influenza. It contains elder flowers, ipecacuanha, poplar, yarrow and cayenne.

Dosage: 1 tablet three times a day.

FRANK ROBERTS HERBAL DISPENSARIES

FRANK ROBERTS COMFREY OINTMENT

An unlicensed simple ointment containing comfrey.
• External use only.

FRANK ROBERTS HERBAL DISPENSARIES

FRANK ROBERTS CONSTIPATION TABLETS

An unlicensed combination of the laxatives aloes, cascara, sagrada and senna with the addition of valerian.

Dosage: 1 or 2 tablets each day; double this quantity if necessary.

FRANK ROBERTS HERBAL DISPENSARIES

*FRANK ROBERTS CRANESBILL COMPOUND TABLETS

This product used to be promoted as a remedy for duodenal ulcers although the current licence only permits it to claim efficacy in the "symptomatic relief of digestive disorders". It contains an American cranesbill, which is an astringent herb, with slippery elm and marshmallow which both act as soothing demulcents for gastric inflammations. Echinacea is included to counter infection.

Dosage: 3 tablets three times a day.

FRANK ROBERTS HERBAL DISPENSARIES

FRANK ROBERTS DEVIL'S CLAW TABLETS

An unlicensed simple containing the equivalent of 820 mg of devil's claw per tablet.

FRANK ROBERTS HERBAL DISPENSARIES

*FRANK ROBERTS DROPS OF LIFE TABLETS

A licensed version of Frank Roberts' liquid "drops of life" remedy for colds and chills. The tablets contain elder flowers, peppermint oil, cayenne and yarrow.

Dosage: 2 or 3 tablets with a hot drink as required. The tablets can also be chewed or allowed to dissolve on the tongue.

FRANK ROBERTS HERBAL DISPENSARIES

*FRANK ROBERTS ECHINACEA TABLETS

Simple echinacea tablets which in this case are licensed as a remedy for minor infections including boils, mouth ulcers and nasal catarrh.

Dosage: 3 tablets, three times a day.

FRANK ROBERTS HERBAL DISPENSARIES

FRANK ROBERTS EPRIMOIL SILVER/GOLD

An unlicensed evening primrose oil supplement in two versions: Eprimoil Silver contains a minimum 8% *gamma*-linolenic acid while Eprimoil Gold has a minimum of 10% GLA. Both are 500 mg capsules.

FRANK ROBERTS HERBAL DISPENSARIES

*FRANK ROBERTS GARLIC OIL CAPSULES

Garlic oil capsules licensed for the relief of colds, catarrh and minor skin conditions.

Dosage: 1 capsule a day.

FRANK ROBERTS HERBAL DISPENSARIES

FRANK ROBERTS GINKGO BILOBA CAPSULES

An unlicensed simple containing 200 mg of ginkgo leaf.

Dosage: 4 tablets daily.

FRANK ROBERTS HERBAL DISPENSARIES

FRANK ROBERTS GINSENG CAPSULES

An unlicensed simple containing ginseng.

Dosage: 2 tablets daily.

FRANK ROBERTS HERBAL DISPENSARIES

FRANK ROBERTS GOLDEN SEAL COMPOUND TABLETS

An unlicensed combination of largely digestive herbs, suitable for various digestive upsets. The mixture contains chamomile – a relaxing carminative; echinacea to counter any infection; golden seal – a digestive stimulant and anti-inflammatory; pokeroot also anti-inflammatory and a stimulant for the immune system; and marshmallow which is a soothing demulcent for the digestive tract.

Dosage: 2 tablets three times a day.

FRANK ROBERTS HERBAL DISPENSARIES

*FRANK ROBERTS KELP AND NETTLE COMPOUND

A licensed product recommended as a slimming aid. Tablets contain kelp, blue flag root and stinging nettle: kelp is a metabolic stimulant while stinging nettles are a good source of minerals and vitamins. Blue flag is generally regarded as a cleansing skin remedy, although experiments with rats suggest that it might encourage a reduced food intake.

Dosage: 2 tablets, three times a day.

FRANK ROBERTS HERBAL DISPENSARIES

*FRANK ROBERTS MOTHERWORT COMPOUND FORMULA

A licensed menopausal remedy with tablets containing motherwort, lime flowers, pasque flower and valerian – a largely sedative mixture to ease emotional stress.

Dosage: 2 tablets, three times a day.

FRANK ROBERTS HERBAL DISPENSARIES

*FRANK ROBERTS NERFOOD TABLETS

Designed to counter stress and tension these licensed tablets contain asafoetida, valerian, wild oats and passion flower.

Dosage: 2 tablets, three times a day.

*FRANK ROBERTS NERVOUS DYSPEPSIA TABLETS

Licensed for the relief of indigestion and nausea these tablets contain ginger, golden seal, myrrh, spearmint oil, dandelion root and rhubarb. Ginger and spearmint are generally carminative while the others are largely digestive stimulants with a laxative action.

Dosage: 1 or 2 tablets four times a day.

FRANK ROBERTS PARSLEY PIERT COMPOUND TABLETS

An unlicensed combination of largely diuretics and kidney herbs that could be suitable for urinary stones and related problems. The mix includes parsley piert, buchu, bearberry and juniper as well as cascara sagrada, a laxative, and cayenne which is generally warming and stimulating.
• As the remedy contains juniper it should not be taken for prolonged periods or in pregnancy.

Dosage: 2 tablets three times a day.

FRANK ROBERTS PHYTOLACCA CREAM

An unlicensed simple cream containing pokeroot.
• External use only.

*FRANK ROBERTS PILEWORT COMPOUND TABLETS – GREEN LABEL

This is a licensed product for treating piles associated with more severe constipation. It contains the laxatives senna and cascara sagrada with astringents pilewort and agrimony. Agrimony is generally avoided in constipation because of its astringency, although in such a strongly laxative mix this is not a problem.

Dosage: 1 tablet three times a day.

*FRANK ROBERTS PILEWORT COMPOUND TABLETS – ORANGE LABEL

This is a rather less laxative combination than Frank Roberts' "Green Label" pile remedy and is licensed as a "stool softener". It contains senna and the astringents pilewort, agrimony and American cranesbill root.

Dosage: 2 tablets three times a day.   FRANK ROBERTS HERBAL DISPENSARIES

*FRANK ROBERTS PILEWORT OINTMENT

A licensed ointment for treating piles containing pilewort as a simple.
• External use only.

FRANK ROBERTS HERBAL DISPENSARIES

*FRANK ROBERTS PRICKLY ASH COMPOUND TABLETS

Under the terms of the licence this is described as "for the symptomatic relief of muscular pain and stiffness, fibrositis and rheumatic pain" although the company used to sell it as an arthritis remedy. It contains a mixture of cleansing herbs regularly used for treating both arthritis and rheumatism: celery, guaiacum, prickly ash and poplar as well as bearberry (a mild diuretic), cayenne as a warming circulatory stimulant and blue flag – generally used in skin remedies but a herb that is also laxative, diuretic and anti-inflammatory.

Dosage: 2 tablets three times a day.

FRANK ROBERTS HERBAL DISPENSARIES

*FRANK ROBERTS PULSATILLA COMPOUND TABLETS

A licensed remedy to counter everyday stress and tension containing valerian, hops, pasque flower and asafoetida, which is a less common herb these days but was once popular for nervous disorders.

Dosage: 2 tablets three times a day.   FRANK ROBERTS HERBAL DISPENSARIES

FRANK ROBERTS RASPBERRY LEAF TABLETS

Unlicensed simple tablets containing 500 mg of raspberry leaf.
• Raspberry leaf should not be taken in early pregnancy.

Dosage: 2 tablets three times a day.   FRANK ROBERTS HERBAL DISPENSARIES

*FRANK ROBERTS REDUCING (SLIMMING) TABLETS

Licensed as a slimming aid, this remedy contains a combination of diuretics, laxatives and metabolic stimulants. It should only be regarded as a short term aid rather than a solution to dieting problems. Herbs include cascara sagrada, boldo, bladderwrack and dandelion root.

Dosage: 2 tablets three times a day.

FRANK ROBERTS HERBAL DISPENSARIES

*FRANK ROBERTS RHEUMATIC PAIN TABLETS

This is a licensed product for the relief of rheumatism which the company has produced for more than 40 years. It contains bogbean, guaiacum, cayenne and celery oil as a cleansing and warming combination.

Dosage: 2 tablets three times a day.

FRANK ROBERTS HERBAL DISPENSARIES

*FRANK ROBERTS ROD-BRON TABLETS

These used to be sold as "Asthma and Bronchitis Tablets" but are now licensed for the symptomatic relief of chestiness and bronchial asthma. The mixture contains the expectorants and antispasmodics: ipecacuanha, Indian tobacco, white horehound and liquorice.

Dosage: 2 tablets twice a day.

FRANK ROBERTS HERBAL DISPENSARIES

FRANK ROBERTS ROSEHIP TABLETS

An unlicensed simple supplement containing rosehips.

Dosage: 3 tablets daily.

FRANK ROBERTS HERBAL DISPENSARIES

*FRANK ROBERTS SCIATICA TABLETS

Licensed as a remedy to relieve the pain of sciatica, this mixture is very similar to other preparations designed to treat arthritis and rheumatism. It contains bogbean, guaiacum, bearberry and celery oil.
• Not recommended during pregnancy or lactation.

Dosage: 2 tablets three times a day.

FRANK ROBERTS HERBAL DISPENSARIES

*FRANK ROBERTS SINUS AND HAY FEVER TABLETS

A licensed mixture of echinacea, elder flowers and garlic which can be sold as suitable for sinus and hay fever problems. Elder is a good anti-catarrhal and both echinacea and garlic will counter infections as well.

Dosage: 2 tablets three times a day.

FRANK ROBERTS HERBAL DISPENSARIES

*FRANK ROBERTS STRENGTH TABLETS

A licensed tonic remedy for temporary fatigue, overwork and feeling "under the weather". It contains a popular combination of tonic herbs – damiana, cola and saw palmetto – and is very similar to a Dorwest product.

Dosage: 2 tablets three times a day.

FRANK ROBERTS HERBAL DISPENSARIES

*FRANK ROBERTS SUPA-TONIC TABLETS

This licensed tonic remedy for "combating the physical effects of overwork" is very similar to Frank Roberts' Strength Tablets but with the addition of rosemary – a good nerve tonic and stimulant.

Dosage: 1 tablet four times a day.

FRANK ROBERTS HERBAL DISPENSARIES

FRANK ROBERTS UVA-URSI COMPOUND TABLETS

An unlicensed combination of largely diuretics and urinary antiseptics which could be helpful for such problems as cystitis. The mixture contains bearberry, shepherd's purse, horsetail, couchgrass, clivers and buchu with the addition of senna as a stimulating laxative.

Dosage: 3 tablets daily.

FRANK ROBERTS HERBAL DISPENSARIES

*FRANK ROBERTS VALERIAN COMPOUND

This remedy is licensed for the symptomatic relief of "nervous dizziness, tension and strain". It contains valerian, lime flowers, Jamaica dogwood and pasque flower which are all sedative herbs.

Dosage: 2 tablets three times a day.

FRANK ROBERTS HERBAL DISPENSARIES

FSC BROMELAIN PLUS

An unlicensed remedy which combines extracts of pineapple and papaya – traditionally used for digestive upsets – with ginger which is a carminative.

Dosage: 1–3 tablets per day with a meal.

FSC QUALITY VITAMINS

FSC CRANBERRY CONCENTRATE TABLETS

An unlicensed combination of 2.4 g of cranberry extract with vitamin C.

Dosage: 2–4 tablets daily with a meal.

FSC QUALITY VITAMINS

FSC DEVIL'S CLAW PLUS

An unlicensed supplement containing devil's claw with the addition of vitamins C, E and B_6, pantothenic acid, zinc, selenium and copper.

FSC QUALITY VITAMINS

FSC FEVERFEW

An unlicensed simple containing 150 mg of feverfew.

Dosage: 1 tablet daily with a meal.

FSC QUALITY VITAMINS

FSC GARLIC GEMS

An unlicensed simple containing 2 mg odourless garlic equivalent per capsule.

Dosage: 1 per day.

FSC QUALITY VITAMINS

FSC GINGER AND TURMERIC

This unlicensed product is based on a traditional Ayurvedic formula used to warm the joints and is said to be suitable for arthritis sufferers. It contains turmeric and ginger and would also stimulate the circulation.

Dosage: 4 capsules daily with meals.

FSC QUALITY VITAMINS

FSC KOREAN GINSENG

Unlicensed simple containing 600 mg of ginseng per tablet.

Dosage: 1 tablet daily.

FSC QUALITY VITAMINS

FSC MILK THISTLE TABLETS

A combination of milk thistle seeds and dandelion root which are both herbs that have a cleansing and tonic effect on the liver.

Dosage: 1–3 tablets per day with a meal.

FSC QUALITY VITAMINS

FSC ORGANIC ECHINACEA

An unlicensed simple tablet containing 500 mg of *Echinacea purpurea*.

Dosage: 1–3 tablets three times a day.

FSC QUALITY VITAMINS

FSC PURE EVENING PRIMROSE OIL COOL PRESSED

Unlicensed simple capsules of evening primrose oil containing either 250, 500 or 1000 mg per capsules, with added vitamin E.

Dosage: 1–6 capsules daily.

FSC QUALITY VITAMINS

FSC SIBERIAN GINSENG

A supplement containing 1 g of Siberian ginseng with safflower oil which contains essential fatty acids.

Dosage: 1 tablet per day.

FSC QUALITY VITAMINS

FSC VALERIAN FORMULA

An unlicensed combination of sedative herbs that could be helpful for nervous tension or insomnia – valerian, passion flower, hops, wild lettuce – with the addition of yellow gentian which is a digestive stimulant and helpful for physical exhaustion.

Dosage: 1 tablet at night before bed.

FSC QUALITY VITAMINS

*FSC WATERFALL

A licensed product to relieve periodic feelings of bloatedness and help maintain a normal fluid balance. It contains the diuretics celery seed, boldo and juniper in a safflower oil base.
• Because of the juniper content, the remedy should not be used for longer than a couple of weeks without a break, or in pregnancy, lactation or kidney disease.

Dosage: 2 capsules in the morning before meals.

FSC QUALITY VITAMINS

FSC WHOLE BULB GARLIC

An unlicensed garlic simple using Pure-Gar® powder which is provided by Pure-Gar Inc. It is a 100% concentrated garlic which claims to be odourless by keeping apart the alliin and allinase – which combine to form allicin – thus delaying the formation of the characteristic smell of garlic's main sulphur-based component. Capsules contain 300 mg of garlic powder equivalent to 750 mg of fresh garlic.

Dosage: 1 or 2 capsules a day with a meal or at bedtime.

FSC QUALITY VITAMINS

FULL POTENCY HERBS VEGICAPS

This is a range of single herbs produced by Solgar Vitamins. All are unlicensed and most are sold in vegetarian capsules although a few are in tablet and gelatin capsule form. The selection includes some common plants, like feverfew, as well as more exotic tonic remedies, such as cat's claw. Information about actions is included in the A–Z of Herbs. The products available are summarised in Table 6 (see below).

SOLGAR VITAMINS

Table 6: Single herbs in the Full Potency Herbs Capsule and Tablet range. (Herbs are in Vegicaps unless otherwise specified.)

Herb	Total herbal content of extract & powder (mg)	Dosage
Aloe Vera Leaf	520 mg	1–3 capsules daily
American Ginseng Root	520 mg	1–3 capsules daily
Astragalus Root	520 mg	1–3 capsules daily

continued

Herb	Total herbal content of extract & powder (mg)	Dosage
Burdock Root	520 mg	1–3 capsules daily
Butcher's Broom	520 mg	1–3 capsules daily
Cat's Claw Tablets	1000 mg	1–3 tablets daily
Cayenne Capsules	520 mg	1–3 capsules daily
Chamomile	520 mg	1–3 capsules daily
Dandelion Root	520 mg	1–3 capsules daily
Devil's Claw	520 mg	1–3 capsules daily
Dong Quai	520 mg (Dang Gui)	1–3 capsules daily
Echinacea	520 mg	1–3 capsules daily
Eyebright	520 mg	1–3 capsules daily
Fenugreek	520 mg	1–3 capsules daily
Feverfew	520 mg	1 or 2 capsules daily
Ginger Root	520 mg	1–3 capsules daily
Ginkgo Biloba	520 mg	1–3 capsules daily
Ginseng (Siberian)	250 mg	1–3 capsules daily
Goldenseal Root	520 mg (golden seal)	1–3 capsules daily
Gotu Kola	520 mg	1–3 capsules daily
Green Tea	520 mg	1–3 capsules daily
Hawthorn Berry	520 mg	1–3 capsules daily
Korean Ginseng	520 mg (ginseng)	1–3 capsules daily
Liquorice Root	520 mg	1–3 capsules daily
Milk Thistle	510 mg	1–3 capsules daily
Pau d'Arco	520 mg	1–3 capsules daily
Sarsparilla Root	520 mg	1–3 capsules daily
Saw Palmetto Berries	520 mg	1–3 capsules daily
Scutellariae	445 mg (skullcap)	1–3 capsules daily
Siberian Ginseng	520 mg	1–3 capsules daily
Super Ginkgo	435 mg (ginkgo)	1–2 capsules daily
Valerian Root	520 mg	1–3 capsules daily
Vegital Silica	520 mg (horsetail)	1–3 capsules daily
Yucca Vegicaps	520 mg	1–3 capsules daily

FULL POTENCY HERBS BILBERRY WITH GINKGO BILOBA VEGICAPS

An unlicensed supplement containing 60 mg of bilberry extract in a base of bilberry and ginkgo leaf powder.

Dosage: 1–3 capsules daily.

SOLGAR VITAMINS

FULL POTENCY HERBS ECHINACEA/GOLDENSEAL/CAT'S CLAW COMPLEX VEGICAPS

An unlicensed combination of echinacea (both *E. angustifolia* and *E. purpurea* extracts) with golden seal and cat's claw: herbs which are generally stimulating for the immune system and could be used to counter recurrent infections.

Dosage: 1–3 capsules daily.

SOLGAR VITAMINS

*FYBOGEL

Fybogel and Fybogel Orange are sachets of granules based on isphaghula husks for use as a bulking laxative.

Dosage: adults and children over 12 years – 1 sachet morning and evening; children six–12 years – ½–1 level 5 ml teaspoonful, depending on age and size, morning and evening.

RECKITT & COLEMAN

GALEN CALENDULA AND VITAMIN E CREAM

An unlicensed cream containing marigold extract with 1% vitamin E.

GALEN HERBAL SUPPLIES

GAMMAOIL PREMIUM

Capsules containing 500 mg or 1000 mg of evening primrose oil plus 10 IU of vitamin E.

Dosage: 1 or 2 capsules three times a day.

QUEST VITAMINS

*GERARD 99

A licensed remedy for the symptomatic relief of tenseness, irritability and stresses and stains of everyday life. It contains a popular combination of sedative herbs: hops, passion flower and valerian.
• Not recommended for children.

Dosage: 2 tablets after meals three times a day.

GERARD HOUSE

GERARD HOUSE AGNACAST

Unlicensed simple chastetree tablets.

GERARD HOUSE

*GERARD HOUSE BIOPHYLIN

A licensed remedy for the symptomatic relief of tenseness, irritability, stresses and strains. It contains valerian, skullcap and Jamaica dogwood which are all largely sedative in action, as well as black cohosh which is more usually found in remedies for coughs, rheumatic pains and menopausal problems, but also has a sedative action.
• Not recommended for children.

Dosage: 2 tablets three times daily after meals.   GERARD HOUSE

*GERARD HOUSE BLUE FLAG ROOT

A licensed remedy for the relief of minor acne, eczema and poor skin conditions. It contains herbs which are all widely used in treating skin problems: blue flag, burdock and sarsparilla.
• Not recommended for children.

Dosage: 1 tablet three times daily after meals.

GERARD HOUSE

*GERARD HOUSE BUCHU COMPOUND

A licensed mixture of diuretics for maintaining normal urinary flow. Like similar mixtures it could also be helpful for cystitis and includes buchu, dandelion, bearberry and clivers.
• Not recommended for children.

Dosage: 2 tablets three times daily after meals.

GERARD HOUSE

GERARD HOUSE CALENDULA OINTMENT

Unlicensed marigold ointment.
• External use only.   GERARD HOUSE

*GERARD HOUSE CELERY

Licensed for the relief of rheumatic pain this is a simple containing celery seed.
The herb is a diuretic and clears uric acid from the system so is also widely used
for arthritis and gout.

Dosage: 1 or 2 tablets three times a day.

GERARD HOUSE

GERARD HOUSE CHAMOMILE OINTMENT

An unlicensed ointment containing chamomile.
• External use only.   GERARD HOUSE

GERARD HOUSE CHICKWEED OINTMENT

An unlicensed ointment containing chickweed.
• External use only.   GERARD HOUSE

GERARD HOUSE COMFREY OINTMENT

An unlicensed ointment containing comfrey.
• External use only.

GERARD HOUSE

GERARD HOUSE CRAMP BARK

Unlicensed simple cramp bark tablets.

GERARD HOUSE

*GERARD HOUSE CRANESBILL TABLETS

Licensed for the treatment of diarrhoea, these tablets contain American cranesbill as a simple.

Dosage: adults – 1 or 2 tablets three times a day; children – 1 tablet twice a day.

GERARD HOUSE

*GERARD HOUSE CURZON

Licensed for the treatment of temporary fatigue, these tablets contain damiana as a simple.
• Not recommended for children.

Dosage: 2 tablets night and morning.

GERARD HOUSE

GERARD HOUSE DEVIL'S CLAW

Unlicensed simple devil's claw bark tablets.

GERARD HOUSE

*GERARD HOUSE DRAGON BALM OINTMENT

A licensed ointment to relieve inflamed or swollen rheumatic joints, this contains oils that are largely rubefacient and warming: camphor, nutmeg, eucalyptus, cassia, pine and Peruvian balsam. It also includes turpentine oil, menthol (a constituent of peppermint oil), thymol which is found in thyme oil, and guaiacol extracted from guaiacum.
• External use only.

Dosage: Apply as required.

GERARD HOUSE

*GERARD HOUSE ECHINACEA

A simple echinacea tablet which in this case is licensed for the symptomatic relief of minor skin conditions, acne and minor eczema – although the same product could also be useful for treating a range of infectious conditions.
• Not recommended for children.

Dosage: 1 or 2 tablets after meals three times a day.

GERARD HOUSE

*GERARD HOUSE ECHINACEA & GARLIC

A licensed remedy for the symptomatic relief of colds and influenza which contains echinacea and garlic. Similar products are licensed for catarrh and coughs.
• Not recommended for children.

Dosage: 1 or 2 tablets three times a day.

GERARD HOUSE

GERARD HOUSE EEZ-A-TEA

A mixture of thyme, common plantain and rosehips sold as a loose tea for "winter comfort" in cold weather. Thyme is a good antiseptic for coughs, rosehips are rich in vitamin C, and common plantain is an anti-microbial useful for catarrh.

GERARD HOUSE

GERARD HOUSE EVENING PRIMROSE

Unlicensed 500 mg capsules of evening primrose oil.

Dosage: 1 to 4 capsules a day.

GERARD HOUSE

GERARD HOUSE FEM-A-TEA

A mixture of herbs sold as a loose tea for women as an aid for the hormonal system. It contains black cohosh, yarrow and chastetree as well as additional vitamins C, B_6 and folic acid. Black cohosh and chastetree are regularly used for menstrual irregularities while yarrow is a diuretic often used for fluid retention.

GERARD HOUSE

*GERARD HOUSE FENULIN

A licensed remedy for the symptomatic relief of digestive upsets containing golden seal, a digestive stimulant, slippery elm which is soothing for the gastric mucosa and fenugreek which is a digestive tonic and very warming for stomach chills.
• Not recommended for children.

Dosage: 2 tablets after meals three times a day.

GERARD HOUSE

GERARD HOUSE FEVERFEW

Unlicensed simple feverfew tablets.

GERARD HOUSE

GERARD HOUSE GARLIC OINTMENT

Unlicensed simple garlic ointment.
• External use only.

GERARD HOUSE

*GERARD HOUSE GARLIC PERLES

These garlic perles are licensed to relieve the symptoms of the common cold and cough, rhinitis and catarrh. Like other garlic capsules they could also be used for a range of other ailments.
• Not recommended for children.

Dosage: 1 capsule three times a day before meals, or 2 to 3 capsules on retiring at night.

GERARD HOUSE

*GERARD HOUSE GINGER

Licensed as a carminative for indigestion, this is a simple ginger tablet that could also be useful for travel sickness and nausea. Like other licensed products this specifies that it should not be used for children although ginger is an ideal remedy for childhood motion sickness.

Dosage: 1 tablet three times a day.

GERARD HOUSE

GERARD HOUSE GINKGO BILOBA

Unlicensed simple ginkgo tablets.

GERARD HOUSE

*GERARD HOUSE GLADLAX

Licensed for the relief of occasional or non-persistent constipation this is a mixture of aloes, which are laxative, with holy thistle – a bitter digestive stimulant. The mixture also includes fennel, which will act as a carminative to counter any griping caused by the aloes, and valerian which is a sedative and carminative and can help relieve intestinal cramps.
• Not recommended for children.

Dosage: 1 or 2 tablets at bed time.   GERARD HOUSE

*GERARD HOUSE GOLDEN SEAL COMPOUND

A licensed remedy for the relief of indigestion, heartburn, flatulence, nausea and gastric irritation this mixture contains golden seal and dandelion root as digestive stimulants along with marshmallow, which helps to protect the gastric mucosa and counter acidity, and American cranesbill – an astringent largely used for diarrhoea.

• Not recommended for children.

Dosage: 2 tablets between meals three times a day.

GERARD HOUSE HAWTHORN

Unlicensed simple hawthorn tablets.

*GERARD HOUSE HELONIAS COMPOUND

Licensed to relieve heavy bloated feelings in women and to maintain normal fluid balance this is largely a combination of diuretics and hormonal herbs. It contains helonias, parsley, black cohosh and raspberry leaf which is sometimes used for period pain. Both black cohosh and helonias are used as menstrual stimulants and to relieve premenstrual syndrome.
• Not recommended for children.

Dosage: 1 tablet after meals three times a day.

*GERARD HOUSE KELP

Licensed as a slimming remedy this is a simple bladderwrack tablet which will act as a metabolic stimulant and can be useful in a range of conditions.
• Not recommended for children, during pregnancy and lactation, or for persons with thyroid disorders.

Dosage: 1 tablet three times a day after meals.

GERARD HOUSE KOREAN GINSENG

Unlicensed simple ginseng tablets.

*GERARD HOUSE LIGVITES

Licensed for the symptomatic relief of rheumatic aches and pains, fibrositis, lumbago, backache and stiffness this is a combination of herbs regularly used for treating both rheumatic and arthritic disorders: guaiacum, black cohosh, white willow and poplar. The mixture also contains sarsparilla which is more often used for skin problems although it is a useful cleansing herb and one used in China for

treating rheumatic disorders.
• Not recommended for children.

Dosage: 2 tablets after breakfast and evening meal.   GERARD HOUSE

*GERARD HOUSE LOBELIA COMPOUND

Licensed for coughs, blocked sinuses and catarrh this remedy is a combination of
squill and Indian tobacco. Squill is a potent expectorant while Indian tobacco is
more often regarded as a respiratory stimulant used to ease asthma, bronchitis
and whooping cough than a product for treating catarrh. The tablets also contain
gum ammoniacum.
• Not recommended for children.

Dosage: 1 tablet, three times a day.   GERARD HOUSE

GERARD HOUSE MARSHMALLOW AND PEPPERMINT

An unlicensed combination of marshmallow and peppermint – a soothing stomach remedy and carminative – suitable for indigestion, heartburn and flatulence.
          GERARD HOUSE

*GERARD HOUSE MOTHERWORT COMPOUND

Licensed for the relief of "modern day stresses and strains" this is a mixture of
gently sedating herbs – passion flower, lime flowers and motherwort. The last
two are also helpful for blood pressure problems and the remedy could thus be
suitable for treating hypertension which is exacerbated by stress.
• Not recommended for children

Dosage: 2 tablets three times a day after meals.   GERARD HOUSE

*GERARD HOUSE PAPAYA PLUS TABLETS

Licensed for the relief of indigestion, heartburn, hyperacidity, flatulence or dyspepsia this mixture contains papaya, slippery elm and golden seal, which would
help to stimulate and normalize digestive function as well as providing protection
for the gastric lining from excessive acidity. The tablets also contain charcoal
which helps to absorb excess acids.
• Not recommended for children.

Dosage: 1 tablet three times a day before meals.   GERARD HOUSE

*GERARD HOUSE PASSIFLORA

A simple passion flower tablet that is licensed as a remedy for insomnia.

Dosage: adults – 1 or 2 tablets two hours before retiring; children five –12 years, one tablet two hours before retiring.

GERARD HOUSE

*GERARD HOUSE PILEWORT COMPOUND

This is a mixture of laxatives and astringents licensed for the relief of constipation and haemorrhoids. It contains senna, cascara sagrada, American cranesbill and pilewort.
• Not recommended for children.

Dosage: 1 or 2 tablets at night before retiring.

GERARD HOUSE

GERARD HOUSE PRICKLY ASH TABLETS

Unlicensed simple prickly ash tablets.

GERARD HOUSE

GERARD HOUSE PULSATILLA

Unlicensed simple pasque flower tablets.

GERARD HOUSE

GERARD HOUSE RASPBERRY LEAF

Unlicensed simple raspberry leaf tablets.

GERARD HOUSE

GERARD HOUSE SEAWEED AND SARSPARILLA TABLETS

A supplement combining kelp and sarsparilla which has traditionally been used as a skin tonic. The combination is also cleansing and stimulating and could be suitable in rheumatic disorders.

GERARD HOUSE

GERARD HOUSE SLEEK-A-TEA

A mixture of silver birch and maté sold as a loose tea for "those on a diet". Birch is diuretic and mildly laxative and more normally used in rheumatic and skin problems, while maté is also a mild diuretic and stimulant thanks to its caffeine and theobromine content. The tea also contains vitamins C and B$_5$.

GERARD HOUSE

*GERARD HOUSE SLIPPERY ELM TABLETS

Licensed to relieve symptoms of gastric disorders and aid the digestion process this is a simple slippery elm tablet.
• Not recommended for children.

Dosage: 1 or 2 tablets after meals three times a day.

GERARD HOUSE

GERARD HOUSE SOOTH-A-TEA

A mixture of herbs suggested as a suitably relaxing drink at bedtime. It contains hops and lemon balm which are both calming and can help insomnia, as well as heather, largely used as a urinary remedy but also mildly sedative, with angelica and peppermint which are both carminatives but are no doubt added to improve the flavour.

GERARD HOUSE

GERARD HOUSE ST JOHN'S WORT

Unlicensed simple St John's wort tablets.

GERARD HOUSE

*GERARD HOUSE VALERIAN COMPOUND TABLETS

Licensed for the relief of restlessness and to promote relaxation and natural sleep this mixture uses a popular combination of herbs: valerian, hops, passion flower, Jamaica dogwood and wild lettuce – all of which are sedating and relaxing.
• Not recommended for children.

Dosage: 2 tablets in the early evening and 2 tablets immediately before bedtime.

GERARD HOUSE

GERARD HOUSE VIG-A-TEA

A combination of largely stimulating herbs sold as a loose tea. The mix includes damiana and rosemary – both good tonic herbs – with maté which is stimulating thanks to the caffeine content and raspberry leaf which is generally astringent and tonifying.
• Because of the raspberry leaf content this tea is probably best avoided in early pregnancy.

GERARD HOUSE

*GERARD HOUSE WATERLEX TABLETS

A licensed remedy "to assist normal urinary flow" this is a combination of diuretic herbs that could be relevant for a number of urinary system disorders including cystitis. It contains dandelion, horsetail and bearberry.
• Not recommended for children.

Dosage: 1 or 2 tablets three times a day. GERARD HOUSE

GERARD HOUSE WILD YAM

Unlicensed simple wild yam tablets.

GERARD HOUSE

GERARD HOUSE WITCH HAZEL OINTMENT

Unlicensed ointment containing witch hazel – a strongly astringent herb that is often used for treating wounds, varicose veins and other skin lesions.
• External use only.

GERARD HOUSE

GINKYO

Unlicensed simple ginkgo tablets each containing 50 mg of standardised extract.

Dosage: 1–3 tablets daily at meal times.

LICTWER PHARMA

GINSENG SLICES

Honey soaked ginseng in slices which can be chewed two or three times a day as a general stimulant and tonic.

ORIENTAL HEALTH

GLANOLIN 500

Capsules containing 500 mg of blackcurrant seed oil as a source of *gamma*-linolenic acid, *alpha*-linolenic acid, linoleic acid, stearidonic acid and vitamin C.

Dosage: 3 or 4 capsules daily with a meal; during menstruation 3 capsules from 14 days before the period is due until it finishes; children under 12 years should take Glanolin 250 which is the same oil in 250 mg capsules.

G R LANE HEALTH PRODUCTS

GOLDEN YELLOW OINTMENT

An unlicensed ointment based on a Chinese formula used for all sorts of toxic swellings including boils, inflamed insect bites and sprains. It includes trichosanthis, phellodendron, turmeric, rhubarb, angelica, arisaema, tangerine peel, liquorice, Chinese golden thread, red paeony and grey atractylodes.
• External use only.

SPRING WIND HERBS (EAST WEST HERBS IN THE UK)

*HACTOS COUGH MIXTURE

A licensed cough mixture first produced more than 50 years ago and containing essential oils of peppermint, anise and cloves with cayenne tincture.

Dosage: 1 or 2 × 5 ml teaspoonfuls, three or four times a day.

HONEYROSE

HARPAGO

Unlicensed simple devil's claw product containing 100 mg of herb per capsule.

Dosage: 1 capsule three times a day before meals, to be taken for three weeks at a time. Double the dose if necessary.

ORTIS

HARPAGO GEL

An unlicensed cream containing devil's claw and juniper – both useful in external rubs for rheumatism and arthritis. It should be massaged into the appropriate area as required and used continuously for a few weeks.
• Do not apply to irritated skin, varicose veins or mucous areas. External use only.

ORTIS

HARTWOOD AROMATICS ESPECIALLY YOURS

A supplement combining 1000 mg of evening primrose oil with calcium for use by menopausal women.

Dosage: 1 or 2 capsules daily.

HARTWOOD AROMATICS

HEALTH AID AMERICAN GINSENG

Phials containing 600 mg of American ginseng extract in 10 ml phials.

PHARMADASS

HEALTH AID BOLDO PLUS

Like a number of other unlicensed products containing boldo and other diuretics, this is designed as a slimming aid. It may help weight loss in the short-term but should not be regarded as a long-term supplement for regular use. As well as boldo this one contains clivers, bearberry, dandelion and bladderwrack (also a metabolic stimulant). The supplement also includes vitamin B_6 and potassium glucontate.
• Not suitable for children under 12.

Dosage: 2 tablets three times a day.

PHARMADASS

HEALTH AID DEVIL'S CLAW WITH ROYAL JELLY

An unlicensed combination of devil's claw and royal jelly.

PHARMADASS

HEALTH AID ECZEM OIL

This contains evening primrose and chamomile oils and is suggested as suitable for dry, itchy or flaking skin, eczema, sunburn, scars, blemishes and wrinkles. It also includes vitamin E with castor, olive, sunflower and grapeseed oils.
• For external use only.

PHARMADASS

HEALTH AID FEMMEVIT

This supplement is described as a "PMS Nutritional Formula" to "help you through difficult days". It is largely a vitamin and mineral mixture containing vitamins B_1, B_2, B_3, B_6, B_{12}, C, and E, with iron, magnesium, chromium, chlorophyll, iodine and titanium oxide. Herbal content is a combination of diuretics (boldo, parsley and juniper), with valerian as a sedative, ginger – warming and carminative – and angelica which is also diuretic and a uterine stimulant sometimes used for menstrual disorders.

• The juniper oil content means that the product should be avoided in pregnancy and kidney disease and should only be taken for short periods at a time.

Dosage: 1 tablet a day.

PHARMADASS

HEALTH AID HERBAL BOOSTER

This supplement contains a number of tonic and stimulant herbs that would be useful to provide an energy boost. This list includes some obvious choices: guarana, Siberian ginseng, gotu kola, cola, hawthorn, echinacea, liquorice, ginger and cayenne, as well as herbs that would not necessarily be thought of as stimulating tonics – mullein (usually regarded as a cough remedy), yellow dock (a laxative) and papaya (normally included in products for stomach upsets).

PHARMADASS

HEALTH AID KOREAN GINSENG

Two versions are available: Korgin Korean Ginseng which contains 250 mg of the herb and Korean Ginseng 600 mg which has the equivalent of 3 g of root.

Dosage: 1 or 2 a day depending on capsule size.

PHARMADASS

HEALTH AID LIQUID HERBAL BOOSTER

A supplement containing some classic tonic herbs regularly used for countering stress and fatigue. The mixture combines guarana, Siberian ginseng, gotu kola, echinacea and muira-puama (also an aphrodisiac).

Dosage: 15 ml daily.

PHARMADASS

HEALTH AID LIVER GUARD FORTE

This product gives a list of not totally accurate botanical names on the packaging which the suppliers have been unable to clarify. It would appear to contain capers, chicory, senna, and yarrow which could be classified as digestive remedies, along with black nightshade *(Solanum nigra)* which is a poisonous plant once

used for insomnia and could be an error for *S. dulcamara* (bittersweet) which can be used for liver problems. The mix also contains *Terminalia arjuna*, which is used in Ayurvedic medicine for ischaemic heart disease although other *Terminalia* spp. *(T. belerica* and *T. chebula)* are used as laxatives and would seem a more suitable choice. Also included in the combination is *Tamarix gallica* which contains liver protecting substances. The supplement is suggested as a liver cleansing remedy or for "people having alcohol-related problems to cleanse the liver" and the suppliers also say it can be given to children to increase appetite and growth.
• There would seem to be some confusion over its precise contents and caution may be necessary until these are clarified.

Dosage: adults – 2 or 3 tablets three or four times a day; children – 1 or 2 tablets four times a day.

PHARMADASS

HEALTH AID MEGA GARLIC OIL

Unlicensed simple garlic capsules containing 2 mg of oil per capsule.

Dosage: 1 per day.

PHARMADASS

HEALTH AID ORGANIC GARLIC OIL

Unlicensed simple garlic capsules.

Dosage: 1 per day.   PHARMADASS

HEALTH AID SIBERIAN GINSENG

Two versions are available: Siberian Ginseng which has 250 mg of herb per capsule and Sibergin-Siberian GR which has the equivalent of 2.5 g of root.

Dosage: 1 or 2 capsules daily depending on size.

PHARMADASS

HEALTH AID SUPER BOLDO

Another of the unlicensed boldo-based combination of diuretics promoted to counter fluid retention. This one also contains dandelion, clivers and bladderwrack – rather similar, in fact, to the company's Boldo Plus product.

Dosage: 2 tablets three times a day during water retention problems, reduce to 3 tablets daily for maintenance.

PHARMADASS

HEALTH AID TRANQUIL CAPSULES WITH VIBURNUM

These unlicensed capsules contain lime flowers, which have a sedative action, with black haw (a relaxant and antispasmodic) and hawthorn normally regarded as a heart tonic but which also has a sedative effect on the nervous system.

Dosage: 1 capsule daily.

PHARMADASS

HEALTH PLUS EVENING PRIMROSE OIL

Unlicensed simple evening primrose capsules each containing 500 mg of oil.

HEALTH PLUS

HEALTHCRAFTS EVENING PRIMROSE OIL

Unlicensed simple evening primrose oil capsules each available in 250 mg, 500 mg and 1,000 mg formats.

FERROSAN HEALTHCARE

HEALTHCRAFTS EVENING PRIMROSE WITH BORAGE OIL

Unlicensed simple capsules containing a mixture of evening primrose and borage oils.

FERROSAN HEALTHCARE

HEALTHCRAFTS GARLIC

Unlicensed simple garlic capsules each containing 2 mg of odourless extract.

Dosage: 1 capsule per day.

FERROSAN HEALTHCARE

HEALTHCRAFTS GEB6 COMBINATION

A combination of 400 mg Siberian Ginseng with vitamins E and B_6 which is suggested as a suitable dietary supplement for menopausal women.

Dosage: 1 capsule a day.

FERROSAN HEALTHCARE

HEALTHCRAFTS HIGH STRENGTH STARFLOWER OIL

Unlicensed simple capsules containing borage oil.

FERROSAN HEALTHCARE

HEALTHCRAFTS KELP

Unlicensed simple kelp tablets.

Dosage: 3 tablets daily with food.

FERROSAN HEALTHCARE

HEALTHCRAFTS KELP PLUS

Unlicensed tablets combining kelp with a turmeric extract, which can help improve digestion, as well as additional iron.

Dosage: 1 tablet daily.

FERROSAN HEALTHCARE

HEALTHCRAFTS KOREAN AND SIBERIAN GINSENG

An unlicensed combination of Siberian and Korean ginsengs which are both useful tonic herbs suitable for tiredness and fatigue.

FERROSAN HEALTHCARE

HEALTHCRAFTS KOREAN GINSENG

Unlicensed simple in two formats, containing either 600 mg or 1200 mg of ginseng per capsule.

FERROSAN HEALTHCARE

*HEALTHCRAFTS NIGHT TIME

A licensed product for use in insomnia containing the popular combination of valerian, hops and passion flower.
• Not recommended for children, avoid in pregnancy.

Dosage: 2 tablets one hour before going to bed.

FERROSAN HEALTHCARE

HEALTHCRAFTS SIBERIAN GINSENG

Unlicensed simple capsules of Siberian ginseng each containing 600 mg of root.

FERROSAN HEALTHCARE

HEALTHWISE EVENING PRIMROSE OIL

Unlicensed simple evening primrose capsules each containing 500 mg of oil.

HEALTH IMPORTS

HEALTHWISE GARLIC PEARLS

Unlicensed simple garlic capsules.

Dosage: 1 a day.

HEALTH IMPORTS

HEALTHWISE GINKGO BILOBA

Unlicensed simple ginkgo tablets each containing the equivalent of 2000 mg of herb.

HEALTH IMPORTS

*HEATH & HEATHER BALM OF GILEAD COUGH MIXTURE

A licensed remedy for the symptomatic relief of coughs and catarrh containing squill and Indian tobacco (cf. *Gerard House Lobelia Compound) with balm of gilead which is a pleasant tasting herb often used for coughs.

FERROSAN HEALTHCARE

*HEATH & HEATHER BALM OF GILEAD COUGH PASTILLES

This has the same formulation as the same company's Balm of Gilead Cough Syrup and is similarly licensed for the symptomatic relief of coughs and catarrh.

FERROSAN HEALTHCARE

*HEATH & HEATHER BECALM

A licensed remedy to aid relaxation from everyday stress this contains the same combination of herbs as a number of other products recommended for both anxiety and insomnia: valerian, hops and passion flower.

FERROSAN HEALTHCARE

*HEATH & HEATHER CATARRH

Licensed for the symptomatic relief of coughs and catarrh this product contains white horehound which is a stimulating expectorant and squill, also expectorant and particularly useful for bronchitis and whooping cough.

FERROSAN HEALTHCARE

*HEATH & HEATHER CELERY SEED

A licensed remedy for the symptomatic relief of lumbago, fibrositis and rheumatic pain this is a simple celery seed product containing 600 mg of seed per tablet.

FERROSAN HEALTHCARE

HEATH & HEATHER FEVERFEW

Unlicensed simple feverfew tablets.

FERROSAN HEALTHCARE

HEATH & HEATHER GARLIC PERLES

Unlicensed simple garlic capsules. The One a Day range contains 2 mg of odourless garlic extract while Odourless Garlic Perles have 0.66 mg and dosage is 3 capsules per day.

FERROSAN HEALTHCARE

*HEATH & HEATHER INDIGESTION & FLATULENCE

Licensed for the symptomatic relief of indigestion and flatulence this product contains fennel and peppermint oils, which are both carminatives, as well as cayenne, which is a warming digestive stimulant.

FERROSAN HEALTHCARE

*HEATH & HEATHER INNER FRESH

A licensed remedy for the relief of occasional constipation this is an alder buckthorn simple.

FERROSAN HEALTHCARE

*HEATH & HEATHER QUIET NIGHT

Licensed as a remedy to soothe and so aid restful sleep this has the same herbal mix (valerian, hops and passion flower) as the same company's Becalm product.

FERROSAN HEALTHCARE

HEATH & HEATHER RASPBERRY LEAF

Unlicensed simple raspberry leaf tablets each containing 640 mg of herb.

FERROSAN HEALTHCARE

*HEATH & HEATHER RHEUMATIC PAIN

Licensed for the symptomatic relief of backache, lumbago, fibrositis and other rheumatic pains this mixture contains herbs that are regularly used by herbalists to treat arthritis as well. These are guaiacum, celery seed and bogbean.

FERROSAN HEALTHCARE

HEATH & HEATHER SKIN TABLETS

Licensed as a remedy for spots, blemishes and dry eczema these tablets contain burdock, which is mildly laxative, diuretic and widely used as a cleansing remedy for the skin, and heartsease – a useful anti-inflammatory for soothing skin eruptions.

FERROSAN HEALTHCARE

*HEATH & HEATHER WATER RELIEF

This mixture is licensed as providing symptomatic relief from premenstrual water retention. It contains clivers and burdock as diuretics, bladderwrack as a metabolic stimulant, and ground ivy which is usually regarded as an astringent anti-catarrhal but also has some diuretic action. Despite the licence, this product could be suitable for a range of urinary problems rather than being a specific for PMS disorders.

FERROSAN HEALTHCARE

HELODERM CT OINTMENT

Unlicensed ointment containing cade oil which is often used in psoriasis treatments. The mixture also contains sulphur tar complex, purified lanolin and Dead Sea mineral salts.

FINDERS INTERNATIONAL

HELODERM CT SHAMPOO

A similar combination to Heloderm CT Ointment only in a shampoo base. It should be massaged into the hair and scalp and left for 5–10 minutes before washing out. Repeat twice a week.

FINDERS INTERNATIONAL

HERBATONE

An unlicensed combination of wild oats, cola, yellow gentian and ginseng in tincture format marketed as a general tonic. The combination of herbs is generally stimulating for the nervous system.

GALEN HERBAL SUPPLIES

HERBCRAFT ALOE LAVENDER SPRAY

This product combines aloe vera juice and lavender oil with comfrey and marigold tinctures in a convenient spray. These herbs are all healing, antiseptic and anti-inflammatory and the mixture would be useful in the first aid box for treating minor cuts, grazes and burns.
• External use only.

FSC QUALITY VITAMINS

HERBCRAFT BURDOCK & NETTLE FORMULA

This unlicensed tincture combines burdock, stinging nettle, yellow dock and sarsparilla, which are all used in treating skin problems, with horsetail, which is astringent and healing, as well as alfalfa and wild oats which are both rich in nutrients to encourage healthy cell growth.

FSC QUALITY VITAMINS

HERBCRAFT CALENDULA & GOLDENSEAL SPRAY

This unlicensed tincture combines herbs that are largely anti-bacterial and antiseptic and would make a useful remedy for a range of infections. The product specifies external use only but the ingredients are all used internally in other products and the same herbs are often used for treating mouth infections, ulcers, sore throats and catarrhal problems. The product includes echinacea, golden seal, marigold, myrrh, cayenne and eucalyptus oil.
• External use only.

FSC QUALITY VITAMINS

HERBCRAFT DANDELION FORMULA

The herbs in this unlicensed combination are largely liver stimulants and restoratives as well as mild laxatives. The combination could be useful for a number of related digestive problems, as well as helping to stimulate a sluggish liver if this is contributing to skin disorders. The mixture contains dandelion, burdock, milk thistle, Oregon grape root and a very small amount of fennel.

FSC QUALITY VITAMINS

HERBCRAFT ECHINACEA, EYEBRIGHT AND BILBERRY FORMULA

This unlicensed combination of tinctures features herbs that are astringent, anticatarrhal, demulcent and anti-bacterial so the combination may be helpful for colds and various catarrhal conditions. The mixture is made up of echinacea, eyebright, bilberry, raspberry and *Usnea* spp. lichens.

FSC QUALITY VITAMINS

HERBCRAFT ECHINACEA FORMULA

This unlicensed combination of tinctures mixes anti-bacterial and antiseptic plants with general tonics and immune stimulants and so could be helpful for colds and recurrent infections. It contains echinacea, St John's wort, American ginseng, osha and cough root – a herb that is rarely found in European herbal products but was popular with Native Americans.   FSC QUALITY VITAMINS

HERBCRAFT FRESH BREATH CINNAMINT SPRAY

As the name implies this mixture is designed as a breath freshener. The herbs it contains are largely astringent and antiseptic to counter any bacterial infection or gum disease that is contributing to the problem, although there are, of course, various other stomach disorders that can lead to bad breath as well. This spray contains wild yam, marigold, silverweed, white oak and myrrh tinctures with very small amounts of cinnamon, peppermint and tea tree oils.

FSC QUALITY VITAMINS

HERBCRAFT GARLIC AND HORSERADISH WINTER FORMULA

This is a warming combination of herbs that would be good to take for colds and chills. The unlicensed product contains garlic, horseradish, onion, ginger, parsley and cayenne in a tincture format.   FSC QUALITY VITAMINS

HERBCRAFT LIQUORICE AND PROPOLIS SPRAY

This unlicensed product is designed as a throat spray. It contains a number of anti-bacterial and demulcent herbs that would be soothing for sore throats, laryngitis, hoarseness and tonsillitis. These are echinacea, liquorice, osha, myrrh, golden seal and *Usnea* spp. lichen with a very small amount of cayenne (often included in herbal gargles and mouth washes). The mixture also contains propolis – an anti-infection bee product.

Dosage: Spray into the back of the throat as required.

FSC QUALITY VITAMINS

HERBCRAFT LIQUORICE FORMULA

This combination is made up of liquorice, gotu kola, borage leaf, American ginseng and cayenne in tincture format. These are largely stimulating tonic herbs with borage and liquorice both useful stimulants for the adrenal glands (this can be helpful for those who have been taking steroids). The mixture could probably be helpful in cases of over-work, stress and exhaustion.

FSC QUALITY VITAMINS

HERBCRAFT MULLEIN FORMULA

This tincture combines a number of expectorant herbs and could be helpful for coughs and bronchitis. The mixture includes mullein, pleurisy root, bloodroot, osha, gumplant, liquorice and ginger.
• As it contains bloodroot the combination should be avoided in pregnancy.

FSC QUALITY VITAMINS

HERBCRAFT PASSIFLORA AND VALERIAN FORMULA

This is largely a soothing combination of relaxing and sedative herbs – passion flower, valerian, chamomile, Jamaica dogwood and wild lettuce – which suggests it could be suitable to ease tension and insomnia. Rather more unusually the mix also includes feverfew, which as an antispasmodic could help ease muscle tension although it is more usually regarded as a treatment for migraine; white willow also an anti-inflammatory normally used for arthritis and rheumatism; and blue vervain, which is a North American herb similar in action to the more familiar vervain used in Europe and is thus another useful sedative.

FSC QUALITY VITAMINS

HERBCRAFT PEPPERMINT FORMULA

This is a mixture of carminative herbs that could be helpful for indigestion and similar minor digestive upsets. It includes peppermint, dill, aniseed, fennel, ginger and cayenne with yellow gentian as a bitter digestive stimulant.

FSC QUALITY VITAMINS

HERBCRAFT REISHI SHIITAKE

In Chinese medicine both the reishi and shiitake mushrooms are regarded as important tonics and modern research has identified them as useful immune stimulants and anti-cancer herbs. This combination would be a useful tonic mix for those suffering from recurrent infections and the herbs can also help to soothe stress and worries.

FSC QUALITY VITAMINS

HERBS OF GRACE ANTI-FUNG

A combination of largely anti-fungal and antiseptic herbs which could be relevant as a supplement in anti-candida diets. The capsules contain marigold, rosemary, thyme, myrrh, hyssop, echinacea, fennel and pau d'arco.
• Avoid during pregnancy.

HERBS OF GRACE

HERBS OF GRACE ARNICA CREAM

An unlicensed cream containing arnica.

HERBS OF GRACE

HERBS OF GRACE BEAT EASY

Capsules containing a mixture of hawthorn, motherwort, ginkgo, dandelion, lime flowers and cayenne promoted for circulatory support. Hawthorn and motherwort are heart tonics, while ginkgo is good for the cerebral circulation and lime flowers help to reduce the risk of arteriosclerosis. Dandelion is possibly there as a diuretic and cayenne as a stimulant for the peripheral circulation.

HERBS OF GRACE

HERBS OF GRACE BTA

Capsules containing the laxative herbs – cascara sagrada and rhubarb – with stimulants, barberry, golden seal, ginger and cayenne, plus Indian tobacco and

raspberry leaf which is suggested as a general bowel tonic.
• Avoid during pregnancy.

HERBS OF GRACE BTB

Offered as a milder version of the same company's BTA product this comprises capsules containing cascara sagrada, rhubarb, chamomile, fennel and ginger (all carminatives), dandelion and wild yam.
• Avoid during pregnancy.

HERBS OF GRACE BTC

A third variation from Herbs of Grace, this one is suggested for use in pregnancy as a general laxative and bowel tonic. The capsules contain yellow dock, dandelion, chamomile and liquorice.

HERBS OF GRACE BULKING AGENT

Capsules containing isphaghula as a bulk laxative with the addition of common plantain (generally soothing for the mucous membranes), onion and dandelion,with cloves and fennel added as carminatives.

HERBS OF GRACE CALENDULA CREAM

An unlicensed cream containing marigold.

HERBS OF GRACE CHAMOMILE CREAM

An unlicensed cream containing German chamomile.

HERBS OF GRACE CHICKWEED CREAM

An unlicensed cream containing chickweed.

HERBS OF GRACE EMOTIONAL BALANCE

Capsules containing herbal nervines which could be suitable for tension and anxiety or as a general uplifting tonic. The mixture includes St John's wort (widely used as an anti-depressant), damiana, borage, ginseng and blue vervain (an American version of vervain and used in similar ways).

• Avoid during pregnancy. HERBS OF GRACE

HERBS OF GRACE EXPECT RELIEF

A warming combination of herbs suggested to ease nasal congestion. The mixture includes pepper, aniseed, cinnamon and ginger.

HERBS OF GRACE

HERBS OF GRACE MENOTUNE

Capsules containing chastetree, motherwort, helonias, *Dang Gui*, liquorice, alfalfa, black haw, black cohosh, sage and St John's wort suggested as a supplement for women in "middle age". Sage, chastetree, helonias, black cohosh and *Dang Gui* are used for a range of menopausal problems while alfalfa and liquorice are generally tonic and supportive herbs. Black haw is a useful uterine relaxant.

HERBS OF GRACE

HERBS OF GRACE PHYTO CALC

Suggested as a useful organic course of calcium, these capsules contain alfalfa, horsetail, chamomile, bladderwrack and marshmallow.

HERBS OF GRACE

HERBS OF GRACE PILEASE

Capsules containing a mixture of American cranesbill, rhubarb, barberry and marshmallow – a combination of laxatives, astringents and demulcents which could be helpful in constipation.

• Avoid during pregnancy. HERBS OF GRACE

HERBS OF GRACE PURE FLOW

Capsules containing a mixture of burdock, Oregon grape, yellow dock, queen's delight, stinging nettles and red clover promoted for circulatory support. These herbs are largely cleansing and diuretic.

• Avoid during pregnancy. HERBS OF GRACE

HERBS OF GRACE SINGLE HERB CAPSULES AND FLUID EXTRACTS

A range of single herbs in capsules, some of which are also available as fluid extracts. The company is currently offering the following capsules (names as listed in the A–Z of Herbs – if different – are given in brackets). Those also available as fluid extracts are indicated †:

Agnus Castus (chastetree)†
Angelica S. (*Dang Gui*)
Bladderwrack†
Cayenne
Dandelion Root (dandelion)†
Echinacea Angustifolia (echinacea)†
Ginger
Golden Seal
Guarana
Panax Ginseng (ginseng)
Passion Flower
Pau d'Arco
Red Clover†
Red Raspberry (raspberry)†
Scullcap (skullcap)†
Siberian Ginseng†
Slippery Elm
Uva Ursi (bearberry)
Valerian†
Wild Yam†
Yellow Dock†

HERBS OF GRACE

HERBS OF GRACE SWEET SLEEP

As the name suggests – a combination of soporific and sedative herbs for use at night. Capsules combine passion flower, skullcap, hops, lime flowers and chamomile with the addition of horsetail, more commonly used as a source of silica.

• Avoid during pregnancy. HERBS OF GRACE

HERBS OF GRACE THYROBAL

Capsules containing a mixture of stimulating herbs which could be relevant for problems associated with a sluggish metabolism or under active thyroid. The mixture includes bladderwrack, stinging nettles, damiana, gotu kola and wormwood (a very bitter digestive stimulant).

• Avoid during pregnancy.

HERBS OF GRACE

HERBS OF GRACE UROTON

Capsules containing diuretic herbs and urinary antiseptics that could be relevant in treating cystitis and similar urinary tract problems. The mixture includes: bearberry, couchgrass, echinacea, yarrow, buchu and marshmallow leaf.

HERBS OF GRACE

HERBS OF GRACE VARI-VN

Capsules containing a mixture of hawthorn, horse chestnut, prickly ash, yarrow and ginger promoted for circulatory support. Horse chestnut is used to treat varicose veins while others in the mix are largely circulatory and heart stimulants.

HERBS OF GRACE

HERBS OF GRACE VITAL FLOW

Capsules containing a mixture of prickly ash, barberry, shepherd's purse, yarrow, golden seal, *Dang Gui* and cayenne promoted for circulatory support. Of these prickly ash and cayenne are circulatory stimulants, while yarrow will relax the peripheral blood vessels and *Dang Gui* is used in Chinese medicine as a blood tonic. Other herbs in the mix are more commonly regarded as digestive stimulants.
• Avoid during pregnancy.

HERBS OF GRACE

HERBS OF GRACE WITCH HAZEL CREAM

An unlicensed cream containing witch hazel.

HERBS OF GRACE

*HERBULAX

A licensed remedy for constipation these tablets contain alder buckthorn and dandelion root which are laxative and bile stimulants.
• Not be used during lactation.

Dosage: adults 1 or 2 tablets before bed; start with 1 tablet and increase to 2 if necessary.

ENGLISH GRAINS HEALTHCARE

HÖFEL'S GINGER PEARLES

Unlicensed simple ginger capsules containing the equivalent of 300 mg of root.

This product is being replaced in mid-1996 with another containing the equivalent of 1200 mg of ginger root and a dosage of one-a-day. Suitable for both adults and children over seven years.

HÖFEL'S PURE FOODS

HÖFEL'S ONE-A-DAY CARDIOMAX GARLIC PEARLES

Capsules containing 4 mg of garlic oil extracted from 400 mg of fresh garlic, with a little peppermint oil to aid digestion.

Dosage: adults and children over seven years – 1 capsule a day.

HÖFEL'S PURE FOODS

*HÖFEL'S ONE-A-DAY GARLIC WITH PARSLEY

Licensed for the symptomatic relief of catarrh, rhinitis, coughs and colds these capsules contain 2 mg of garlic oil, equivalent to 2 g of fresh garlic, plus 15 mg of parsley extract which is traditionally used to reduce garlic odours.

Dosage: adults and children over seven years – 1 capsule a day.

HÖFEL'S PURE FOODS

HÖFEL'S ONE-A-DAY NEO-GARLIC PEARLES

Unlicensed simple garlic capsules containing 2 mg of garlic oil and reputedly tasteless and odourless.

Dosage: adults and children over seven – one a day.

HÖFEL'S PURE FOODS

*HÖFEL'S ORIGINAL ONE-A-DAY GARLIC PEARLES

Licensed for the symptomatic relief of catarrh, rhinitis, coughs and colds these capsules contain 2 mg of garlic oil equivalent to 2 g of fresh garlic.

Dosage: adults and children over seven years – 1 capsule a day.

HÖFEL'S PURE FOODS

HONEYROSE HERBAL CIGARETTES

A range of nicotine-free cigarettes which can be substituted for tobacco and thus could help smokers break the habit. Several flavours are available based on a mixture of herbs including marshmallow, red clover, rose and ginseng sometimes flavoured with honey and apple juice.

For smokers used to more than five tobacco cigarettes a day, the company recommends gradually replacing them with its herbal versions over a two week period and then phasing out the herbal products over the following week.

HONEYROSE.

*HRI CALM LIFE TABLETS

Licensed for restlessness and irritability this remedy contains a combination of popular sedative herbs – valerian, hops, Jamaica dogwood, skullcap and chamomile.
• Not to be taken during pregnancy unless under professional guidance.

Dosage: 1 or 2 tablets three times a day.

JESSOP MARKETING

*HRI CLEAR COMPLEXION TABLETS

Licensed for minor skin disorders and acne this product contains cleansing herbs widely used in skin remedies – sarsparilla, blue flag and burdock.
• Not to be taken in pregnancy or lactation unless prescribed.

Dosage: adults – 1 tablet two or three times a day; children over 12 years – 1 tablet, twice a day.

JESSOP MARKETING

*HRI GOLDEN SEAL DIGESTIVE

A licensed remedy for digestive problems, flatulence, irritable bowel, constipation and stomach disorders this remedy contains herbs that are stimulating for the digestion, laxative and carminative: ginger, myrrh, golden seal, rhubarb and valerian. The tablets also contain lactose.
• Not to be taken in pregnancy or lactation or by children under 12 years. Not to be taken by those with severe kidney disorders.

Dosage: 1 tablet three times a day. JESSOP MARKETING

*HRI HERBAL CATARRH AND RHINITIS TABLETS

This is a garlic simple containing 150 mg of garlic and 1 mg of garlic oil which is licensed for recurrent colds, hayfever and other nasal inflammations and respiratory infections. Like all garlic products it does have a wider spectrum of potential use.

• Not to be taken in pregnancy or lactation.

Dosage: adults – 1 tablet three times a day; children over eight years – 1 tablet night and morning.

JESSOP MARKETING

HRI NIGHT TABLETS

Although currently unlicensed, an application for this remedy is being processed by the Medicines Control Agency and a licence may be issued soon. It is a mixture of sedative herbs suitable for insomnia or general tension and includes wild lettuce, vervain, hops, passion flower and valerian.
• Not to be taken in pregnancy or lactation unless under professional guidance.

Dosage: 2 tablets early evening plus 2 or 3 tablets at bedtime.

JESSOP MARKETING

HRI WATER BALANCE TABLETS

Another product currently the subject of a licence application to the Medicines Control Agency, this is a combination of diuretic herbs that could be suitable for a number of urinary tract problems although the actual wording of the licence will probably simply specify fluid retention or slimming. It contains parsley piert, buchu, bearberry and dandelion root.
• Not to be taken in pregnancy or lactation unless under professional guidance.

Dosage: 2 tablets night and morning.   JESSOP MARKETING

IDOLOBA

Unlicensed ginkgo extract optimised to focus on flavonglycosides, ginkgolides A, B, C and bilobalide.

Dosage: 1 tablet two or three times daily, reduce to 1 or 2 tablets daily after two to six weeks.

FERROSAN HEALTHCARE

IMUNO-STRENGTH

This supplement is designed to boost the immune system and counter recurrent infections. It contains vitamins A, E, C and B_6 with iron, zinc, manganese and selenium, and the herbs echinacea, Siberian ginseng and more unusually, devil's claw which is anti-inflammatory rather than having an obvious tonic action on the immune system.

LAMBERTS HEALTHCARE

JAY-VEE TABLETS

An unlicensed combination of largely sedative herbs that could be helpful for anxiety and tension. The mix includes valerian, hops, lemon balm, hawthorn and passion flower with the addition of zinc.

Dosage: 1 or 2 tablets after meals, three times a day.

LAMBERTS HEALTHCARE

KELP PLUS 3

Food supplement containing 50 mg of kelp along with vitamin B_6, cider vinegar and lecithin.

Dosage: 2 tablets 30 minutes before main meals.

LARKHALL GREEN FARM

KIRA

Unlicensed simple tablets of St John's wort each containing 30 µg of hypericin.

Dosage: 1 tablet three times a day.

LICTWER PHARMA

KORDEL'S CELERY 3000 PLUS

An unlicensed combination of herbs which are generally used for treating arthritis and rheumatism – celery, white willow, feverfew and devil's claw – with the addition of yucca, rarely used in the UK, but an anti-inflammatory herb useful in the treatment of muscle and joint pains.

HEALTH IMPORTS

KORDEL'S CELERY AND JUNIPER

A mixture of diuretic herbs with additional potassium which can easily be depleted by use of such remedies. The combination includes celery, juniper, parsley and horsetail.
• Because of the juniper content it would be best avoided in pregnancy or by those with kidney disease, and should only be taken for short periods.

Dosage: 1 or 2 tablets three times a day.

HEALTH IMPORTS

KORDEL'S FEVERFEW AND WILLOW

An unlicensed combination of feverfew and white willow which could be suitable for headaches or joint pains.

Dosage: 1 or 2 tablets daily with food.

HEALTH IMPORTS

KORDEL'S GARLIC 3000

Unlicensed simple garlic capsules with an enteric coating flavoured with lemon-grass oil.

Dosage: 1 capsule a day.

HEALTH IMPORTS

KORDEL'S HORSERADISH, ODOURLESS GARLIC AND VITAMIN C

This unlicensed product is suggested as a supplement for hayfever and catarrh. It contains horseradish and garlic which are both warming and can be helpful for colds and catarrh as well as fenugreek – another warming herb which is also expectorant and a digestive stimulant – and marshmallow a soothing demulcent that can be helpful for coughs and catarrh. The tablets also contain potassium salts and vitamin C.

Dosage: adults – 1 or 2 tablets four times a day; children up to half the adult dose.

HEALTH IMPORTS

KORDEL'S I-VISTA

A combination of vitamins A, B_1, B_2 and C with eyebright designed as a tonic for the eyesight.

Dosage: 1 tablet daily.

HEALTH IMPORTS

KORDEL'S KALM-EX

Sedative combination of valerian, passion flower, hops and wild oats plus dolomite and vitamin B_1. The tablets also contain celery seed which is generally regarded as a rheumatic remedy but is also antispasmodic and carminative.

Dosage: 1–3 tablets daily.

HEALTH IMPORTS

KORDEL'S QUIET TIME

A combination of largely sedative herbs designed as a night-time supplement to aid sleep. The mixture comprises valerian, skullcap, chamomile, hops and passion flower with yellow gentian (a bitter digestive herb with some tonic action) and cayenne which is warming and stimulating.

Dosage: 1 or 2 half an hour before bedtime.

HEALTH IMPORTS

KORDEL'S WOMEN'S MULTI

An unlicensed combination of vitamins and minerals, with evening primrose oil, bearberry, horsetail, raspberry leaf, black cohosh, St John's wort and ginkgo designed as a general purpose tonic supplement. Bearberry and horsetail are diuretics while raspberry leaf, St John's wort and black cohosh are all used for menstrual irregularities.

Dosage: 1 tablet daily.

HEALTH IMPORTS

KWAI

Probably the top selling garlic product, these unlicensed tablets each contain the equivalent of 300 mg of herb. The product claims a particularly high proportion of allicin and alliin produced by using Chinese garlic.

Dosage: 1–2 tablets three times a day. A one-a-day version is also available.

LICTWER PHARMA

KYOLIC

An odourless garlic tablet produced from Japanese "aged garlic" which the suppliers claim breaks down the allicin content into equally beneficial but less smelly compounds. A number of strengths are available: Kyolic 100 tablets contain 300 mg of garlic powder, Kyolic 102 have 350 mg and Kyolic Reserve has 600 mg of garlic. Kyolic 100 also contains whey powder said to encourage gut bacteria.

Dosage: 1–4 tablets daily depending on tablet strength.

QUEST VITAMINS

KYOLIC LIQUID

A liquid version of the Kyolic garlic tablets.

Dosage: 4 ml a day mixed with a fruit drink, or used for topical application.

QUEST VITAMINS

LA GELEE ROYALE

A tonic combination of ginseng, damiana, saw palmetto, cayenne and borage oil with vitamin E which could be a help for fatigue and tiredness. The damiana and saw palmetto content could also be helpful for impotence. The product is supplied in 15 ml phials.

Dosage: 2 phials each morning.

ORTIS

LADIES MENO-LIFE FORMULA

An unlicensed product suggested as a supplement for menopausal women and containing a combination of sedatives, diuretics and tonic herbs. The mix includes kava kava, kelp, bearberry, black haw and wild lettuce, as well as life root which is now rarely used internally because of concerns over its toxicity. The tablets also contain vitamin B_6.
• Not to be taken in pregnancy.

Dosage: 1 tablet three times daily.

GALEN HERBAL SUPPLIES

LADYCARE: FOR WOMEN GOING THROUGH THE MENOPAUSE

This is basically a vitamin and mineral supplement with Siberian ginseng, which is a useful tonic for countering stress. The tablets contain vitamins A, D, E, C and B_6, with calcium, iodine and iron.

Dosage: 1 tablet a day.

FERROSAN HEALTHCARE

LADYCARE: FOR WOMEN WITH MONTHLY PERIODS

A vitamin and mineral supplement with the addition of bearberry as a diuretic. The tablets contain vitamins E, C, B_6, B_{12} and folic acid, as well as calcium, copper, iodine and iron.

FERROSAN HEALTHCARE

LAMBERTS ALFALFA EXTRACT

Unlicensed simple alfalfa tablets containing 450 mg equivalent of herb.

LAMBERTS HEALTHCARE

LAMBERTS CHEWABLE BROMELAIN WITH PAPAIN

A combination of bromelain and papain derived, respectively, from pineapple and papaya. These enzymes hydrolyse digestive products including amides and polypeptides so improving function.

Dosage: 1 or 2 capsules daily.

LAMBERTS HEALTHCARE

LAMBERTS EVENING PRIMROSE

Capsules of evening primrose oil containing 8% *gamma*-linolenic acid and available in 250, 500 and 1,000 mg.

Dosage: 1–3 capsules.

LAMBERTS HEALTHCARE

LAMBERTS FLAX SEED OIL

Capsules containing 1000 mg of linseed oil as a source of *cis*-linoleic and *alpha*-linolenic acid.

Dosage: 1–3 capsules daily.

LAMBERTS HEALTHCARE

LAMBERTS GARLIC OIL

Unlicensed simple garlic capsules containing 2 mg of oil said to be equivalent to 1 g of garlic.

Dosage: 1–3 capsules daily.

LAMBERTS HEALTHCARE

LAMBERTS GARLIC & PARSLEY

A combination of 574 mg garlic and 110 mg parsley which can help to reduce garlic smells.

Dosage: 1–3 capsules daily.   LAMBERTS HEALTHCARE

LAMBERTS GINKGO BILOBA EXTRACT

Unlicensed simple ginkgo capsules each containing 40 mg of herb.

Dosage: 1–3 capsules daily

LAMBERTS HEALTHCARE

LAMBERTS HIGH GLA

Unlicensed capsules containing 754 mg of borage oil which has a higher percentage of *gamma*-linolenic acid than evening primrose oil.

Dosage: 1 capsule daily.

LAMBERTS HEALTHCARE

LAMBERTS KELP TABLETS

Unlicensed simple kelp tablets using the seaweed *Ascophyllum nodosum.*

Dosage: 1–3 capsules daily.

LAMBERTS HEALTHCARE

LAMBERTS PEPPERMINT OIL CAPSULES

Capsules containing 50 mg of peppermint oil in a sunflower oil base.
• Excessive use of peppermint can damage the stomach lining and lead to ulceration.

Dosage: 1 capsule after meals three times a day.

LAMBERTS HEALTHCARE

LAMBERTS PURE-GAR

Capsules containing 500 mg of Pure-Gar® garlic powder (See: FSC Whole Bulb Garlic).

Dosage: 1–3 capsules daily.

LAMBERTS HEALTHCARE

LAMBERTS SILYMARIN EXTRACT

Unlicensed simple milk thistle tablets containing 50 mg of herb.

Dosage: 1–3 capsules daily.

LAMBERTS HEALTHCARE

*LANE'S CUT-A-COUGH

A licensed remedy for the relief of coughs, colds and chestiness based on squill as an expectorant with cayenne, peppermint, aniseed, clove and eucalyptus oil as warming and anti-catarrhal additions.

Dosage: adults and children over 7 years – 1 × 5 ml teaspoon three or four times a day.

RICKARD LANE'S & W H BOX

*LANE'S NUMBER 44 SKIN OINTMENT

An ointment containing a small amount of tea tree which is licensed for the relief of eczema, pimples and skin irritation. The product also contains zinc oxide, potassium hydroxyquinoline sulphate, and coal tar solution, which is often used in psoriasis treatments.

Dosage: adults and children over 8 years – apply 2–3 times a day.

RICKARD LANE'S & W H BOX

*LANE'S SAGE AND GARLIC CATARRH REMEDY

This is a licensed remedy for the symptomatic relief of colds, nasal and bronchial catarrh and to soothe chesty coughs. It contains liquorice (an expectorant) with garlic and sage which are both anti-bacterial, pine (decongestant and expectorant) and juniper oils. The mixture also contains chloroform spirit, tragacanth gum, menthol (a peppermint extract) and syrup.
• Not recommended in pregnancy and when breast feeding.

Dosage: adults 1 × 5 ml teaspoon three or four times a day and during the night; children 8–15 years – 1 × 5 ml teaspoon every six hours.

RICKARD LANE'S & W H BOX

*LANES ATHERA

A licensed remedy for the relief of minor symptoms associated with the menopause. This product contains the diuretics and laxatives parsley, senna and clivers along with vervain which is an effective nervine.
• Not to be taken in pregnancy.

Dosage: 2–3 tablets three times a day.

METABASIC PRODUCTS/G R LANE HEALTH PRODUCTS

*LANES BIOBALM

Licensed for the symptomatic relief of indigestion, flatulence and stomach upsets, this remedy is a combination of soothing demulcents, that would combat stomach acidity and carminatives. The mixture includes slippery elm, marshmallow, Irish moss and chamomile.
• Not suitable for children under five years.

Dosage: 1 or 2 teaspoons in half a cup of cold water. Add hot water or juice. Reheat for one or two minutes.

MODERN HEALTH PRODUCT/G R LANE HEALTH PRODUCTS

*LANES CASCADE

Licensed to "assist in the elimination of excess water" this is a mixture of diuretic herbs including bearberry, clivers and burdock root with some parsley root powder.
• Not suitable in pregnancy, while breast feeding or for children under 12 years.

Dosage: 2 tablets three times a day.

MODERN HEALTH PRODUCTS/G R LANE HEALTH PRODUCTS

*LANES DIGEST

A licensed remedy for the relief of indigestion and flatulence this mixture combines centaury – a bitter digestive stimulant – with marshmallow which would help to protect the stomach lining. It also includes parsley (which is carminative and slightly laxative) and chamomile, also carminative.
• Not suitable in pregnancy, while breast feeding, or for children under 12 years.

Dosage: 2 tablets three times a day before meals.

MODERN HEALTH PRODUCTS/G R LANE HEALTH PRODUCTS

*LANES DUAL-LAX EXTRA STRONG

This mixture of potent laxatives – aloin (an extract of aloes), cascara sagrada and senna – is licensed for the relief of temporary constipation.
• Not recommended for children, during early pregnancy or when breast feeding.

Dosage: 1 or 2 tablets at night.

G R LANE HEALTH PRODUCTS

*LANES GARLODEX

Licensed for the symptomatic relief of colds and catarrh this remedy combines

garlic oil with marshmallow which is a soothing demulcent that can ease coughs and catarrh. The product also contains parsley which may be there to reduce the smell of garlic.
• Not suitable in pregnancy, during breast feeding or for children under five years.

Dosage: 1 tablet three times a day.

MODERN HEALTH PRODUCTS

*LANES HEEMEX

A licensed remedy for treating piles, this ointment contains distilled witch-hazel with zinc oxide and benzoin which is a useful herb for various skin irritations.
• Not recommended for children or if there is benzoin allergy; for external use only.

Dosage: Apply night and morning and after emptying the bowels.

G R LANE HEALTH PRODUCTS

*LANES HERBELIX SPECIFIC

The main herbs in this mixture are Indian tobacco and tolu balsam which although they can relieve catarrh, are both also expectorants ideal for stubborn coughs, although the licence for this remedy suggests that it is suitable for the symptomatic relief of catarrh, hay fever, rhinitis, head colds and mucous congestion. It also contains sodium bicarbonate, and small amounts of cayenne, peppermint oil, ginger, yellow gentian, quassia and rhubarb which are are largely bitter digestive stimulants rather than anti-catarrhal herbs.
• Not recommended for children under seven years, not suitable in pregnancy or during breast feeding.

Dosage: adults – 1 × 5 ml teaspoon in a little water at night; children over seven years – 2.5 ml in a little water at night.

MODERN HEALTH PRODUCTS/G R LANE HEALTH PRODUCTS

*LANES HONEY AND MOLASSES COUGH MIXTURE

This remedy combines a number of expectorant and anti-catarrhal herbs and is licensed for the symptomatic relief of coughs, colds, hoarseness, sore throats and catarrh. It includes ipecacuanha, white horehound, squill and tolu with a little cayenne, peppermint and anise oil which will improve the flavour.
• Not to be used in pregnancy, while breast feeding or if there is heart or kidney disease.

Dosage: adults – 1 × 5 ml teaspoon, three times a day; children seven to 14 years

– 2.5 ml three times a day; children two to seven years – 2.5 ml once a day.

*LANES KALMS

Licensed for relieving symptoms of stress, tension or insomnia, this mixture contains the sedatives valerian and hops with yellow gentian which is useful for physical exhaustion.
• Not recommended for those suffering from clinical depression, during pregnancy or lactation, or for children.

Dosage: 2 tablets three times a day after meals.

G R LANE HEALTH PRODUCTS

*LANES KLEER

A licensed remedy for skin conditions and eczema this mixture combines antibacterial echinacea with stinging nettle and burdock which are both cleansing herbs popular for skin problems. The mixture also includes a little parsley powder which may be there purely as a colourant rather than for therapeutic purposes.

Dosage: adults – 2 tablets three times a day before meals; children aged five to 12 years – 1 tablet three times a day before meals.

MODERN HEALTH PRODUCTS/G R LANE HEALTH PRODUCTS

*LANES KLEER TI-TREE AND WITCH HAZEL CREAM

As its name implies, this product combines tea tree and witch hazel with the addition of eucalyptus oil and is licensed for the relief of minor skin conditions, cuts and wounds. Tea tree and eucalyptus are antiseptic while the distilled witch hazel is astringent and healing.
• Not to be used with creams containing benzyl penicillan; for external use only.

Dosage: Use as required and at night.   G R LANE HEALTH PRODUCTS

*LANES NATUREST

This is a simple passion flower tablet which is licensed for the treatment of temporary or occasional sleeplessness caused by everyday problems.
• Not recommended for children under 12 years, or during pregnancy and lactation.

Dosage: Adults and children over 12 – two tablets, three times a day and up to 3 more at bedtime.

G R LANE, HEALTH PRODUCTS

*LANES PILEABS

Licensed for the temporary relief of constipation and for itching and discomfort due to piles, this remedy actually contains the laxative cascara sagrada combined with slippery elm which is a soothing demulcent normally used in such conditions as gastritis and indigestion rather than as a pile remedy.
• Not recommended for children or during pregnancy.

Dosage: 2 tablets three times a day.

G R LANE HEALTH PRODUCTS

*LANES QUIET LIFE TABLETS

This licensed remedy for nervous tension and insomnia contains a popular combination of sedative herbs – hops, valerian, wild lettuce, motherwort and passion flower – with the addition of vitamins B_1, B_2 and B_3. Supplements of vitamins B_1 and B_3 are sometimes given for nervous problems.
• Not recommended during pregnancy, lactation or for children. High doses may cause headaches or sickness in sensitive individuals.

Dosage: 2 tablets twice a day after meals and 2 or 3 tablets at bedtime.

G R LANE HEALTH PRODUCTS

LANES SHEN

A simple garlic tablet using Chinese garlic powder and a slow air drying technique which is said to reduce odours. The tablets are enteric coated and contain the equivalent of 300 mg of fresh garlic.

Dosage: adults – 1 or 2 tablets three times a day; children – 1 tablet three times a day to be taken with food. Do not chew.

G R LANE HEALTH PRODUCTS

*LANES SINOTAR

This is a licensed remedy to provide symptomatic relief from blocked up sinuses and catarrh. It contains echinacea which is anti-bacterial, anti-catarrhal elder flowers and marshmallow which is a soothing demulcent for the mucous membranes.
• Not for use in pregnancy, while breast feeding or for children under five.

Dosage: adults – 2 tablets three times a day before meals; children five to 12 years – 1 tablet three times a day.

MODERN HEALTH PRODUCTS/G R LANE HEALTH PRODUCTS

*LANES VEGETEX

A licensed remedy for the symptomatic relief of muscular rheumatic pain, lumbago and fibrositis this mixture contains anti-inflammatory herbs that are also often used for arthritic problems. The mixture includes celery leaf, bogbean, black cohosh and celery, with horseradish and cayenne which would stimulate the circulation.
• Not recommended for children under 12 years, during pregnancy or breast feeding.

Dosage: 3 tablets three times a day.

MODERN HEALTH PRODUCTS/G R LANE HEALTH PRODUCTS

LIQUID IRON

An iron tonic using extracts of bilberry in mistella wine with the addition of "vegetable iron" This is based on apple juice to which iron has been added so that the acidity of the fruit naturally dissolves and absorbs a small amount of iron.

Dosage: 1 × 5 ml teaspoon in the morning, diluted in fruit juice if preferred. In severe cases the dose can be increased to 10 or 15 ml for a week or two.

ORTIS

*LUSTY'S GARLIC PERLES

A licensed simple garlic product recommended for coughs, colds and catarrh. Each capsule contains 0.66 mg of garlic oil.
• Not recommended for children under five years.

Dosage: adults – 1 capsule three times a day, or up to 3 at night; children five to 12 years – 1 capsule twice a day with food.

G R LANE HEALTH PRODUCTS

*LUSTY'S HERBALENE

A licensed laxative mixture for temporary or occasional constipation which combines senna, alder buckthorn, and elder leaves (a strong purgative but now rarely used) with fennel as a carminative to counter griping. The mixture is sold as a dried herbal powder to be taken in infusion and is flavoured with maté.

Dosage: adults – ½–1 × 5 ml teaspoon on the tongue washed down with warm water first thing in the morning or last thing at night or the same dose infused in a cup of boiling water; children seven to 14 years – half the adult dose.

G R LANE HEALTH PRODUCTS

MAN POWER

A tonic supplement containing ginseng and evening primrose oil with the addition of lecithin and vitamin E.

Dosage: 1 or 2 capsules daily.

POWER HEALTH

MELBROSIA EXECUTIVE

A tonic mixture for men containing flower pollen, royal jelly and ginseng.

CEDAR HEALTH

MELBROSIA PLD

This supplement is sold as a menopause product and contains flower pollen, royal jelly and acerola.

CEDAR HEALTH

*MUIR'S CATARRH

A licensed product for the symptomatic relief of nasal catarrh, throat catarrh and the catarrh of hay fever, this mixture combines echinacea and myrrh (both strongly anti-bacterial) with boneset, which is often used for treating colds and influenza, and black catechu a strongly astringent herb.
• Avoid in early pregnancy.

Dosage: adults – 2 tablets three times a day; children over eight years – 1 tablet three times a day.

WILLIAM MUIR/HEALTH IMPORTS

*MUIR'S ECHINACEA

A simple echinacea product which in this case is licensed for the symptomatic relief of minor skin conditions and blemishes although the herb is also effective for a wide range of infectious conditions.
• Not recommended for use in pregnancy or lactation.

Dosage: 2 tablets, three times a day.

WILLIAM MUIR/HEALTH IMPORTS

*MUIR'S GASTRIC-ESE

A combination of digestive stimulants and astringents which is licensed for the

symptomatic relief of stomach pain and discomfort. The mixture includes golden seal and barberry which are both bitter liver stimulants, agrimony, American cranesbill and liquorice (also laxative).
• Not recommended for use in pregnancy or lactation.

Dosage: 1 tablet an hour before breakfast; 1 two hours after each meal, and 1 at bedtime.

WILLIAM MUIR/HEALTH IMPORTS

*MUIR'S HEAD-ESE

This combination of nervines is licensed for the symptomatic relief of tenseness and agitation. The mix includes wild lettuce, Jamaica dogwood, valerian, vervain, passion flower and wild oats which is a sedative and restoring combination.
• Not recommended for use in pregnancy or lactation.

Dosage: 2 tablets three times a day.

WILLIAM MUIR/HEALTH IMPORTS

*MUIR'S PICK-ME-UP

A tonic combination of stimulants, sedatives and digestive remedies which is licensed for debility in convalescence and to aid recovery after periods of stress and strain. The mix comprises lime flowers, motherwort, skullcap and valerian which are all basically sedating, with cola (a stimulant rich in caffeine), agrimony and Oregon grape which are both liver stimulants to improve the digestion.

Dosage: adults – 2 tablets three times a day; children over eight years – 1 tablet three times a day.

WILLIAM MUIR/HEALTH IMPORTS

*MUIR'S RHEUMATIC PAIN

A licensed remedy for the symptomatic relief of rheumatic pain, lumbago and fibrositis this mixture combines cleansing, diuretic herbs with circulatory stimulants and anti-inflammatories. The mix could also be suitable for arthritis and is made up of bogbean, prickly ash, black cohosh, yellow dock, buchu and cayenne.
• Not recommended for use in pregnancy or for children.

Dosage: 2 tablets three times a day.

WILLIAM MUIR/HEALTH IMPORTS

*MUIR'S SCIATICA

Although licensed as a remedy for the symptomatic relief of sciatica and lumbago, this is a combination of diuretic herbs which would be suitable if the back pain was related to kidney or urinary dysfunction rather than stemming from the sciatic nerve. It contains shepherd's purse, juniper, wild carrot, bearberry and clivers.

• Because of the juniper content the remedy should be avoided during pregnancy or in kidney disease and should not be taken for long periods without a break.

Dosage: 2 tablets three times a day. The last dose at 6pm.

WILLIAM MUIR/HEALTH IMPORTS

*MUIR'S STRESS-ESE

Licensed for the relief of nervous restlessness and tension due to the stresses and strains of modern life, this is a combination of sedative and restoring nervine herbs very similar to Muir's Head-Ese combination. This product includes vervain, wild lettuce, wild oats, passion flower, valerian and Jamaica dogwood.

• Avoid in early pregnancy.

Dosage: 2 tablets three times a day.

WILLIAM MUIR/HEALTH IMPORTS

*MUIR'S WATER-ESE

A combination of diuretic herbs licensed "to balance natural body fluids" but which could be helpful for cystitis as well. The remedy comprises buchu, juniper, parsley piert and bearberry which are also urinary antiseptics and astringents.

• Because of the juniper content the remedy should be avoided during pregnancy or in kidney disease and should not be taken for long periods without a break.

Dosage: 2 tablets three times a day, the last dose at 6pm.

WILLIAM MUIR/HEALTH IMPORTS

MYCOHERB MYCO FORTE

This liquid extract combines extracts of five fungi used in traditional Chinese medicine: cordyceps, reishi, shiitake, maitake and snow fungus. These have all been shown to have significant effects on the immune system and can be useful as a general tonic or for combating recurrent infection. Research also suggests the herbs may have anti-cancer activity.

EAST WEST HERBS

MYCOHERB REI SHI GEN

This is a combination of reishi and shiitake mushrooms which are immune stimulants and also have an uplifting effect on the emotions (cf. Herbcraft Reishi Shiitake). The mixture is available in liquid extract, capsules and powder formats.

Dosage: 1–6 capsules daily.

EAST WEST HERBS

MYCOHERB TRI MYCO GEN

This is a combination of three traditional Chinese medicinal fungi – cordyceps, reishi and shiitake. It is reputedly immune stimulating and anti-bacterial, useful for tonifying blood and *Qi* and given for general weakness and debility. The product is available in both liquid extract and powdered in capsules.

EAST WEST HERBS

*NATRACALM

This is a simple passion flower tablet which is licensed for nervous tension, stress and strain.

Dosage: 1 tablet three times a day with an additional tablet at night if required.

ENGLISH GRAINS HEALTHCARE

*NATRALEZE

This licensed remedy combines slippery elm, meadowsweet and liquorice for the symptomatic relief of heartburn, dyspepsia and indigestion. It also contains peppermint oil as a flavouring although this herb is also a carminative. Meadowsweet is an effective remedy for a variety of gastric upsets while slippery elm is a useful demulcent for protecting the stomach lining. Liquorice is used in various digestive disorders ranging from constipation to stomach ulcers.
• Not recommended for use in pregnancy.

Dosage: adults and children over 12 years – chew 2 tablets after meals; children seven to 12 years – chew 1 tablet after meals.

ENGLISH GRAINS HEALTHCARE

*NATRASLEEP

A licensed combination of hops and valerian which can be used for insomnia.

Dosage: 1–3 tablets as required half an hour before bedtime.

ENGLISH GRAINS HEALTHCARE

NATURAL FLOW CITRIMAX FAT CONTROL NUTRITIONAL COMPLEX

This is a slimming aid using a 500 mg extract of the Malabar tamarind (a source of (-)-hydroxycitric acid – HCA) which has been shown to reduce the appetite. The product also includes 20 mg vitamin C which helps to stabilise HCA.

Dosage: 2–4 tablets, three times a day, preferably 30–60 minutes before meals.
LARKHALL GREEN FARM

NATURAL FLOW COLONITE

From the Nature Flow range of cleansing digestive products, this contains a mixture of holy thistle, butternut, cloves, corn silk, red clover and yellow dock. These are mainly laxative, liver stimulants and diuretics. Colonite is recommended to be taken with a bulking laxative (such as isphaghula) as part of a colon cleansing programme.

Dosage: 1 or 2 tablets two to four times a day.
LARKHALL GREEN FARM

NATURAL FLOW EVENING PRIMROSE OIL

Evening primrose oil with 10% of *gamma*-linolenic acid in 500 mg and 1000 mg capsules

Dosage: 1–6 capsules daily.   LARKHALL GREEN FARM

NATURAL FLOW PSYLLIUM HUSKS

Isphaghula husks sold loose in packs and also available in a capsule format. They should be taken with large amounts of water.
LARKHALL GREEN FARM

NATURAL FLOW REGULAR TEN POWDER

Like other Natural Flow products this is aimed at improving digestive function. It is largely a combination of laxative herbs, with garlic as an anti-bacterial to help normalize gut flora, slippery elm, which is soothing and protective for the gastric mucosa, and alfalfa which also stimulates bowel action. Other herbs in the mix are isphaghula, burdock, cascara sagrada and clove; it also includes *Lactobacillus acidophilus*.

Dosage: 1 heaped teaspoon up to twice a day in water.
LARKHALL GREEN FARM

NATURAL FLOW TRIPLE GINSENG

An unlicensed combination of Korean, Siberian and American ginsengs which could provide a stimulating energy tonic.

LARKHALL GREEN FARM

NATURE'S PLUS GARLITE

A simple garlic capsule containing 500 mg of cool dried herb in an enteric coating to reduce odour.

LARKHALL GREEN FARM

NATURE'S PLUS GINKGO COMBO

A tonic combination of ginkgo and gotu kola with a little cayenne and vitamin E which could be a useful stimulating supplement for the elderly.

LARKHALL GREEN FARM

NATURE'S PLUS IMMUNFORTE

A supplement to boost the immune system containing vitamins A, C, and E with zinc and selenium, echinacea and ginseng.

LARKHALL GREEN FARM

NATURE'S PLUS PROST-ACTIN

A mixture of saw palmetto extract, zinc and vitamins suggested to maintain a healthy prostate gland.

LARKHALL GREEN FARM

NATURE'S VYRBRIT

This unlicensed lip salve has been available in Germany for 10 years but was only recently launched in the UK. It contains "melpan 5" which is a lemon balm extract, and also contains allantoin (a healing substance also found in comfrey). It is marketed as a product for chapped lips and cold sores.
• External use only.

Dosage: apply two to four times a day.

BRITANNIA HEALTH

NEAL'S YARD ALOE VERA JUICE

A simple aloe vera juice extract.

NEAL'S YARD REMEDIES

NEAL'S YARD ANTI-OXIDANT HERBS ELIXIR

The herbs in this mixture have been shown to have anti-oxidant properties which can combat free radicals and counter the ageing of cells. The mixture contains rosemary, marjoram, oregano, peppermint, sage and thyme and each capsule is said to provide anti-oxidant activity equivalent to at least 60 mg of *beta*-carotene. (cf Pure-fil Romagen).

• Consult your doctor if pregnant or taking medicines.

Dosage: 1 capsule daily.

NEAL'S YARD REMEDIES

NEAL'S YARD ARNICA OINTMENT

Unlicensed ointment containing arnica.
• External use only.

NEAL'S YARD REMEDIES

NEAL'S YARD BALM OF GILEAD

Neal's Yard Remedies says this is Potter's Balm of Gilead product repackaged under a different brand name. The mix of herbs is, however, slightly different to those listed by Potter's (q.v.) and in this case is balm of gilead, squill, Indian tobacco, ipecacuanha and lungmoss ("lungwort lichen"). It is not sold as a licensed remedy although Potter's version is, of course, licensed as a cough remedy.

Dosage: adults – 2 × 5 ml teaspoons three or four times a day; children – 1 × 5 ml teaspoon three times a day, diluted in water if preferred.

NEAL'S YARD REMEDIES

NEAL'S YARD BLADDERWRACK CAPSULES

An unlicensed simple containing 500 mg of ground bladderwrack per capsule.

Dosage: 2 capsules three times a day.

NEAL'S YARD REMEDIES

NEAL'S YARD BUCHU COMPOUND CAPSULES

Unlicensed capsules containing a combination of diuretics and urinary anti-septics that would be useful for cystitis and other types of urinary problems. Herbs used are buchu, bearberry and dandelion.

Dosage: 1 or 2 capsules three times a day.

NEAL'S YARD REMEDIES

NEAL'S YARD CALENDULA OINTMENT

An unlicensed ointment containing marigold.
• External use only.

NEAL'S YARD REMEDIES

NEAL'S YARD CASCARA COMPOUND

This is a combination of the laxatives cascara sagrada and senna with fennel added as a carminative to counter any griping pains they may produce.
• Seek professional advice for chronic constipation.

Dosage: 1 or 2 capsules before retiring.

NEAL'S YARD REMEDIES

NEAL'S YARD CELLULITE OIL

This combination of lemon, juniper and pepper oils with frankincense is pro-moted as a massage treatment for cellulite. This is largely a rubefacient mix to encourage blood flow, although frankincense is also traditionally used to improve skin quality.
• External use only.

NEAL'S YARD REMEDIES

NEAL'S YARD COMFREY OINTMENT

Unlicensed ointment containing comfrey.
• External use only.

NEAL'S YARD REMEDIES

NEAL'S YARD ECHINACEA AND PROPOLIS OINTMENT

An unlicensed ointment containing echinacea and propolis (a bee product) which are both effective at combating infections, so this preparation may be useful for cuts, pimples and boils, for example.

• External use only.

NEAL'S YARD REMEDIES

NEAL'S YARD ECHINACEA CAPSULES

Unlicensed capsules containing 300 mg of echinacea *(E. angustifolia)* as a simple.

Dosage: 1 or 2 capsules three times a day.

NEAL'S YARD REMEDIES

NEAL'S YARD ECHINACEA & MALLOW LINCTUS

A cough syrup containing marshmallow and aniseed, which are soothing and gentle expectorants, with echinacea in a base of Canadian clover honey and glycerine.

Dosage: adults – 2 × teaspoons three times a day; children – 1 teaspoon three times a day.

NEAL'S YARD REMEDIES

NEAL'S YARD ELDERFLOWER, PEPPERMINT & COMPOSITION ESSENCE

This is a Potter's product which is repackaged by Neal's Yard Remedies. It contains the same mix of herbs: elder flowers, peppermint, bayberry, hemlock spruce, cayenne, ginger, cassia, clove and pimento *(Pimenta dioica)* as a warming brew for colds and chills. (cf. *Culpeper's Elder Flower and Peppermint Mixture.)

Dosage: adults – 2 teaspoons in half a cup of hot water, three times a day and at bedtime; children over five years – half the adult dose.

NEAL'S YARD REMEDIES

NEAL'S YARD EUCALYPTUS & MENTHOL LOZENGES

A mixture of essential oils, herbal macerates and honey produced in France for Neal's Yard. The mix is largely anti-catarrhal, astringent and antiseptic and the lozenges may thus be helpful for colds and nasal congestion. It includes eucalyptus, lemon and peppermint oil with golden seal and additional menthol (an active constituent of peppermint).

NEAL'S YARD REMEDIES

NEAL'S YARD EVENING PRIMROSE OIL CAPSULES

Unlicensed capsules containing 500 mg of evening primrose oil.

Dosage: 1–8 capsules a day with food.

NEAL'S YARD REMEDIES

NEAL'S YARD EVENING PRIMROSE OIL DROPS

Evening primrose oil for external use and for those who do not want to take gelatin capsules.

NEAL'S YARD REMEDIES

NEAL'S YARD FEVERFEW CAPSULES

Unlicensed capsules containing 500 mg of feverfew as a simple.
• Not to be taken in pregnancy.

Dosage: 1 capsule three times a day.

NEAL'S YARD REMEDIES

NEAL'S YARD GARLIC CAPSULES

Unlicensed simple garlic capsules using powdered garlic rather than oil.

Dosage: 1 capsule three times a day.

NEAL'S YARD REMEDIES

NEAL'S YARD GINGER AND JUNIPER WARMING OIL

A warming rub for use after sports or when over-exerted containing essential oils often used for muscular aches and pains and stiffness. These are ginger, juniper, rosemary, lavender and sage oils.
• External use only.

NEAL'S YARD REMEDIES

NEAL'S YARD GINSENG CAPSULES

Unlicensed capsules containing 500 mg of powdered ginseng root as a simple.

Dosage: 1 capsule a day.

NEAL'S YARD REMEDIES

NEAL'S YARD HOREHOUND & ANISEED LINCTUS

Neal's Yard Remedies says that this is a Potter's product repackaged under its name (cf. *Potter's Horehound & Aniseed Linctus) which is licensed as a cough remedy.

Dosage: adults – 2 × 5 ml teaspoons three to four times a day; children – 1 teaspoon, three times a day, diluted in water if preferred.

NEAL'S YARD REMEDIES

NEAL'S YARD HOREHOUND & HONEY LOZENGES

A mixture of essential oils, herbal macerates and honey produced in France for Neal's Yard and containing white horehound, coltsfoot and aniseed with thyme and cypress oils. These herbs are expectorant, antispasmodic or anti-catarrhal and the lozenges could thus be helpful for coughs and bronchial congestion.

NEAL'S YARD REMEDIES

NEAL'S YARD HYPERCAL OINTMENT

An unlicensed ointment containing marigold and St John's wort which are both antiseptic and healing herbs used for treating minor wounds.
• External use only.

NEAL'S YARD REMEDIES

NEAL'S YARD HYPERICUM AND URTICA OINTMENT

An unlicensed ointment containing stinging nettles and St John's wort. Nettles are sometimes used in creams for skin eruptions and eczema although the herb is more usually taken internally for such conditions. St John's wort is antiseptic and healing.
• External use only.

NEAL'S YARD REMEDIES

NEAL'S YARD KELP TABLETS

Unlicensed tablets containing unspecified seaweed extracts.
• Not to be taken with thyroid problems or during pregnancy or lactation.

Dosage: adult – 1 × tablet four times a day; children – 1 tablet twice a day.

NEAL'S YARD REMEDIES

NEAL'S YARD LEMON & HONEY LOZENGES

A mixture of essential oils, herbal macerates and honey produced in France for Neal's Yard and containing ginger and lemon oils with echinacea and sage. These last two herbs are often used for treating sore throats and laryngitis. The mixture also contains propolis.

NEAL'S YARD REMEDIES

NEAL'S YARD PASSIFLORA TABLETS

Unlicensed tablets containing passion flower as a simple.

Dosage: adult – 2 tablets at tea-time and 2 at bedtime; children – 1 tablet at bedtime.

NEAL'S YARD REMEDIES

NEAL'S YARD RASPBERRY LEAF CAPSULES

Unlicensed capsules containing 500 mg of organically grown raspberry leaf as a simple.

Dosage: 1 capsule three times a day.

NEAL'S YARD REMEDIES

NEAL'S YARD RHUS TOX AND RUTA OINTMENT

An unlicensed ointment containing rue and poison ivy – both herbs used in homoeopathy for treating muscular pains, sprains and bruising.
• External use only.

NEAL'S YARD REMEDIES

NEAL'S YARD SCULLCAP COMPOUND CAPSULES

A combination of sedative and relaxing herbs – valerian, skullcap and vervain suitable for anxiety, mild depression, and insomnia.

Dosage: for day time use take 1 capsule three times a day; for night time use take 1 or 2 capsules at bedtime.

NEAL'S YARD REMEDIES

NEAL'S YARD SLIPPERY ELM TABLETS

Chewable tablets containing mainly slippery elm which has been flavoured by the carminative oils cinnamon, clove and peppermint. The combination would be suitable to indigestion and various stomach upsets.

Dosage: adults – 1 or 2 tablets after meals; children – 1 tablet after meals up to four times a day.

NEAL'S YARD REMEDIES

NEAL'S YARD SPORTS SALVE

A rub for use after sports or for over-exertion containing primarily rubefacient oils to improve circulation with healing herbs to help any damaged tissues. The salve contains ginger, rosemary and lavender oils with arnica and comfrey.
• External use only.

NEAL'S YARD REMEDIES

NEAL'S YARD STELLARIA OINTMENT

An unlicensed ointment containing chickweed.
• External use only.

NEAL'S YARD REMEDIES

*NELSONS ARNICA 6×

Homoeopathic tablets containing arnica which can be used for accidents, shock, traumatic injuries or to improve recovery after surgery and childbirth.

A NELSON & CO

*NELSONS ARNICA CREAM

A licensed cream containing arnica which can be used for all types of bruises resulting from injuries, knocks and falls.
• External use only.

Dosage: apply gently to bruised areas.

A NELSON & CO

*NELSONS BURNS OINTMENT

Licensed to relieve pain, prevent blistering and promote rapid healing, this ointment is suitable for minor burns and contains St John's wort with marigold, echinacea and annual nettle which is used in homoeopathic treatments for burns.
• External use only.

Dosage: Apply the ointment immediately to cover more than the affected area. Cover with a dry dressing and bandage lightly if necessary.

A NELSON & CO

*NELSONS CALENDULA CREAM

A licensed marigold cream sold as a multi-purpose skin salve and suitable for use on cuts, grazes, sore nipples, eczema or for nappy rash in babies.
• External use only.

Dosage: apply gently to sore and rough skin, repeat as necessary.

A NELSON & CO

*NELSONS CHILBLAIN OINTMENT

This is a homoeopathic remedy using the potent herb bryony in small quantities. It is licensed to give soothing relief from chilblains. Bryony is also used externally for rheumatic pain.
• External use only.

Dosage: gently apply to unbroken chilblains and the surrounding area as often as necessary.

A NELSON & CO

NELSONS EVENING PRIMROSE CREAM

Unlicensed cream containing evening primrose oil.
• External use only.

Dosage: apply gently to the affected dry or tired skin area, repeat if necessary.

A NELSON & CO

*NELSONS HAEMORRHOID CREAM

This is largely an astringent mixture of herbs which is licensed as a remedy to relieve the discomfort of piles. It contains horse chestnut, marigold and witch hazel with the rather unusual addition of paeony which is anti-inflammatory and was once more widely used as a remedy for piles, anal fissure and ulceration of the perineum.
• Sufferers from persistent haemorrhoids should consult a doctor; external use only.

Dosage: wash the affected area with warm water then apply the cream.

A NELSON & CO

*NELSONS HEALING OINTMENT

Licensed for the relief for cuts and grazes and to soothe and heal sore, sensitive and roughened skin this is a simple marigold ointment.

• External use only.

Dosage: apply the ointment gently to cover more than the affected area. Cover with a plaster or dry dressing and bandage if required.

A NELSON & CO

*NELSONS HYPERCAL CREAM

This is a licensed combination of St John's wort and marigold which is popularly used for cuts and sores. Marigold is a good antiseptic while St John's wort also helps to relieve pain.
• External use only.

Dosage: apply gently to the affected area and cover with a plaster or dry dressing and bandage if required.

A NELSON & CO

*NELSONS HYPERCAL TINCTURE

Similar to *Nelson's Hypercal Cream this mixture can also be used for cuts and grazes.
• External use only.

Dosage: apply neat to small cuts and abrasions; for larger cuts dilute one part in ten of water and bathe.

A NELSON & CO

*NELSONS PYRETHRUM SPRAY

This spray is licensed as a remedy to relieve all types of insect bites and stings. It contains some familiar antiseptic and healing herbs – St John's wort, echinacea, marigold, yellow dock and arnica – along with the rather less common pyrethrum (an insecticide) and wild rosemary which is an astringent and insect repellent.
• External use only.

A NELSON & CO

*NELSONS RHUS TOX CREAM

Licensed for the relief of rheumatic aches and pains this cream contains poison ivy which is used in homoeopathy for sprains and joint inflammations.
• External use only.

Dosage: massage gently into the affected areas as required.

A NELSON & CO

*NELSONS STRAINS OINTMENT

A licensed ointment which can be used for sprains and to relieve strained tendons, this contains rue, which is a specific in homoeopathy for injuries to the shinbone and can also be used for sprains and bruising.
• External use only.

Dosage: massage gently into the affected area as required.

A NELSON & CO

NELSONS TEA TREE CREAM

An unlicensed cream containing tea tree as a simple.
• External use only.

Dosage: apply gently to affected area, repeat as necessary.

A NELSON & CO

*NURSE HARVEY'S GRIPE WATER

A mixture containing dill oil, caraway oil, ginger tincture and sodium bicarbonate for the relief of colicky pain and wind in babies.

Dosage: birth–1 month, 2.5 ml; 1–2 months, 5 ml; 2–6 months, 10 ml; 6–12 months, 10–15 ml; over 12 months, 15–20 ml given after or during feeds up to eight doses in 24 hours.

HARVEY SCRUTON

OBBEKJAERS PEPPERMINT

Unlicensed capsules each containing 200 mg peppermint oil suspended in sunflower oil.
• Excessive use of peppermint can irritate the stomach lining.

Dosage: 1 or 2 capsules a day before the main meal.

BENDIX FOODS (IMPORTED BY BENNETT NATURAL PRODUCTS)

*OLBAS OIL

This is a very widely used licensed remedy for the symptomatic relief of muscular pain, stiffness including backache, sciatica, lumbago, fibrositis, or rheumatic pain when used topically, while as an inhalant the licence extends to include the relief of bronchial and nasal congestion caused by colds, catarrh, influenza, hay fever, rhinitis and upper respiratory tract infections. The mixture contains cajuput, clove, eucalyptus, juniper and wintergreen oils with the addition of menthol and "dementholised mint oil" which is said to make the product safe for use in babies and children. Normally peppermint should not be give to young children because of its irritant effect.

• Possible side-effects – rash on skin contact in sensitive individuals; stinging if in contact with the eyes.

Dosage: adults – 3 or 4 drops inhaled from a handkerchief or tissue; several drops rubbed into a painful joint; children over two years – 1 or 2 drops inhaled from a handkerchief; infants three months to two years – 1 drop on a tissue placed out of the child's reach or on a bed sheet or nightwear.

G R LANE HEALTH PRODUCTS

*OLBAS PASTILLES

This contains similar oils to the company's *Olbas Oil but in this case the product licence extends only to providing symptomatic relief of colds, coughs, catarrh, sore throats, and influenza, catarrhal headaches and nasal congestion. The pastilles contain peppermint, eucalyptus, wintergreen, juniper and clove oils with additional menthol.

Dosage: adults and children over seven years – 1 pastille as required, up to 8 pastilles in any 24 hour period.

G R LANE HEALTH PRODUCTS

OMEGA 3

These capsules contain a mixture of evening primrose and salmon oils with vitamin E. Salmon oil is rich in eicosapentaenoic acid (EPA) and docosahexaenic acids (known as omega-3 acids) which are needed to produce the PGE_3 family of prostaglandins.

Dosage: 2 capsules daily.

HEALTH PERCEPTIONS

ORTILAX

Unlicensed tablets containing the laxatives senna and alder buckthorn for use in constipation.

Dosage: 2 tablets in the evening; increase as need be.

ORTIS

ORTIS FRESH DEVIL'S CLAW DRINK

This liquid product combines devil's claw with blackcurrant buds in a wine base.

Blackcurrant buds are used in parts of Europe as a remedy for rheumatism and to treat urinary problems so this combination could be helpful for various arthritic and rheumatic complaints.

Dosage: 10 ml twice a day to be taken for three weeks without interruption, then stop for a week and start another three week course. For full maintenance take a week on followed by a week off; double the dose if necessary.

ORTIS

ORTIS FRESH GINSENG

A fresh ginseng preparation in a wine base.

Dosage: 1 × 5 ml teaspoon daily.

ORTIS

ORTIS FRESH GINSENG IN SOLUTION

This combination mixes ginseng with royal jelly and vitamin E in a wine base.

Dosage: A measuring cup is included in the pack and will take around 15 ml of the liquid which provides 750 mg of ginseng; the dose can be doubled if required.

ORTIS

ORTIS FRUIT & FIBRES

A supplement for constipation combining a mixture of fruits and fibres: figs, rhubarb, tamarind pulp and dates in a chewable fruit cube. The tamarind is said to help hold water in the intestines and thus keep the stool soft.
• Not advisable during pregnancy, or for children under eight years.

Dosage: chew half a cube in the evening with a glass of water; increase if necessary.

ORTIS

ORTIS GINSENG + E

Capsules combining ginseng with wheatgerm oil as a source of vitamin E.

Dosage: 2 capsules a day before breakfast or 1 capsule daily as a maintenance dose.

ORTIS

ORTIS PANAX GINSENG

A combination of 500 mg of ginseng and 150 mg of royal jelly in 15 ml phials.

Dosage: 1 per day.

ORTIS

ORTISAN

Sold as a food supplement these chewable fruit cubes are similar to Ortis' Fruit and Fibres product, only in this case the mixture combines fig and tamarind pulp as a rather more potent laxative for use in more chronic conditions.
• Not advised during pregnancy, or for children under eight years.

Dosage: chew half a cube in the evening with a glass of water; increase if necessary.

ORTIS

ORTISAN LIQUID

A mixture of fruit fibres (fig, tamarind and prunes) with the laxative senna in a liquid preparation for use in constipation.

Dosage: adults – 1 × 5 ml teaspoon in the evening; increase as required; children from 8 years upwards – half a teaspoon a day.

ORTIS

PANAX GINSENG AND ROYAL JELLY

A combination of ginseng and royal jelly sold in 15 ml phials.

Dosage: 1 phial per day.

EAST-WEST HERBS

PHOENIX NUTRITION CITRIMAX

Another of the slimming products based on CitriMax™ a standardized herbal extract of (-)-hydroxycitric acid produced from the Malabar tamarind which creates a feeling of fullness and thus reduces appetite.

PHOENIX NUTRITION

PHOENIX NUTRITION ECHINACEA ACES

A combination of 250 mg of echinacea *(E. angustifolia)* combined with *beta*-carotene, selenium, and vitamins C and E as an immune-enhancing supplement.

Dosage: 1–3 tablets daily in 15-day cycles with 10 days taking the tablets and five days not, as research suggests that after 10 days its efficiency wears off.

PHOENIX NUTRITION

PHOENIX NUTRITION OMEGA 3–6

An essential fatty acid combination of 500 mg of combined evening primrose and borage oils plus fish lipid concentrates and vitamin E.

PHOENIX NUTRITION

PHYTORHUMA

An unlicensed massage oil containing devil's claw and myrtle oil sold as a warming and relaxing gel. Devil's claw is useful for treating rheumatic and arthritic disorders while myrtle is more normally regarded as a urinary antiseptic and anti-microbial.

Dosage: massage into painful areas two or three times a day; treatment should be continued for at least a month.

ARKOPHARMA

PHYTOVARIX

An unlicensed massage oil sold for "tired legs" although the herbs included in the oil are often used for varicose veins. Phytovarix contains: red vine, butcher's broom, witch hazel and horse chestnut with the addition of menthol (from peppermint oil) and cypress and lavender oils.

Dosage: massage from knee to ankle two or three times a day.

ARKOPHARMA

*POTTER'S ACIDOSIS

A licensed remedy for the symptomatic relief of indigestion, stomach ache, heartburn and acid stomach. This contains a mixture of largely carminative and antacid herbs – meadowsweet with aniseed, caraway, cardamom and cinnamon oils – as well as rhubarb, which has a laxative and stimulating action, and charcoal which helps to absorb stomach acids.

Dosage: 2 tablets three times a day after meals.

POTTER'S

*POTTER'S ADIANTINE

A licensed hair rub for dandruff and to improve general hair condition, this mixture combines West Indian bay oil (once a very popular and widely used hair treatment) with rosemary and southernwood (both traditionally used to improve hair growth) and witch hazel.

Dosage: massage into the scalp night and morning.

POTTER'S

*POTTER'S ANASED PAIN RELIEF TABLETS

A licensed remedy for the symptomatic relief of minor aches, tenseness and irritability, this product contains a combination of herbs widely used in generally sedating mixtures: hops, Jamaica dogwood, wild lettuce, passion flower and pasque flower. Both pasque flower and Jamaica dogwood have analgesic properties useful for tension headaches.

Dosage: 1 or 2 tablets three times daily and 2 at bedtime.

POTTER'S

*POTTER'S ANTIBRON TABLETS

A licensed remedy for the symptomatic relief of coughs, this mixture combines a number of expectorants (coltsfoot, pill-bearing spurge, pleurisy root, senega and liquorice) with Indian tobacco which is antispasmodic and helpful in asthma and bronchitis, wild lettuce – a suppressant for persistent tickling coughs, and cayenne which is generally warming and stimulating.

Dosage: adults – 2 tablets three times a day; children over seven years – 1 tablet three times a day.

POTTER'S

*POTTER'S ANTIFECT

A licensed remedy for the symptomatic relief of catarrh, rhinitis and nasal congestion this is a combination of garlic and echinacea which could also be relevant for a range of infectious conditions such as colds and influenza. The mixture also contains vegetable charcoal which can help reduce any stomach irritation caused by garlic.

Dosage: adults – 2 tablets three times a day; children – half the adult dose.

POTTER'S

*POTTER'S ANTIGLAN TABLETS

A licensed remedy for the symptomatic short-term relief of mild bladder discomfort this product largely focuses on herbs generally used to tackle prostate enlargement – these include kava kava, saw palmetto, and hydrangea as well as horsetail, which is both diuretic and healing for the urinary tract.

Dosage: 2 tablets three times a day. Increase to 3 tablets, three times a day in severe cases.

POTTER'S

*POTTER'S ANTISMOKING TABLETS

A licensed remedy "to reduce addiction to tobacco smoking" these are tablets of Indian tobacco which contain the alkaloid lobeline which is similar to nicotine so it is thought to act as a temporary replacement.
• High doses will cause nausea although very small amounts of Indian tobacco are included in the tablets and up to 10 tablets a day can usually be tolerated.

Dosage: 1 tablet to be taken every hour all day. Each tablet to be sucked for half a minute and then swallowed whole.

POTTER'S

*POTTER'S ANTITIS TABLETS

A licensed remedy used for the symptomatic relief of urinary or bladder discomfort; the herbs in this mixture are largely diuretic and urinary antiseptics so would be suitable for cystitis and urinary tract infections. The mixture includes buchu, clivers, couchgrass, horsetail, shepherd's purse (also helpful to reduce bleeding in severe cystitis) and bearberry.
• Increase fluid intake.

Dosage: 2 tablets three times a day.

POTTER'S

*POTTER'S APPETISER MIXTURE

This product was at one time known as "Tonic and Nervine Essence" and combines chamomile, which is sedative and carminative, with yellow gentian and calumba which both stimulate the appetite. It could be helpful in convalescence as well as for the flatulence and poor appetite problems covered in the licence.
• Best avoided in pregnancy and lactation.

Dosage: 1 × 5 ml teaspoon three times a day, in a little water before meals.

POTTER'S

*POTTER'S BACKACHE TABLETS

A licensed remedy for the symptomatic relief of backache this is really a mixture of diuretic and urinary antiseptic herbs which would be relevant if the backache related to urinary or kidney problems rather from some muscular or joint cause. The mixture contains gravel root, hydrangea, buchu and bearberry.
• Not recommended during pregnancy.

Dosage: 2 tablets, three times a day.

POTTER'S

*POTTER'S BALM OF GILEAD

A classic Potter's remedy licensed for the symptomatic relief of coughs this mixture includes squill, Indian tobacco, balm of gilead and lungwort which is expectorant and antispasmodic. The mixture is sweetened with apple juice.
• Not recommended during pregnancy.

Dosage: adults – 2 × 5 ml teaspoon three to four times a day; children – 1 × 5 ml teaspoon three to four times a day. Dilute in water if necessary.

POTTER'S

*POTTER'S BOLDO AID TO SLIMMING TABLETS

This remedy is licensed as a slimming aid – like others on the market – combines diuretics, laxatives and metabolic stimulants. It has been sold since the 1930s although is best regarded as a short-term supplement rather than an effective solution for over-eating. It includes dandelion, boldo, butternut and bladderwrack – which is a thyroid stimulant so best avoided by those suffering from thyroid disorders.

Dosage: adults – 1 or 2 tablets three times a day; elderly – one tablet three or four times a day.

POTTER'S

POTTER'S BUCKWHEAT TABLETS

Unlicensed buckwheat tablets as a source of rutin.

POTTER'S

*POTTER'S CATARRH MIXTURE

Licensed for the symptomatic relief of nasal catarrh and catarrh in the throat, this is a combination of herbs used for treating coughs and colds (hyssop and boneset) with blue flag and burdock which are more usually regarded as cleansing remedies for skin problems or rheumatic pain. The mix also includes cayenne which is a warming stimulant.

Dosage: adults – 1 × 5 ml teaspoon three times a day; children over seven years – 1 × 5 ml teaspoon morning and evening.

POTTER'S

*POTTER'S CHEST MIXTURE

A licensed remedy for the symptomatic relief of coughs and catarrh in the upper respiratory tract this combines expectorants – white horehound, squill, pleurisy root and senega – with Indian tobacco which is antispasmodic and also expectorant. White horehound can be helpful for soothing the mucous membranes in colds and sore throats.
• Not recommended in pregnancy.

Dosage: 1 × 5 ml teaspoon every three hours.

POTTER'S

*POTTER'S CHLOROPHYLL TABLETS

This combination of cola and chlorophyll is licensed as a remedy for temporary tiredness. Cola is rich in caffeine so is very stimulating while chlorophyll (the green part of plants) is regarded by some as energy giving and has also been used for such diverse problems as bad breath, sore throats and slow-healing wounds

Dosage: 1 or 2 tablets three times a day.

POTTER'S

*POTTER'S CLEANSING HERB

Licensed as a remedy for the prevention and relief of occasional constipation this is a combination of the laxatives alder buckthorn and senna which are both rich in anthraquinones to irritate the gut and isphaghula which is a mucilaginous bulking laxative. The mixture is sold as a granular powder.

Dosage: half a level teaspoon night and morning when required. Add boiling water and allow the mixture to stand for 15 minutes before drinking the lot.

POTTER'S

*POTTER'S COMFREY OINTMENT

A licensed simple comfrey ointment which can claim efficacy in the symptomatic relief of bruises and sprains.

• Because of concerns over the pyrrolizidine alkaloids contained in comfrey, Potter's now recommend limiting use to no more than ten days. External use only; do not apply to broken skin.

POTTER'S

POTTER'S COMFREY TABLETS

Unlicensed comfrey tablets as a simple.

POTTER'S

*POTTER'S DERMACREME OINTMENT

This ointment – licensed as a mild antiseptic for cuts, grazes and minor burns – is now produced from methyl salicylate (as originally extracted from wintergreen) and menthol which is an active constituent of peppermint oil. Methyl salicylate can help relieve pain while, although cooling, menthol or peppermint oil is more usually used in rubs for aches and muscle stiffness.
• External use only.

POTTER'S

*POTTER'S DIURETABS

Licensed "to balance natural body fluids" this is another of the products aimed at treating problems associated with premenstrual syndrome but which usually describe their role as reducing fluid retention. The mixture is largely diuretic – buchu, juniper, parsley piert and bearberry – so could actually be relevant for various urinary tract disorders including kidney stones.
• The juniper content could be irritating so should be avoided in kidney disease and the remedy not taken for more than two or three weeks.

Dosage: 2 tablets three times a day.

POTTER'S

*POTTER'S ECZEMA OINTMENT

A licensed eczema remedy, this ointment combines chickweed with zinc oxide, salicylic acid and benzoic acids, lanolin. Chickweed can often help ease the irritation of dry eczema.

Dosage: apply twice daily to affected areas.
• External use only.

POTTER'S

*POTTER'S ELDERFLOWERS, PEPPERMINT AND COMPOSITION ESSENCE

This is one of Potter's oldest remedies produced in its current form for at least 55 years. It is licensed to relieve fevers and the discomforts of colds, chills and sore throats and contains – as the name implies – elder flowers, peppermint and Potter's Composition Essence which is mainly bayberry and hemlock spruce.

Dosage: adults – 2 × 5 ml teaspoons in warm water three times a day; children over five years – half the adult dose.

POTTER'S

*POTTER'S ELIXIR OF DAMIANA AND SAW PALMETTO

Licensed as "a traditional restorative" this product has been sold by Potter's for around 60 years and was once more actively promoted as an aphrodisiac for elderly men. It contains damiana and saw palmetto – tonic and helpful for prostate problems – as well as corn silk which would similarly ease urinary problems in the elderly.

Dosage: 2 × 5 ml teaspoons three times a day for one week, then 1 × 5 ml teaspoon three times a day.

POTTER'S

*POTTER'S GARLIC TABLETS

Simple garlic tablets which in this case are licensed for the symptomatic relief of common colds, rhinitis and catarrh. Garlic does, of course, have a number of other properties (including helping to reduce cholesterol and combating arteriosclerosis) for which these tablets could be just as relevant.

Dosage: adults – 2 tablets three times a day; children over eight years – 1 tablet three or four times a day.

POTTER'S

*POTTER'S GB TABLETS

The "GB" in this name used to stand for gall bladder and the tablets were promoted as a stimulating liver remedy. Modern licensing laws have rather modified this application and the tablets are now promoted "for the symptomatic relief of short-term discomfort in the upper abdomen following meals". The tablets contain liver and bile stimulants and antispasmodics – black root, wahoo, and kava kava – as well as burdock root which is laxative and cleansing. The product could be helpful for the sort of abdominal discomfort associated with gall bladder disorders.

Dosage: 2 tablets three times a day.

POTTER'S

POTTER'S GINGER ROOT TABLETS

Unlicensed tablets containing ginger as a simple.

POTTER'S

*POTTER'S HERBHEAL OINTMENT

An ointment licensed for irritating skin conditions which contains chickweed (often used for eczema) and marshmallow which is soothing and drawing. The ointment also contains colophony, a resin derived from *Pinus palustris* (long-leaf pine), and used for treating boils, ulcers and fungal skin problems, as well as sulphur, starch and lanolin.
• External use only.

Dosage: Apply night and morning.

POTTER'S

*POTTER'S HOREHOUND AND ANISEED COUGH MIXTURE

Licensed for the symptomatic relief of coughs this mixture combines the expectorants pleurisy root, elecampane, white horehound, skunk cabbage and Indian tobacco with wild cherry which is a cough suppressant, anise oil and cayenne – warming and stimulating for cold conditions. The mixture has been sold for more than 60 years and is a well-established household standby.
• Not recommended during pregnancy or lactation.

Dosage: adults – 2 × 5 ml teaspoon three times a day; children over five years – 1 × 5 ml teaspoon three times a day.

POTTER'S

*POTTER'S INDIAN BRANDEE

A traditional warming digestive mix which is licensed to give symptomatic relief from digestive discomfort. It combines cayenne and ginger which are both warming and will help to stimulate the digestion and relieve wind, with rhubarb added as a laxative.
• Not recommended during pregnancy.

Dosage: adults – 1 × 5 ml teaspoon in a little warm water. Repeat once or twice if necessary.

*POTTER'S INDIGESTION MIXTURE

A combination of meadowsweet, yellow gentian and wahoo, licensed – as the name implies – for the symptomatic relief of indigestion, heartburn and flatulence. Meadowsweet is a good antacid stomach remedy for all sorts of upsets and gastritis while yellow gentian is a very bitter digestive stimulant. Wahoo is normally regarded as a liver herb, useful to stimulate bile flow and ease any congestion.
• Not recommended during pregnancy and lactation, and not really suitable for children.

Dosage: 1 × 5 ml teaspoon after meals, three or four times daily.

*POTTER'S JAMAICAN SARSPARILLA

This is a sarsparilla simple which is licensed for symptomatic treatment of complexion and skin blemishes, minor skin complaints and rashes.

Dosage: 2 × 5 ml teaspoons in water three times a day.

*POTTER'S KAS-BAH HERB

This is a mixture of dried, largely diuretic herbs which can be used as an infusion. The mix includes buchu, clivers, couchgrass, horsetail and bearberry with the addition of senna, a laxative. It is licensed for the short-term symptomatic relief of urinary and bladder discomfort and associated backache.

Dosage: 3 level teaspoonfuls (about 6 g) infused in 500 ml of boiling water and taken in daily portions when cool enough.

*POTTER'S LIFE DROPS

Licensed as suitable to relieve the discomfort of influenza, fever, colds, chills and sore throats this mixture contains elder flowers (an anti-catarrhal) with peppermint (warming and antiseptic) and cayenne – also warming and stimulating.

Dosage: adults – 11 drops (0.2 ml) in one or two tablespoons of warm water every hour when required; children over seven years, adult dose every two hours.

*POTTER'S LIGHTNING COUGH REMEDY

A combination of liquorice and anise oil which is expectorant and soothing for the respiratory tract that is licensed for the symptomatic relief of coughs.

Dosage: adults – 2 × 5 ml teaspoon three or four times a day; children over five years – 1 × 5 ml teaspoon every five or six hours.

POTTER'S

*POTTER'S MALTED KELP TABLETS

These are kelp tablets flavoured with anise oil and malt which are licensed as a traditional supplementary source of minerals, an aid to convalescence, and as an adjunct in the management of rheumatic pain.

Dosage: adults – 1 tablet three times a day after meals; children over five years – one tablet twice a day.

POTTER'S

*POTTER'S MEDICATED EXTRACT OF ROSEMARY

Rosemary is a traditional hair remedy used for dandruff and to improve lustre. In this remedy it is combined with West Indian bay oil and rose geranium which is used in aromatherapy for acne and fungal problems and will also improve the scent of the mixture. The product also contains methyl salicylate and is licensed as a general hair tonic.

Dosage: gently massage into the scalp twice daily.

POTTER'S

*POTTER'S NEWRELAX

Licensed for the symptomatic relief of tenseness, irritability or agitation due to the stresses and strains of modern life this remedy contains the popularly used nervines – hops, skullcap, valerian and vervain – which can all be useful for a range of nervous problems.

Dosage: 2 tablets three times a day.

POTTER'S

*POTTER'S NINE RUBBING OILS

A licensed rub for the relief of muscular pain and stiffness including backache, sciatica, lumbago, fibrositis, rheumatic pain and strains this mixture contains clove, eucalyptus, linseed, mustard, thyme and peppermint oils with amber, methyl salicylate and turpentine – all extensively used for treating various muscular aches and pains.

• Apply only to unbroken skin; external use only.

Dosage: rub into the affected part as required.

POTTER'S

*POTTER'S NODOFF MIXTURE

A suitably named licensed product for insomnia, this remedy contains passion flower, skullcap, hops, valerian and Jamaica dogwood – all useful relaxing herbs.

• Not recommended in early pregnancy.

Dosage: 1 × 5 ml teaspoon after the last meal of the day and 2 × 5 ml teaspoons at bedtime.

POTTER'S

*POTTER'S OUT OF SORTS TABLETS

A licensed remedy for the symptomatic relief of occasional constipation and feelings of bloatedness this product is a potent combination of laxatives – senna, aloes and cascara sagrada – with dandelion root (also a bile stimulant) and fennel seed to act as a carminative for any griping pains such a brew may cause.

• Not recommended during pregnancy or lactation. If symptoms persists seek professional advice.

Dosage: adults – 1 or 2 tablets at bedtime as necessary.

POTTER'S

*POTTER'S PARASOLV OINTMENT

An ointment combining clivers and poke root which is licensed for the treatment of mild psoriasis. The mixture also contains starch to protect and prevent bacterial infection, sulphur as a mild antiseptic and zinc oxide to soothe and protect.

• External use only.

Dosage: apply up to four times a day; do not apply on top of any other product.

POTTER'S

*POTTER'S PASSIFLORA

A simple passion flower tablet which is licensed as an aid to promote natural sleep and is also useful as a daytime remedy for tension and anxiety. The product comprises chewable tablets, suitable for infants and the elderly.

Dosage: for sleep aid, 2 tablets at tea-time and 2 at bedtime; for daytime use – 1 or 2 tablets four times a day.

POTTER'S

*POTTER'S PEERLESS COMPOSITION ESSENCE

One of Potter's well-established traditional remedies which is licensed to relieve colds and chills. It includes a number of astringent and warming herbs tradition-ally used for catarrh and to stimulate the circulation. The mixture includes oak, hemlock, spruce, poplar, prickly ash, bayberry and cayenne.
• Not recommended during pregnancy or lactation.

Dosage: adults – 1 or 2 × 5 ml teapoons every three hours when necessary; chil-dren over eight years – 1 × 5 ml teaspoon every three hours when necessary.

POTTER'S

*POTTER'S PILETABS

A licensed remedy to relieve the discomfort of haemorrhoids aggravated by con-stipation which contains a mix of laxatives (cascara sagrada and stone root) with agrimony and pilewort which are both astringent and popularly used for piles.
• Not recommended during pregnancy.

Dosage: adults – 2 tablets three times a day; elderly – 2 tablets morning and night.

POTTER'S

*POTTER'S PILEWORT OINTMENT

An ointment containing pilewort as a simple which is licensed for the relief of the discomfort of piles.
• External use only.

Dosage: apply to affected parts twice a day.

POTTER'S

*POTTER'S PREMENTAID

This is a combination of sedating and diuretic herbs licensed for the sympto-matic relief of the discomforts of a bloated, heavy feeling. It is (as the name sug-gests) primarily aimed at relieving premenstrual syndrome and contains herbs which are known to be effective for this problem. The combination includes ver-vain, motherwort, pasque flower, bearberry and valerian.
• Not recommended in pregnancy.

Dosage: 2 tablets three times a day on uncomfortable days. Take regularly for several days.

POTTER'S

*POTTER'S PROTAT

Licensed for the short-term relief of bladder discomfort, this is the sort of product which may also be helpful in prostate treatment. It includes kava kava which is generally tonifying for the urinary-genital organs and cornsilk, a soothing diuretic.

Dosage: 1 × 5 ml teaspoon three times a day.

POTTER'S

*POTTER'S RASPBERRY LEAF

Raspberry leaf tablets as a simple which in this case are licensed for relieving painful menstrual cramps.
• Although the herb is popular and safe to use in the last few weeks of pregnancy this licensed product cautions that it can no longer be recommended for use in pregnancy except where labour has begun.

Dosage: 2 tablets three times a day after meals.

POTTER'S

*POTTER'S RHEUMATIC PAIN TABLETS

These tablets contain a combination of diuretic, cleansing and anti-inflammatory herbs used for treating both arthritis and rheumatism although the licence for this remedy only covers the aches and pains of rheumatism. The product contains yarrow, burdock, guaiacum and nutmeg.

Dosage: 2 tablets, three times a day.

POTTER'S

*POTTER'S SCIARGO

This is a diuretic mixture which is actually licensed for the symptomatic relief of sciatica and lumbago, although it would seem to be a more relevant choice where urinary or kidney problems were a contributory cause of the back pain. The mixture includes shepherd's purse, wild carrot, clivers, bearberry and juniper oil.
• With juniper used in the mix it should be avoided in kidney disease, during pregnancy and for long-term use.

Dosage: 2 tablets three times a day.

POTTER'S

*POTTER'S SCIARGO HERB

This is the same combination of herbs as in Potter's Sciargo (only with juniper berries rather than the oil) which is sold in tea bags for use in infusions. It is similarly licensed for symptomatic relief of sciatica, lumbago and muscular backache.
• Unsuitable during pregnancy, lactation or for those with poor kidney function.

Dosage: use 1 tea bag, infused, five times a day.

POTTER'S

*POTTER'S SENNA TABLETS

Laxative senna tablets with a little fennel added as a carminative. The product is licensed for the relief or prevention of occasional constipation.

Dosage: adults – 2 tablets at bedtime when required; children – 1 tablet in the morning when required.

POTTER'S

*POTTER'S SKIN CLEAR OINTMENT

A tea tree ointment which in this case is licensed for mild acne and the relief of mild dry eczema and difficult skin affections. It also contains starch, sublimated sulphur and zinc oxide and soft yellow paraffin.
• Not for children under five years; external use only.

Dosage: apply night and morning.

POTTER'S

*POTTER'S SKIN CLEAR TABLETS

Simple echinacea tablets which are licensed for the symptomatic relief of minor skin conditions and blemishes although the herb is, of course, equally useful in a range of infection conditions including colds and cystitis.

Dosage: 2 tablets three times a day.

POTTER'S

*POTTER'S SKIN ERUPTIONS MIXTURE

Licensed for the symptomatic relief of mild eczema, psoriasis and other skin diseases, this mixture contains diuretics, laxatives and traditional cleansing herbs often used for treating skin problems. The combination includes blue flag, burdock, yellow dock, sarsparilla, cascara sagrada and buchu.

Dosage: sage: adults – 1 × 5 ml teaspoon three times a day; children over eight years – 1 × 5 ml teaspoon every 12 hours.

POTTER'S

*POTTER'S SLIPPERY ELM STOMACH TABLETS

Slippery elm tablets licensed as a remedy for indigestion, dyspepsia, heartburn and flatulence which are flavoured with cinnamon, clove and peppermint oils.

Dosage: 1 or 2 tablets to be chewed after each meal, up to five times a day. Regular use is said to be the best.

POTTER'S

*POTTER'S SPANISH TUMMY MIX

A useful astringent combination for the relief of non-persistent diarrhoea: as the name implies this is an ideal remedy for holiday stomach upsets. It contains blackberry root and pale catechu.

Dosage: 1 × 5 ml teaspoon every hour (sold in 50 ml bottles for convenience when travelling).

POTTER'S

*POTTER'S STOMACH MIXTURE

A mixture of largely laxative and bile stimulating herbs which is licensed for stomach ache and stomach upsets. The mixture comprises dandelion, yellow gentian and rhubarb which is an extremely bitter combination so buchu is added to help improve the flavour. The mix also includes bismuth ammonium citrate – a traditional antacid.
• Not recommended in pregnancy or suitable for children.

Dosage: 1 × 5 ml teaspoon three times a day.

POTTER'S

*POTTER'S STRENGTH TABLETS

A classic combination of tonic and stimulating herbs which is marketed by some suppliers as an aphrodisiac mixture although the Potter's product is sold as a remedy to aid convalescence after illness. It contains cola, damiana and saw palmetto.

Dosage: 2 tablets three times a day. Use regularly for two or three months.

POTTER'S

*POTTER'S TABRITIS

A licensed remedy for the symptomatic relief of rheumatic pain and stiffness this mixture contains cleansing diuretic herbs and circulatory stimulants: elder flowers, prickly ash, yarrow, burdock, clivers, poplar and bearberry – all of which are often included in remedies for rheumatism and arthritis. The product is also available as Potter's Tabritis Plus which additionally contains kelp (another regular rheumatism supplement).
• Not recommended in pregnancy.

Dosage: 2 tablets three times a day.

POTTER'S

*POTTER'S VARICOSE OINTMENT

A combination of cade oil and witch hazel which is licensed for "the relief of lower limb skin conditions where there is irritation due to varicosity". Distilled witch-hazel is an astringent regularly used for varicose veins although cade oil (a juniper extract) is more widely used for psoriasis so this product may also be helpful for varicose eczema. It also contains zinc oxide.
• External use only.

Dosage: apply to affected areas night and morning.

POTTER'S

*POTTER'S VEGETABLE COUGH REMOVER

An impressive combination of expectorants licensed for the symptomatic relief of coughs. The list includes ipecacuanha, pleurisy root, elecampane, white horehound, hyssop, liquorice and anise with the addition of skullcap (antispasmodic) and black cohosh, which is usually considered anti-inflammatory and antispasmodic but which can also help counter coughs. The product has been sold in this format since at least 1930.

Dosage: adults – 2 × 5 ml teaspoons three or four times a day; children over eight years – 1 × 5 ml teaspoon three times a day; children aged five to seven years – 1 × 5 ml teaspoon every 12 hours.

POTTER'S

*POTTER'S WATERSHED MIXTURE

A diuretic combination which is now licensed "to promote normal fluid balance and the symptomatic relief of heavy and bloated feelings in women" but would also be useful for a wide range of urinary tract disorders including cystitis. The

mixture includes wild carrot, pellitory-of-the-wall, juniper, clivers and buchu.
• The juniper content suggests it should only be used for short periods and not in kidney disease or during pregnancy.

Dosage: 1–2 × 5 ml teaspoons three or four times daily.

POTTER'S

*POTTER'S WELLWOMAN HERBS

A herbal mixture sold in tea bags for infusion of herbs that are largely calming and diuretic and would also ease anxiety and palpitations. The mixture comprises motherwort, skullcap, yarrow and bearberry and it is licensed as suitable for menopausal women.
• Not recommended during early pregnancy.

Dosage: infuse 2 tea bags three times a day.

POTTER'S

*POTTER'S WELLWOMAN TABLETS

Like Potter's Wellwomen Herbs, this is licensed "to help the well-being of middle aged women". It comprises relaxing herbs often used for menopausal problems but also generally helpful for anxiety and tension. Tablets contain yarrow, motherwort, lime flowers, skullcap and valerian.
• Not recommended in pregnancy.

Dosage: 2 tablets three times a day.

POTTER'S

POWER GINSENG

Unlicensed ginseng capsules.

Dosage: 1 capsule a day with food.

POWER HEALTH

POWER HEALTH ALFALFA

Unlicensed simple alfalfa capsules.

Dosage: 1 or 2 daily.

POWER HEALTH

POWER HEALTH ALFALFA, KELP & YEAST

An unlicensed combination of alfalfa, kelp and yeast which provides a broad spectrum of minerals and vitamins as a food supplement.

POWER HEALTH

POWER HEALTH ALOE VERA

Power Health markets a range of simple aloe vera extracts in both liquid and capsule form. Aloe Vera 5000 is available in capsules with Aloe Vera Juice Drink and Aloe Vera Double Strength.

POWER HEALTH

POWER HEALTH BORAGE OIL

Unlicensed capsules containing 250 mg of borage oil.

POWER HEALTH

POWER HEALTH CARROT OIL

Unlicensed capsules containing 250 mg of carrot oil as a source of pro-vitamin A.

POWER HEALTH

POWER HEALTH CIRCULATING COMPOUND

An unlicensed combination of mistletoe, hawthorn and garlic which are heart tonics and anti-cholesterol remedies to improve circulation. The mixture also includes additional bioflavanoids.

Dosage: 2–4 tablets three times a day.   POWER HEALTH

POWER HEALTH CRANBERRY JUICE

Power Health produces cranberry juice extract in 140 mg capsules as well as Cranberry Juice Concentrate powder and Cranberry Juice Double Strength tablets. Cranberry has recently been shown to be helpful in the treatment of cystitis.

POWER HEALTH

POWER HEALTH ECHINACEA STANDARDISED

Unlicensed simple echinacea tablets.   POWER HEALTH

POWER HEALTH EVENING PRIMROSE OIL

Unlicensed evening primrose oil capsules containing 250 mg of oil per capsule. A combination "Super Evening Primrose Oil and Borage Oil" which contains 50 mg of *gamma*-linolenic acid is also supplied by the company.

POWER HEALTH

POWER HEALTH GARLIC OIL

Unlicensed capsules containing 250 mg equivalent of garlic extract.

POWER HEALTH

POWER HEALTH HARD GEL CAPSULES

A range of unlicensed simple powdered herbs in gelatin capsules. Table 7 summarises details of herbs available and the weights of powder they contain.

• *Dosage:* 1–3 capsules daily.

POWER HEALTH

Table 7: Power Health "Pure Herb" Hard Gel Capsules range

Name	*Herb (as listed in the A to Z)*	*Powder content (mg)*
Agnus Castus	chastetree	200
Celery Seed	celery	200
Dandelion	dandelion	250
Devils Claw	devil's claw	250
Feverfew	feverfew	200
Ginger	ginger	280
Ginkgo biloba	ginkgo	180
Guarana	guarana	500
Isphaghula	isphaghula	350
Milk thistle	milk thistle	100
Nettle Leaf	stinging nettle	200
St John's Wort	St John's wort	200
Uva Ursi	bearberry	200
Valerian	valerian	270
White Willow	white willow	200

POWER HEALTH HAWTHORN

Unlicensed simple hawthorn tablets.

POWER HEALTH

POWER HEALTH HEAD CLEAR

Capsules containing eucalyptus, menthol and camphor which are designed as an inhalant in colds, catarrh and nasal congestion.
• External use only.

Dosage: 1 or 2 capsules dissolved in 500 ml of boiling water as a steam inhalation or else put the capsule contents on a handkerchief or pillow at night and inhale.

POWER HEALTH

POWER HEALTH KELP

Unlicensed simple kelp tablets.

POWER HEALTH

POWER HEALTH OLIVE OIL

Unlicensed capsules containing 300 mg olive oil.

POWER HEALTH

POWER HEALTH OMEGA OIL

Unlicensed capsules containing 250 mg of linseed oil.

POWER HEALTH

POWER HEALTH PASSION FLOWER OIL

Unlicensed simple capsules containing 250 mg passion flower in an oil base.

POWER HEALTH

POWER HEALTH PEPPERMINT OIL

Unlicensed capsules containing peppermint oil as a simple.

POWER HEALTH

POWER HEALTH PUMPKIN SEED OIL

Unlicensed capsules containing 300 mg pumpkin seed extract as a simple.

POWER HEALTH

POWER HEALTH SAFFLOWER OIL

Unlicensed capsules containing 300 mg safflower oil as a simple.

POWER HEALTH

POWER HEALTH SIBERIAN GINSENG

Unlicensed capsules containing 500 mg Siberian ginseng as a simple.

POWER HEALTH

PRIMROSA MARINE

Capsules containing a blend of evening primrose oil concentrates that can contain 20% *gamma*-linolenic acid with fish lipid concentrate offering a high proportion of eicosapentaenoic acid and docasahexaenoic acid totalling 800 mg of oil.

Dosage: 1 or 2 capsules daily.

PHOENIX NUTRITION

PROFESSIONAL HERBS CASCARA AND RHUBARB

Capsules containing a mix of butternut, cascara sagrada, rhubarb, and liquorice – all laxatives – with ginger as a carminative, Irish moss (a soothing demulcent for the digestive system) and cayenne, a warming stimulant. The combination would be suitable for constipation.

Dosage: 3–6 capsules at bedtime as required.

QUEST VITAMINS

PROFESSIONAL HERBS CAYENNE & GINGER

Gelatin capsules containing cayenne, kelp, yellow gentian, ginger and blue vervain and suggested as a mixture of herbs traditionally used for circulatory disorders. Cayenne and ginger will certainly stimulate the peripheral circulation, although yellow gentian is more normally regarded as a digestive stimulant and kelp as a metabolic stimulant. Blue vervain is a North American herb which is largely similar to vervain – both a liver stimulant and relaxing nervine rather than a circulatory stimulant.

• To be avoided by hypoglycaemics.

Dosage: 1 or 2 capsules with each meal.

QUEST VITAMINS

PROFESSIONAL HERBS FEVERFEW

Capsules containing 150 mg of feverfew with parsley added as a filler.

Dosage: one capsule daily.

QUEST VITAMINS

PROFESSIONAL HERBS UVA URSI AND PARSLEY

Unlicensed capsules containing a lengthy mixture of diuretic herbs: cornsilk, bearberry, clivers, parsley, buchu, juniper berries, and gravel root with the addition of kelp (a metabolic stimulant) and cayenne, a warming digestive and circulatory stimulant. The combination is suggested as relevant for "maintaining fluid balance" although, given the number of urinary antiseptics, it is a potent enough brew to be effective in a wide range of urinary tract infections and inflammations.

• Not to be used during pregnancy or in kidney inflammation.

Dosage: 1 or 2 capsules with each meal.

QUEST VITAMINS

PROFESSIONAL HERBS VALERIAN

Unlicensed gelatin capsules containing a popular combination of sedating herbs that could be relevant for insomnia or, indeed, for a daytime treatment for anxiety and nervous tension. The capsules contain valerian, skullcap, hops and passion flower.

Dosage: 2 capsules at bedtime.

QUEST VITAMINS

PROSTEX

A vitamin and mineral supplement that also contains saw palmetto and could thus be useful for elderly men or in the treatment of prostate problems.

Dosage: 1 or 2 capsules, daily.

LAMBERTS HEALTHCARE

PURE-FIL AQUA-VITE SUPER KELP

Capsules containing 525 mg sea kelp harvested in Norway and derived from *Ascophyllum nodosum* seaweed with additional vitamins A, B_1, B_2, B_6, B_{12}, C, D, E, calcium pantothenate, niacinamide, biotin, folic acid and inosotil.

Dosage: 1–3 capsules daily.

BIO-HEALTH

PURE-FIL ECHINACEA ROOT

Simple echinacea capsules containing 250 mg of *E. purpurea* and 150 mg of *E. angustifolia*.

Dosage: 1 or 2 capsules up to three times daily.

BIO-HEALTH

PURE-FIL EVENING PRIMROSE OIL

Unlicensed capsules containing 500 mg of evening primrose oil.

BIO-HEALTH

PURE-FIL FEVERFEW LEAF

Unlicensed capsules containing 100 mg of organically-grown feverfew leaves as a simple.

Dosage: 1 capsule daily.

BIO-HEALTH

PURE-FIL LOW ODOUR WHOLE GARLIC CONCENTRATE

Unlicensed capsules containing 250 mg of dried garlic concentrate prepared from 2 g of fresh garlic cloves, reduced odour using drying techniques which reputedly preserve allicin content.

Dosage: 1 or 2 capsules daily.

BIO-HEALTH

PURE-FIL ROMAGEN HERBAL ANTIOXIDANT

A 250 mg combination of herbs which have recently been found to display considerable anti-oxidant properties. The mixture includes rosemary, sage, thyme, marjoram, oregano and peppermint all grown in the Mediterranean and equivalent to 60 mg *beta*-carotene. This product is very similar to Neal's Yard Anti-Oxidant Herbs Elixir.

Dosage: 1 capsule daily.   BIO-HEALTH

PURE-FIL RUTIN

Capsules containing 60 mg of a standard rutin extract recombined with 120 mg of buckwheat herb. Rutin has been used as a food supplement for a range of circulatory and heart disorders.

Dosage: 1 capsule daily.   BIO-HEALTH

PURE-FIL SUPER PANAX KOREAN GINSENG

Capsules containing 500 mg of four-year old Korean *Panax ginseng* root certified by the Korean government as a simple.

Dosage: 1 capsule daily.

BIO-HEALTH

PURE-FIL TRAVELLERS FRIEND

Unlicensed simple ginger capsules containing 500 mg of the herb.

Dosage: adults and children over 10 years – 1–2 capsules 20 minutes before travelling, repeat every two hours up to 6 capsules a day; children under ten years – 1 capsule every two hours up to 3 capsules daily.

BIO-HEALTH

PYCNOGENOL

An anti-oxidant supplement containing 20 mg of a pine extract which French research has suggested can be good at combating free radicals and cell ageing.
• Not recommended during pregnancy.

Dosage: 1 or 2 capsules daily.

LAMBERTS HEALTHCARE

RED GINSENG IN HONEY

A mixture of ginseng in honey sold in 15 ml phials.

Dosage: 1 phial daily.   EAST-WEST HERBS

RED KOOGA BETALIFE CAPSULES

Capsules combining ginseng with fish oils, vitamins C and E, *beta*-carotene and selenium as a general tonic supplement.

Dosage: adults and children over 12 – 1 capsule daily.

ENGLISH GRAINS HEALTHCARE

RED KOOGA ELIXIR

A liquid ginseng extract sold as a simple.

Dosage: adults and children over 12 – 2 × 5 ml teaspoon daily.

ENGLISH GRAINS HEALTHCARE

RED KOOGA GINSENG AND GINKGO BILOBA

A combination of ginseng and ginkgo which would be a useful tonic supplement for the elderly.

Dosage: adults and children over 12 years – 1 or 2 tablets daily.

ENGLISH GRAINS HEALTHCARE

RED KOOGA GINSENG CAPSULES AND TABLETS

Unlicensed ginseng capsules and tablets sold as a simple.

Dosage: adults and children over 12 years – 1 capsule or tablet daily.

ENGLISH GRAINS HEALTHCARE

REEVECREST GINSENG – RED ROOTS

Unlicensed ginseng tablets sold as a simple.

POWER HEALTH

REEVECREST BOM-DIA

Unlicensed simple guarana capsules each containing 500 mg of herb.

Dosage: 3–5 capsules a day half an hour before meals.

POWER HEALTH

REEVECREST FEVERFEW FORTE

Unlicensed simple feverfew tablets each containing 150 mg of herb.

Dosage: 1 tablet per day.   POWER HEALTH

REEVECREST GUM THYME

Tablets designed to be sucked or chewed after brushing the teeth and combining thyme, which is strongly antiseptic, with silver birch, an astringent herb. The mix also includes peppermint to improve the flavour with co-enzyme Q10 and silica.

Dosage: 1 tablet after brushing the teeth.   POWER HEALTH

REEVECREST LIBIDEX 5

Marketed "for loving adults" this product contains the aphrodisiac muira-puama with Siberian ginseng – a good tonic to counter stress. The tablets also contain vitamin E with zinc and selenium.

Dosage: 2 capsules daily.   POWER HEALTH

REEVECREST NUTRIMENTAL PLUS

Unlicensed simple buckwheat capsules.
                                                             POWER HEALTH

REEVECREST SUPER EVENING PRIMROSE OIL AND BORAGE OIL

A combination of evening primrose oil and borage oil which increases the proportion of *gamma*-linolenic acid.

Dosage: 1 or 2 capsules daily.
                                                             POWER HEALTH

*REGULAN

Satchets of isphaghula husks suitable as a bulking laxative and stool softener.

Dosage: adults – 1–3 sachets daily; children six to 12 years – $^1/_2$–1 level 5 ml teaspoon one to three times daily.

                                                     PROCTOR & GAMBLE

*REVITONIL

Licensed for the symptomatic relief of colds and upper respiratory tract infections these are chewable tablets containing 40 mg of echinacea *(E. purpurea)* equivalent to 260 mg of root which are flavoured with small amounts of liquorice, eucalyptus, aniseed, fennel, peppermint and cloves – herbs which are also helpful for clearing nasal congestion.

Dosage: adults – 2 or 3 tablets, three times a day; children 10 to 15 years – 2 tablets three times a day; children six to ten years – 1 tablet three times a day.

MEDIC HERB

*RHEUMASOL

Licensed for symptomatic relief of muscular pain and stiffness associated with sciatica, backache, lumbago, fibrositis, rheumatism and painful joints, these tablets basically combine guaiacum, which is anti-inflammatory and diuretic and extensively used for both rheumatism and arthritis, and prickly ash, which is a warming circulatory stimulant and anti-rheumatic.

Dosage: 1 tablet three times a day.

ENGLISH GRAINS HEALTHCARE

*RICKARD'S SLIMWELL HERBAL ANTI-FAT TABLETS

Licensed as an aid to slimming, this product combines the metabolic stimulant bladderwrack, with clivers as a diuretic.
• Not recommended during pregnancy and when breast feeding, or for children.

Dosage: 2 tablets, three times a day.

RICKARD LANE'S & W H BOX

*RICKARD'S WOODSAP OINTMENT

Licensed for symptomatic relief of eczema and temporary relief of psoriasis, this ointment contains the demulcents marshmallow and slippery elm with rosemary oil (often added to eczema creams to help local circulation) and eucalyptus oil (also rubefacient). The mixture also contains zinc oxide and sulphur. It could be helpful for a variety of skin irritations and inflammations.
• External use only.

Dosage: adults and children over eight years – apply to the affected skin night and morning.

RICKARD LANE'S & W H BOX

*RICOLA SWISS HERB LOZENGES

Licensed for "the discomforts of irritating coughs, sore throats and stuffy noses", these popular cough lozenges come in a variety of flavours (not all of them with the full product licence of the original Swiss Cough Herb Lozenges). The basic mixture includes common plantain, marshmallow, peppermint, thyme, sage, lady's mantle, elder flowers, cowslip, yarrow, burnet, speedwell, mallow and white horehound, which are all herbs that can be used as astringents, expectorants or anti-catarrhals, in a sugar free base. Total herbal extract is around 0.97% by weight so these are quite gentle remedies.

Other flavoured varieties include "Lemon Mint" which also includes lemon balm, "Blackcurrant" and "Orange Mint".
• Not suitable for children under four years.

Dosage: adults – not more than 24 lozenges in 24 hours; children – not more than 10 lozenges in 24 hours.

CEDAR HEALTH

RIO AMAZON GUARANA

Unlicensed capsules containing 500 mg of guarana as a simple. Also available under the Rio Amazon brand are a tablet version, a powder for adding to drinks or sprinkling on cereals, and a "guarana stick" said to be traditionally used by the Maues Sateres Indians.

Dosage: 2 capsules before breakfast, or an additional 2 or 3 during the day as well.

RIO TRADING COMPANY (HEALTH)

RIO AMAZON GUARANA BUZZ GUM

A chewing gum with guarana.

RIO TRADING COMPANY (HEALTH)

RIO AMAZON GUARANA JUNGLE ELIXIR

Liquid containing guarana macerated in wine and wheatgerm oil.

RIO TRADING COMPANY (HEALTH)

RIO D'AMOR CATUABA

Unlicensed capsules containing 500 mg of catuaba as a simple. Rio Trading also markets the same herb in tea bag form.

Dosage: 2 or 3 capsules daily.

RIO TRADING COMPANY (HEALTH)

RIO PARATUDO PFAFFIA

Unlicensed capsules containing 500 mg of paratudo as a simple.

Dosage: 2 or 3 capsules daily.

RIO TRADING COMPANY (HEALTH)

RIO VITALIS LAPACHO

Unlicensed capsules containing 500 mg of pau d'arco as a simple. Rio Trading also markets the same herb in tea bag form.

Dosage: 2 or 3 capsules daily.

RIO TRADING COMPANY (HEALTH)

RUTIVITE

Unlicensed capsules containing buckwheat as a simple and source of rutin.

POWER HEALTH

*SABALIN

Licensed as providing symptomatic relief for male urinary discomfort, the remedy is actually a saw palmetto simple containing 95 mg of berries per tablet so could be ideal for benign prostate enlargement.
• The tablet base contains lactose.

Dosage: 2 tablets three times a day.

MEDIC HERB

SCHOENENBURGER PLANT JUICES

A range of freshly pressed plant juices mostly derived from the whole plant which is widely used in Germany and other parts of Europe for a range of ailments (see the A–Z of Herbs). Herbal juices never taste particularly pleasant but good therapeutic results have been reported using these sorts of extracts. Most of the juices are sold in 160 ml bottles. Details are given in Table 8 (below).

Dosage: 1 × tablespoon of the juice diluted in water, milk or tea to be taken three or four times a day.

PHYTO PRODUCTS (IN THE UK)

Table 8: Schoenenberger Fresh Plant Juices

Brand	Herbal content (as listed in the A to Z)
Acerola Cherry	acerola
Artichoke	globe artichoke
Asparagus	asparagus
Bean	beans
Beetroot Red	red beet
Birch	silver birch
Black Radish	black radish
Borage	borage
Carrot	wild carrot
Celery	celery
Chamomile	chamomile
Coltsfoot	coltsfoot
Dandelion	dandelion
Echinacea	echinacea
Elderberry	elder
Fennel	fennel
Garlic	garlic
Ginkgo	ginkgo
Hawthorn	hawthorn
Horsetail	horsetail
Horse Radish	horseradish
Manna Fig	fig
Melissa	lemon balm
Mistletoe	mistletoe
Oat	wild oats
Onion	onion
Parsley	parsley
Potato	potato
Pumpkin	pumpkin
Ramson	ramsons
Ribwort Plantain	ribwort plantain
Rosemary	rosemary
Sage	sage

continued

Brand	Herbal content (as listed in the A to Z)
Sauerkraut	cabbage
Silverweed	silverweed
Stinging Nettle	stinging nettle
St Johns Wort	St John's wort
Thyme	thyme
Valerian	valerian
Watercress	watercress
White Cabbage	cabbage
Wormwood	wormwood
Yarrow	yarrow

SEREDRIN

An unlicensed simple ginkgo product, this contains the ginkgo flavonglycosides and 120 mg of ginkgo "phytosome" which is formed by combining flavonoids from the ginkgo leaf with molecules of phosphatidylcholine. This chemical is an essential component of the cell membranes within the body and the phytosome is believed to be more effectively absorbed into the system and increases its biological activity. The phytosome development is by Indena in Italy and research information from this laboratory suggests that the extract is a useful remedy for Raynaud's phenomenon and peripheral vascular disease as well as for the more usual cerebral insufficiency which ginkgo is used to treat.

Dosage: 2 or 3 tablets daily.

HEALTH PERCEPTIONS

SERENOA-C

A supplement combining 160 mg of saw palmetto with vitamins D, E, C, B_1, B_2, B_6, magnesium, zinc, manganese, copper, selenium and chromium which would be a suitable supplement for men (the pack says those aged 35 years or older) likely to be suffering from prostate problems.

Dosage: 1 tablet a day.

WASSEN INTERNATIONAL

SEVEN SEAS COD LIVER OIL AND EVENING PRIMROSE OIL

Capsules combining evening primrose oil and cod liver oil with the addition of vitamins A, D and E as a dietary supplement.

SEVEN SEAS

SEVEN SEAS COD LIVER OIL AND STARFLOWER OIL

Capsules combining cod liver oil and borage oil with the addition of vitamins A, D and E as a dietary supplement.

SEVEN SEAS

SEVEN SEAS EVENING PRIMROSE AND STARFLOWER OIL

Capsules containing a mixture of evening primrose and borage oils in 250, 500 and 1,000 mg version giving respectively 33, 67 and 130 mg of *gamma*-linolenic acid. Each capsule also contains additional vitamin E.

SEVEN SEAS

SEVEN SEAS EVENING PRIMROSE OIL

Capsules of evening primrose oil in 250, 500, and 1,000 mg versions and also as a chewable lemon flavoured "berry" version.

SEVEN SEAS

SEVEN SEAS GARLIC OIL PERLES

An unlicensed capsule containing garlic oil as a simple.

Dosage: 1 a day.

SEVEN SEAS

SEVEN SEAS KOREAN GINSENG

An unlicensed capsule containing 250 mg of ginseng as a simple.

Dosage: 1 a day.

SEVEN SEAS

SEVEN SEAS ODOURLESS GARLIC PERLES

An unlicensed capsule containing garlic as a simple.

Dosage: 1 a day.   SEVEN SEAS

SEVEN SEAS PURE STARFLOWER OIL

Unlicensed capsules containing 500 mg of borage oil giving 102 mg of *gamma*-linolenic acid. Capsules also contain 10 mg of vitamin E.

Dosage: 1 capsule a day.

SEVEN SEAS

SOLGAR ALFALFA TABLETS

Unlicensed tablets each containing 600 mg of alfalfa as a simple.

Dosage: 1–9 tablets daily.

SOLGAR VITAMINS

SOLGAR BROMELAIN TABLETS

Unlicensed tablets each containing 500 mg bromelain from fresh pineapple.

SOLGAR VITAMINS

SOLGAR CERTIFIED ORGANIC GARLIC OIL VEGICAPS

Capsules each contain 500 mg of garlic in a non-gelatin capsule suitable for vegetarians.

Dosage: 1 or 2 capsules daily.

SOLGAR VITAMINS

SOLGAR CRANBERRY EXTRACT

An unlicensed combination of 400 mg of cranberry extract and 60 mg of vitamin C.

Dosage: 1 or 2 capsules daily.

SOLGAR VITAMINS

SOLGAR EVENING PRIMROSE OIL SOFTGELS

Evening primrose oil in either 500 mg or 1300 mg capsules which also contain vitamin E.

Dosage: 3–6 of the 500 mg capsules daily or 1 of the 1300 mg capsules.

SOLGAR VITAMINS

SOLGAR GARLIC PERLES SOFTGELS

Capsules containing garlic oil from 500 mg of fresh herb in a reduced odour format.

Dosage: 1 capsule daily.

SOLGAR VITAMINS

SOLGAR HERBAL WATER FORMULA CAPSULES

A diuretic combination of buchu, bearberry, juniper berry and parsley extracts with the addition of barberry – a bitter digestive and liver stimulant. The combination could be helpful for various urinary tract disorders.

Dosage: 1–3 capsules daily.

SOLGAR VITAMINS

SOLGAR LINSEED OIL SOFTGELS

Unlicensed capsules containing 1250 mg linseed oil as a simple.

Dosage: 2 capsules daily.

SOLGAR VITAMINS

SOLGAR MAXGAR GARLIC SOFTGELS

Capsules each containing the 280 mg of garlic extract (equivalent of 672 mg of fresh garlic) which is described as a garlic oil macerate rich in allicin.

Dosage: 1 capsule daily.

SOLGAR VITAMINS

SOLGAR PSYLLIUM SEED HUSKS

Isphaghula husks sold loose and in capsules as a source of dietary fibre and useful as a bulking laxative. The capsules are non-gelatin so are suitable for vegetarians.

SOLGAR VITAMINS

SOLGAR SAFFLOWER OIL

Unlicensed simple capsules of safflower oil as a source of unsaturated fatty acids.

Dosage: 6 capsules daily to provide 6.9 g of safflower oil.

SOLGAR VITAMINS

SOLGAR SUPER GLA

Unlicensed capsules each containing 300 mg of *gamma*-linolenic acid derived from borage oil.

Dosage: 1 a day.

SOLGAR VITAMINS

SPRING WIND OINTMENT

A combination of Chinese herbs traditionally used to relieve dry itching skin. The mixture includes Chinese foxglove, lithospermum, Chinese gold thread, saf-flower, *Dang Gui,* peach seeds and liquorice.

Dosage: apply two to four times a day.

SPRING WIND HERBS (EAST WEST HERBS IN THE UK)

ST HILDEGARD EBERRAUTEM CREAM AND JUICE

Extracts of southernwood recommended by Hildegard of Bingen as a massage rub for rheumatism while the juice was reputedly useful for skin problems of the scalp.

Dosage: half a wine glass before and after meals, up to three times a day.

ST HILDEGARD-POSCH (VIA S SCHERNDAL IN THE UK)

ST HILDEGARD ENZIAN WINE

A simple of yellow gentian for digestive problems.

Dosage: Drink a small glass during and after meals.

ST HILDEGARD-POSCH (VIA S SCHERNDAL IN THE UK)

ST HILDEGARD GALANGAL AND FENNEL TABLETS

One of Hildegard of Bingen's traditional remedies combining galangal and fennel which is traditionally used as a stimulant for the circulation and digestion.

Dosage: 1 or 2 tablets three times a day.

ST HILDEGARD-POSCH (VIA S SCHERNDAL IN THE UK)

ST HILDEGARD HART'S TONGUE FERN ELIXIR

This is one of Hildegard of Bingen's traditional remedies produced by St Hildegard-Posch in Austria. The product is now available in the UK and was recommended by Hildegard for chronic coughs and asthma as well as liver and gall bladder problems.

Dosage: half a wine glass before and after meals, up to three times a day.
ST HILDEGARD-POSCH (VIA S SCHERNDAL IN THE UK)

ST HILDEGARD STINGING NETTLE OIL

A simple infused oil of stinging nettle, often used as a skin remedy for irritant eruptions, but recommneded by Hildegard as a massage remedy for forgetfulness.

ST HILDEGARD-POSCH (VIA S SCHERNDAL IN THE UK)

ST HILDEGARD VIOLET SALVE

An ointment using sweet violet which Hildegard suggested for skin problems and swellings. This herb was once a mainstay of herbal treatments for breast cancer.

Dosage: rub the cream gently into the skin; do not massage.
ST HILDEGARD-POSCH (VIA S SCHERNDAL IN THE UK)

ST HILDEGARD WACHOLDER ELIXIR

A juniper-based liquid which Hildegard recommended as a remedy for bronchial asthma, although we more normally regard this herb as an external treatment for aches and pains or as a diuretioc and urinary antiseptic.

Dosage: half a wine glass before and after meals, up to three times a day.
ST HILDEGARD-POSCH (VIA S SCHERNDAL IN THE UK)

STARFLOWER OIL

An unlicensed supplement containing 250 mg of borage oil which include 23% of *gamma*-linolenic acid. The capsules also contain additional vitamins C and E.

Dosage: 2 or 3 capsules a day for 12 weeks if taking a GLA supplement for the first time; 1 or 2 capsules a day as a maintenance dose.

ROCHE

SUPER GARLIC PERLES FOR MEN

A tonic combination of garlic and pumpkin seed oil with lecithin and vitamin E. Pumpkin seed is rich in zinc which can be helpful for the prostate gland.

Dosage: 1 capsule twice a day before meals.   POWER HEALTH

SUPER GARLIC PERLES FOR WOMEN

A tonic supplement combining garlic with evening primrose oil and cod liver oil.

Dosage: 1 capsule twice a day.   POWER HEALTH

SUPER GRE-CAPS

A supplement sold as a general pick-me-up combining 600 mg of Siberian ginseng root, with royal jelly and 200 IU of vitamin E.

JESSOP MARKETING

SX FORMULA

A tonic combination sold as a liquid extract containing ginseng, celery, damiana, ginger, wheatgerm, oysters, royal jelly and wine. These are generally tonic and stimulating herbs or extracts (oysters were once thought to be aphrodisiac) and the mix is suggested for menopausal problems (which possibly explains the presence of celery as a diuretic) impotence and fatigue.

Dosage: drink 2 × 15 ml phials daily.   ORTIS

THREE G'S

A tonic product combining ginseng, garlic and ginkgo which is suggested to combat fatigue and strengthen the immune system.

Dosage: 2 tablets a day.

HEALTH PERCEPTIONS

THURSDAY PLANTATION ANTISEPTIC CREAM

An unlicensed simple tea tree cream.
• External use only.

HEALTH IMPORTS

THURSDAY PLANTATION THROAT LOZENGES

These lozenges combine tea tree which is antiseptic, wild cherry (a cough suppressant), white horehound – expectorant and soothing for the mucous membranes – and lemon balm, a useful healing herb but one that is generally regarded as a carminative and antidepressant. The lozenges could be suitably for both throat infectious and minor coughs.

HEALTH IMPORTS

THURSDAY PLANTATION WALKABOUT

An insect repellent spray combining tea tree and lemon oils which are both effective at keeping bugs away.
• External use only.

HEALTH IMPORTS

TRIMULINA ISPHAGHULA

Capsules containing isphaghula as a simple which are promoted as a slimming aid. The herb is known to help reduce fat consumption and create a feeling of fullness although it is usually considered a bulking laxative.

Dosage: 5 capsules half an hour before meals with plenty of water.

POWER HEALTH

ULTRA PREMIUM EVENING PRIMROSE

Capsules containing 500 mg of evening primrose oil (10% *gamma*-linolenic acid) with vitamin E added as an anti-oxidant.

Dosage: 2 or 3 capsules daily.

PHOENIX NUTRITION

ULTRA PREMIUM PRIMROSA

Capsules containing either 600 mg or 1200 mg of variety of evening primrose oil which reputedly contains 20% *gamma*-linolenic acid – a considerably higher percentage than normal evening primrose oil plants. The tablets also contain vitamin E and lecithin.

Dosage: 1200 mg daily.

PHOENIX NUTRITION/ENEREX NUTRACEUTICALS

ULTRA PREMIUM STARFLOWER OIL

Unlicensed capsules containing borage oil with 24% *gamma*-linolenic acid.

PHOENIX NUTRITION

*UVACIN

Licensed as a suitable remedy for short term female bladder discomfort (a description which clearly suggests cystitis without actually saying so). These tablets basically combine diuretic dandelion leaf with bearberry – a urinary

antiseptic. The tablets also include peppermint which is not normally regarded as a remedy for the urinary tract but will improve the flavour.
• Not recommended for children; the tablet base contains lactose.

Dosage: 2 tablets three times a day.

MEDIC HERB

*VALERINA – DAY-TIME

Licensed to ease tension, irritability, and stress. this remedy contains valerian and lemon balm – respectively tranquillizing and antidepressant.
• Not recommended for children; the tablet base contains lactose.

Dosage: 2 tablets three times a day.

MEDIC HERB

*VALERINA – NIGHT-TIME

Licensed as a remedy for the symptomatic relief of tension, irritability and insomnia this is similar to the Valerina – Day-Time product, but contains hops – a soporific – as well.
• Not recommended for children; the tablet base contains lactose.

Dosage: 2–4 tablets at night.

MEDIC HERB

WASSEN GARLIC TABLETS

Unlicensed tablets containing the equivalent of 968 mg of garlic, spray dried to give a more odourless product.

Dosage: 1 a day.

WASSEN INTERNATIONAL

WEIGHT LOGIC

Another of the Malabar tamarind extracts sold as a slimming aid. This one contains 500 mg of the herb with 500 mg of chromium and vitamin B_3.

Dosage: 2 capsules one hour before each meal.

HEALTH PERCEPTION

*WELEDA ARNICA 6×

Homoeopathic tablets containing arnica which can be used for accidents, shock, traumatic injuries or to improve recovery after surgery and childbirth.

Dosage: 1 or 2 tablets every two hours in acute cases or else three times a day.

WELEDA

*WELEDA ARNICA OINTMENT

A licensed simple arnica ointment to relieve sprains and bruises. Weleda also produces an arnica ointment which can be diluted in water to bathe injuries.
• Do not use on unbroken skin; external use only.

Dosage: apply as required.

WELEDA

*WELEDA AVENA SATIVA COMP

An anthroposophical combination licensed as of right as an aid to peaceful relaxation. The mixture contains wild oats, hops, passion flower and valerian (all useful sedatives for the nervous systems) along with homoeopathic Coffea 60× which is similarly used as a remedy for restlessness and nervous agitation.

Dosage: adults and children over 12 years – 10–20 drops in water half an hour before retiring; children over two years – half the adult dose.

WELEDA

*WELEDA BALSAMICUM OINTMENT

An anthroposophical ointment, licensed as of right as a healing remedy for abrasions, boils, nappy rash and slow-healing minor wounds. It contains marigold – widely used in such preparations – along with the more unusual dog's mercury (a remedy for toxic inflammations little used these days), Peruvian balsam – useful for itching skin – and antimony.
• External use only.

Dosage: apply to the affected part or on a dry dressing several times a day.

WELEDA

WELEDA BIRCH ELIXIR

An unlicensed anthroposophical preparation, suggested as a spring and autumn tonic and as an aid to the symptomatic relief of muscular rheumatism. As well as birch it contains lemon juice and cane sugar.

Dosage: 2 × 5 ml teaspoon (10 ml) in water, two or three times a day.

WELEDA

WELEDA BLACKTHORN ELIXIR

An unlicensed anthroposophical tonic which is suggested for use in convalescence. It contains blackthorn fruit juice with cane sugar and lemon juice.

Dosage: 2 × 5 ml teaspoon (10 ml) in water, two or three times a day.

*WELEDA CALENDOLON OINTMENT

Given a full product licence as a treatment of cuts, minor wounds and abrasions this ointment is a marigold simple.
• External use only.

Dosage: apply to affected areas two or three times daily or on a dressing.

WELEDA

*WELEDA CALENDULA LOTION

A simple marigold lotion licensed for the treatment of cuts, grazes, minor wounds and abrasions.
• External use only.

Dosage: dilute with cooled boiled water to cleanse wounds.

WELEDA

*WELEDA CARMINATIVE TEA

This tea has a full product licence as a remedy for the relief of flatulence. It combines some traditional carminative herbs – aniseed, fennel, caraway and chamomile – with yarrow which is antispasmodic and helpful for relieving stomach cramps.

Dosage: adults – 1 × 5 ml teaspoon in a cup of boiling water, simmer for one minute and filter. Drink one cup, twice a day; children – half the adult dose.

WELEDA

*WELEDA CATARRH CREAM

An anthroposophical remedy licensed for the relief of catarrhal congestion and inflammation of the nasal mucosa. It contains a combination of herbal and homoeopathic extracts including largely anticatarrhals, antiseptics and astringents as well as echinacea which is anti-bacterial. The mixture also includes barberry, blackthorn, Bryonia 3×, camphor and eucalyptus, peppermint and thyme

oil, as well as aesculin (a saponin found in horse chestnut) and a homoeopathic mineral extract Merc. Sulph. 5×.
• Not for children under the age of three; external use only.

Dosage: insert a small quantity in each nostril as required.

WELEDA

*WELEDA CHAMOMILLA 3× PILLULES AND DROPS

Licensed homoeopathic chamomile extracts which are suitable for the relief of colicky pain and teething troubles in infants.

Dosage: pillules – 1–5 pillules to be dissolved in the mouth every half hour (the pillules can be crushed for children under six months); drops – 5–10 drops in a little water, to be given three times a day, or five drops every half hour until the condition improves for up to four hours.

WELEDA

*WELEDA CLAIRO TEA

This remedy has a full product licence for the symptomatic relief of occasional or non-persistent constipation. It combines senna with the carminatives aniseed and clove and also contains a high proportion of peppermint, which is both carminative for the digestive system and will improve the flavour.

Dosage: adults, half a 5 ml teaspoon in a cup of boiling water, simmer for one minute and filter, then take one cup twice a day; for milder action pour boiling water on half a teaspoon of the mixture in a cup, leave for five minutes and take at night; children over six years, half a cupful in the morning.

WELEDA

*WELEDA COMBURDORON OINTMENT

An anthroposophical remedy with a full product licence for the relief of minor burns and scalds. It combines arnica and annual nettle (a standard homoeopathic remedy for burns) and the same combination is also available in a spray format for use on insect bites.
• External use only.

Dosage: apply to affected part directly or on a dry dressing as directed.

WELEDA

*WELEDA COUGH DROPS

An anthroposophical remedy, licensed as of right, for use in relieving coughs. These drops contain angelica, which is expectorant, with a number of carminative and warming extracts – cinnamon, climes, coriander, lemon and nutmeg. The mixture also contains lemon balm which is normally used for nervous upsets but is also helpful in feverish conditions.

Dosage: 10–12 drops in a little water every four hours.

WELEDA

*WELEDA COUGH ELIXIR

An anthroposophical remedy licensed as of right for the symptomatic relief of coughs. It combines several expectorants and respiratory antiseptics either as herbal extracts or in homoeopathic doses. The mixture includes thyme, anise, white horehound, marshmallow, Drosera 2× (homoeopathic sundew); Ipecac. Rad. 1× (homoeopathic ipecacuanha) and Pulsatilla 3× (homoeopathic pasque flower).

Dosage: adults and children of 12 and over – 2 × 5 ml teaspoon every three or four hours undiluted or in a little water, up to four doses daily; children six to 12 years – half the adult dose.

WELEDA

*WELEDA DERMATODENDRON OINTMENT

An anthroposophical remedy licensed as of right for the relief of eczema which contains bittersweet flowers and creeping Jenny.
• External use only.

Dosage: apply to affected areas three or four times a day.

WELEDA

*WELEDA DIGESTODORAN TABLETS

An anthroposophical remedy licensed as of right for the symptomatic relief of indigestion, heartburn, flatulence and non-persistent constipation. As well as white willow (anti-inflammatory and sometimes used for gastric upsets) it contains an unusual mixture of little-used ferns – male fern, polypody and hart's tongue – which have some tradition as digestive remedies, especially in mainland Europe.

Dosage: 2–4 tablets to be taken with water three times a day, 15 minutes before meals.

WELEDA

*WELEDA FRAGADOR TABLETS

Licensed as a remedy for the relief of occasional edginess brought about by every-day stress and strains this is an original anthroposophical combination of both herbs and homoeopathic extracts. It includes wild strawberry, horseradish, aniseed, lovage, sage, stinging nettle, honey, wheatgerm and homoeopathic minerals Conchae 10×, Nat. Carb. 1× and Ferr. Phos. 4×.

Dosage: 2 tablets to be taken with water three times a day.

WELEDA

*WELEDA FROST CREAM

An anthroposophical remedy licensed as of right for the symptomatic relief of chilblains. It includes southernwood, arnica (a widely used herb for unbroken chilblains), Peruvian balsam and rosemary – both used to relive skin itching – and antimony.
• External use only.

Dosage: apply several times a day or on a dry dressing.

WELEDA

*WELEDA GENCYDO OINTMENT

An anthroposophical remedy licensed as of right for the symptomatic relief of hay fever symptoms. The mixture includes cydonia seeds which are produced from the Japanese quince and are not generally regarded as a medicinal herb, along with lemon juice.
• External use only.

Dosage: insert a small quantity into each nostril twice a day and before retiring, treatment can be repeated every four hours if required.

WELEDA

*WELEDA HERB AND HONEY COUGH ELIXIR

A fully licensed remedy for the symptomatic relief of dry and irritating coughs it combines glycerol and honey (favourite for soothing coughs) with herbal demul-cents, expectorants anticatarrhals and antiseptics. The list includes marshmallow, elder flowers, white horehound, Iceland moss, thyme and anise.
• Not to be taken by diabetics because of the sugar content and probably best avoided in pregnancy.

Dosage: adults – 2 × 5 ml teaspoons in a little water every three or four hours; children over six years – half the adult dose.

WELEDA

*WELEDA HYPERICUM/CALENDULA OINTMENT

A licensed remedy for treating painful cuts and minor wounds, this is a popular combination of pain-killing St John's wort and antiseptic marigold.
• External use only.

Dosage: apply as required.

WELEDA

*WELEDA LARCH RESIN LOTION

An anthroposophical remedy licensed as of right for the relief of tired or strained eyes and suggested as refreshing to use while driving or studying. The mixture includes extracts of pineapple, larch and lavender oil.
• Do not use to treat inflamed conditions of the eye; external use only.

Dosage: apply sparingly to a piece of cotton wool around the eye and temple area but not in the eye.

WELEDA

*WELEDA LAXADORON TABLETS

An anthroposophical mixture of herbal and homoeopathic extracts licensed as of right as a mild laxative for occasional non-persistent constipation. The mixture includes the laxative senna, with centaury (a bitter digestive stimulant) and some carminative and antispasmodic herbs to ease griping and flatulence: caraway, cloves, peppermint, aniseed and yarrow.

Dosage: 2–4 tablets before retiring.

WELEDA

*WELEDA MASSAGE BALM WITH ARNICA

A gentle massage oil licensed for the relief of sprains, bruises, muscular aches and rheumatic pain which contains arnica.
• External use only.

WELEDA

*WELEDA MASSAGE BALM WITH CALENDULA

A gentle massage oil for muscular tension, stiffness, cramp and aches and pains of physical pursuits and containing marigold.
• External use only.

WELEDA

*WELEDA MEDICINAL GARGLE

An anthroposophical remedy licensed as of right as a gargle and mouthwash for the symptomatic relief of sore throats, mouth ulcers and tender gums. It contains largely antiseptic and astringent oils and herbal extracts – myrrh plus sage, clove, lavender, rose geranium, eucalyptus and peppermint oils – plus the little used herb rhatany, which is an astringent, helpful for piles, sore throats and gum disease, and a homoeopathic extract of horse chestnut (Aesculus 19×) which is also astringent. The product includes a number of other homoeopathic mineral extract: Argent Nit. 14×; Calc. Fluor. 10×, and Mag. Sulph. 10×.
• Not to be swallowed in large quantities.

Dosage: as a gargle for sore throats – 20 drops in warm water; as a mouthwash for daily freshness and oral hygiene, 10 drops in warm water; apply undiluted to soothe sore gums and mouth ulcers.

WELEDA

*WELEDA MELISSA COMP

A fully licensed herbal remedy for the symptomatic relief of nausea, stomach ache, stomach upsets and occasional diarrhoea this product combines herbal carminative and antispasmodic in a pleasantly tasting mixture. The combination includes: lemon balm, nutmeg, cinnamon, angelica, lemon oil, coriander and cloves.
• Not for children below eight because of the alcohol content.

Dosage: adults – 10–20 drops in a little water, every hour as required, up to eight times a day or as directed; children over eight years – half the adult dose.

WELEDA

*WELEDA OLEUM RHINALE

An anthroposophical remedy licensed as of right for the relief of catarrh, sinus congestion and dry rhinitis. It combines peppermint and eucalyptus oil (a combination once much favoured by traditional herbalists as an inhalant for catarrh) with marigold which is antiseptic and astringent.
• Not for infants because of the peppermint content; external use only.

Dosage: 2–4 drops in or around the opening of each nostril, twice a day.

WELEDA

*WELEDA RHUS TOX OINTMENT

Poison ivy is a standard external homoeopathic remedy for rheumatic pains and sprains. This licensed product also contains rosemary oil which can also help to

ease rheumatism and arthritis.
• External use only.

Dosage: massage into the affected area morning and evening.

WELEDA

*WELEDA RUTA OINTMENT

In homoeopathy, rue is a specific for injuries to the shinbone and also for strains
and bruising – which covers the licence of this remedy which is a rue simple.
• External use only.

Dosage: massage into the affected area morning and evening.

WELEDA

*WELEDA WCS DUSTING POWDER

An anthroposophical remedy licensed as of right for the treatment of minor
burns, soreness and slow-healing wounds which need to be kept dry. The product combines arnica, marigold and echinacea. Arnica is useful as a tissue healer in
trauma while both marigold and echinacea are antiseptic and anti-bacterial. The
product also include antimony and silica.

Dosage: dust the affected part liberally and cover with a dry dressing; change the
dressing twice a day or as directed.

WELEDA

*WOODWARD'S GRIPE WATER

A combination of dill seed oil and sodium bicarbonate for the symptomatic relief
of the distress associated with wind in infants up to one year.
• Not suitable for babies under one month.

Dosage: children one to six months – 1 × 5 ml teaspoon; aged six to 12 months
– 2 × 5 ml teaspoon; all to be given during or after feeds or up to six times in any
24 hour period.

LRC PRODUCTS

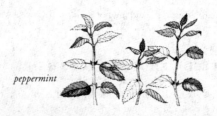

peppermint

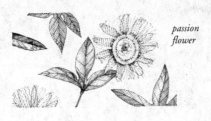

passion flower

Glossaries

BOTANICAL NAMES AND SYNONYMS

Herbs in the A–Z section are listed by common name and referred to by such throughout the text. The following list provides an alphabetical cross reference of botanical names and other common synonyms of those plant names used in the book and listed in the index.

Aaron's rod	Mullein
Abele	Poplar
Acacia catechu	Black catechu
Achillea millefolium	Yarrow
Aesculus hippocastanum	Horse chestnut
Agathosma betulina	Buchu
Agnus castus	Chastetree
Agrimonia eupatoria	Agrimony
Agropyron repens	Couchgrass
Alchemilla arvensis	Parsley piert
Alchemilla vulgaris	Lady's mantle
Alchemilla xanthoclora	Lady's mantle
Alehoof	Ground ivy
Alexandrian senna	Senna
Allium cepa	Onion
Allium sativa	Garlic
Allium ursinum	Ramsons
Aloe barbadiensis	Aloe vera
Aloe ferox	Aloes
Aloe perryi	Aloes
Aloe vera	Aloe vera

Alpinia galanga	Galangal
Althaea officinalis	Marshmallow
Alum root	American cranesbill
Ananas comosus	Pineapple
Ananas sativa	Pineapple
Anemopaegma arvense	Catuaba
Anethum graveolens	Dill
Angelica archangelica	Angelica
Angelica polymorpha var. *sinensis*	*Dang Gui*
Angelica sinensis	*Dang Gui*
Aniba parviflora	Rosewood
Aniseed	Anise
Aphanes arvensis	Parsley piert
Apium graveolens	Celery
Arctium lappa	Burdock
Arctostaphylos uva-ursi	Bearberry
Arisaema consanguineum	Arisaema
Armoracia rusticana	Horseradish
Arnica montana	Arnica
Artemisia abrotanum	Southernwood
Artemisia absinthum	Wormwood
Artemisia annua	Sweet Annie
Asclepias tuberosa	Pleurisy root
Ascophyllum nodosum	Kelp
Asparagus officinalis	Asparagus
Aspidium filix-mas	Male fern
Asthma weed	Indian tobacco
Asthma weed	Pill-bearing spurge
Astragalus membranaceus	Astragalus
Atractylodes lancea	Grey atractylodes
Atropa belladonna	Deadly nightshade
Avena sativa	Wild oats
Bai Mu Er	Snow fungus
Bai Mo Gu	Maitake
Bai Shao Yao	Paeony
Balm	Lemon balm
Balsam of Peru	Peruvian balsam
Balsam poplar	Balm of gilead
Bambusa arundinacea	Bamboo
Barbados aloe	Aloe vera
Barbados cherry	Acerola
Barosma betulina	Buchu
Bayberry tree	West Indian bay
Bay laurel	Bay
Bear's garlic	Ramsons

Bee's nest plant	Wild carrot
Beggar's buttons	Burdock
Benne	Sesame
Berberis vulgaris	Barberry
Bergamot	Bitter orange
Beta conditiva alef	Red beet
Betula alba	Silver birch
Betula pendula	Silver birch
Betula verrucosa	Silver birch
Bissy nuts	Cola
Bitter aloes	Aloes
Black bryony	Bryony
Black cherry	Wild cherry
Black mint	Peppermint
Black pepper	Pepper
Black poplar	Poplar
Black snakeroot	Black cohosh
Black tang	Bladderwrack
Blazing star	Helonias
Blessed thistle	Holy thistle
Blood root	Tormentil
Blueberry	Bilberry
Blue gum	Eucalyptus
Blue mallow	Mallow
Bola	Myrrh
Borago officinalis	Borage
Boswellia sacra	Frankincense
Bottlebrush	Horsetail
Box holly	Butcher's broom
Bramble	Blackberry
Brassica nigra	Mustard
Brassica oleracea	Cabbage
Brazilian cocoa	Guarana
Brazilian ginseng	Paratudo
Breakstone parsley	Parsley piert
Bryonia dioica	Bryony
Buckbean	Bogbean
Burnet saxifrage	Burnet
Bugbane	Black cohosh
Burning bush	Wahoo
Butterfly weed	Pleurisy root
Calendula	Marigold
Calendula officinalis	Marigold
Calluna vulgaris	Heather
Camellia sinensis	Tea
Cammock	Restharrow

Cananga odorata	Ylang ylang
Candleberry	Bayberry
Cang Zhu	Grey atractylodes
Cape aloes	Aloes
Capparis spinosa	Capers
Capsella bursa-pastoris	Shepherd's purse
Capsicum spp.	Cayenne
Caragheen	Irish moss
Carbenia benedictus	Holy thistle
Cardamine pratensis	Bitter cress
Carduus marianus	Milk thistle
Carica papaya	Papaya
Carthamus tinctorius	Safflower
Carum carvi	Caraway
Cassia angustifolia	Senna
Cedrus atlantica	Cedar
Centaurium erythraea	Centaury
Centella asiatica	Gotu kola
Cephaelis ipecacuanha	Ipecacuanha
Cereus	Night-blooming cactus
Cetraria islandica	Iceland moss
Chamaelirium luteum	Helonias
Chamaemelum nobile	Chamomile
Chamomilla recutita	Chamomile
Checkerberry	Wintergreen
Chelidonium majus	Greater celandine
Chen Pi	Tangerine
Chicorium intybus	Chicory
Chili	Cayenne
Chinese angelica	*Dang Gui*
Chinese caterpillar fungus	Cordyceps
Chinese rhubarb	Rhubarb
Chionanthus virginianum	Fringe Tree
Chi Shao Yao	Paeony
Chondrus crispus	Irish moss
Church steeple	Agrimony
Cimicifuga racemosa	Black cohosh
Cinnamonum camphora	Camphor
Cinnamomum cassia	Cassia
Cinnamomum zeylanicum	Cinnamon
Citrus aurantium	Bitter orange
Citrus limon	Lemon
Citrus medica	Citron
Citrus reticulata	Tangerine
Citrus × paradisis	Grapefruit
Cleavers	Clivers

Cnicus benedictus	Holy thistle
Cochlearia armoracia	Horseradish
Cocklebur	Agrimony
Coffea arabica	Coffee
Cola vera	Cola
Colchicum autumnale	Autumn crocus
Colic root	Wild Yam
Collinsonia canadensis	Stone root
Colombo	Calumba
Colorado cough root	Osha
Commiphora molmol	Myrrh
Commiphora mukul	Gugulon
Commiphora myrrha	Myrrh
Common mallow	Mallow
Coptis chinensis	Chinese gold thread
Cordyceps sinensis	Cordyceps
Coriandrum sativum	Coriander
Cramp weed	Silverweed
Crataegus laevigata	Hawthorn
Crataegus monogyna	Hawthorn
Crataegus oxycantha	Hawthorn
Creosote bush	Chaparral
Cuckoo flower	Bitter cress
Cucurbita maxima	Pumpkin
Culver's root	Black root
Cupressus sempervirens	Cypress
Curaçao aloe	Aloes
Curaçao aloe	Aloe vera
Curled dock	Yellow dock
Curcuma longa	Turmeric
Cydonia japonica	Japanese quince
Cymbopogon citratus	Lemongrass
Cynara scolymus	Globe artichoke
Cyprepedium parviflorum var. *pubescens*	American valerian
Daemonorops draco	Dragon's blood
Da Huang	Rhubarb
Daucus carota	Wild carrot
Dalmatian pellitory	Pyrethrum
Deer fungus	Cordyceps
Dendranthema × grandiflorum	Chrysanthemum
Dendrobium nobile	Suk gok
Devil's bit	Helonias
Devil's dung	Asafoetida
Dewberry	Blackberry
Dew plant	Sundew

Dioscorea villosa	Wild yam
Dong Chong Xia Cao	Cordyceps
Drimia maritima	Squill
Drosera rotundifolia	Sundew
Dryopteris filix-mas	Male fern
Dulacia inopiflora	Muira-puama
Dwale	Deadly nightshade
Dyer's saffron	Safflower
Echinacea angustifolia	Echinacea
Echinacea pallida	Echinacea
Echinacea purpurea	Echinacea
Elettaria cardamomum	Cardamom
Eleutherococcus senticosus	Siberian ginseng
Elymus repens	Couchgrass
English lavender	Lavender
English mandrake	Bryony
Equisetum arvense	Horsetail
Erythraea centaurium	Centaury
Eschscholzia californica	Californian poppy
Eucalyptus globulus	Eucalyptus
Euonymous atropurpureus	Wahoo
Eupatorium perfoliatum	Boneset
Eupatorium purpureum	Gravel root
Euphorbia hirta	Pill-bearing spurge
Euphorbia pilulifera	Pill-bearing spurge
Euphrasia officinalis	Eyebright
Fagopyrum esculentum	Buckwheat
False saffron	Safflower
False unicorn root	Helonias
Featherfew	Feverfew
Ferula assa-foetida	Asafoetida
Feverwort	Boneset
Feverwort	Centaury
Ficus carica	Fig
Filipendula ulmaria	Meadowsweet
Fish poison tree	Jamaica dogwood
Flax seed	Linseed
Flea seed	Isphaghula
Fleawort	Isphaghula
Fluellen	Speedwell
Foeniculum vulgare	Fennel
Fo ti	Gotu kola
Fragaria vesca	Wild strawberry
Fragrant sumach	Sweet sumach
Frangula bark	Alder buckthorn
French jujube	Chinese date

Fucus vesiculosis	Bladderwrack
Fu Ling	Tuckahoe
Fu Shen	Tuckahoe
Galeopsis segetum	Hemp nettle
Galium aparine	Clivers
Ganoderma lucidem	Reishi
Gao Liang Jiang	Galangal
Garcinia	Malabar Tamarind
Garcinia cambogia	Malabar Tamarind
Garden mint	Spearmint
Gaultheria procumbens	Wintergreen
Ge Gen	Kudzu
Ge Hua	Kudzu
Gentiana lutea	Yellow gentian
Geranium maculatum	American cranesbill
Geranium Bourbon	Rose geranium
German chamomile	Chamomile
Gingili	Sesame
Ginkgo biloba	Ginkgo
Glechoma hederacea	Ground ivy
Glycyrrhiza glabra	Liquorice
Goora nut	Cola
Goosegrass	Clivers
Goraka	Malabar Tamarind
Gospel herb	Amachazuru
Greater plantain	Common plantain
Grifola frondosa	Maitake
Grindelia camporum	Gumplant
Groats	Wild oats
Guaiacum officinale	Guaiacum
Guaiac	Guaiacum
Guelder rose	Cramp bark
Guggulu	Gugulon
Gumweed	Gumplant
Gynostemma pentaphyllum	Amachazuru
Hamamelis virginiana	Witch Hazel
Harpagophytum procumbens	Devil's claw
Heath speedwell	Speedwell
Hedera helix	Ivy
Helianthus tuberosus	Jerusalem artichoke
Hen of the woods	Maitake
Herb of grace	Rue
Hilba	Fenugreek
Hoarhound	White horehound
Horehound	White horehound
Horse balm	Stone root

Horsehoof	Coltsfoot
Hot pepper	Cayenne
Huang Bai	Phellodendron
Huang Lian	Chinese gold thread
Huang Qi	Astragalus
Huckleberry	Bilberry
Humulus lupulus	Hops
Hydrangea arborescens	Hydrangea
Hydrastis canadensis	Golden seal
Hydrocotyle asiatica	Gotu kola
Hypericum perforatum	St John's wort
Hyssopus officinalis	Hyssop
Ilex paraguariensis	Maté
Indian bread	Tuckahoe
Indian date	Tamarind
Indian pennywort	Gotu kola
Indian plum	Chinese date
Indian rhubarb	Rhubarb
Indian squill	Squill
Inula helenium	Elecampane
Ipecac	Ipecacuanha
Ipê-roxa	Pau d'arco
Iris versicolor	Blue flag
Jack-in-the-pulpit	Arisaema
Jasminum officinale	Jasmine
Jateorhiza palmata	Calumba
Jerusalem cowslip	Lungwort
Jew's myrtle	Butcher's broom
Joe Pye Weed	Gravel root
Juglans cinerea	Butternut
Juglans regia	Walnut
Ju Hua	Chrysanthemum
Juniperis communis	Juniper
Kava	Kava kava
Kelpware	Bladderwrack
Kidney bean	Beans
Knitbone	Comfrey
Knotgrass	Knotweed
Kola	Cola
Krameria triandra	Rhatany
Lactuca virosa	Wild lettuce
Lad's love	Southernwood
Lady's slipper orchid	American valerian
Lady's smock	Bitter cress
Laminaria spp	Kelp
Lapacho	Pau d'arco

Laquered bracket fungus	Reishi
Larix decidua	Larch
Larrea tridentata	Chaparral
Laurus nobilis	Bay
Lavandula angustifolia	Lavender
Lavandula officinalis	Lavender
Ledum palustre	Wild rosemary
Lemon walnut	Butternut
Lentinus edodes	Shiitake
Leonurus cardiaca	Motherwort
Leopard's bane	Arnica
Leptandra virginica	Black root
Lesser celandine	Pilewort
Lettuce opium	Wild lettuce
Lignum vitae	Guaiacum
Ligusticum porteri	Osha
Linden	Lime
Ling	Heather
Ling Zhi	Reishi
Linum usitatissimum	Linseed
Lion's foot	Lady's mantle
Lion's tail	Motherwort
Lithospermum erythrorhizon	Lithospermum
Lobaria pulmonaria	Lungmoss
Lobelia	Indian tobacco
Lobelia inflata	Indian tobacco
Lomatium dissectum	Cough root
Lucerne	Alfalfa
Lungwort lichen	Lungmoss
Lysimachia nummularia	Creeping Jenny
Lythrum salicaria	Purple loosestrife
Macrocysris pyrfera	Kelp
Mad dog herb	Skullcap
Mahonia aquifolia	Oregon grape
Maidenhair tree	Ginkgo
Malpighia punicifolia	Acerola
Malva sylvestris	Mallow
Marian thistle	Milk thistle
Marrubium vulgare	White horehound
Marsh cistus	Wild rosemary
Marsh tea	Wild rosemary
Marybud	Marigold
Matricaria recutita	Chamomile
Matto grosso	Ipecacuanha
May	Hawthorn
Maypops	Passion flower

Mayweed	Chamomile
Marsh trefoil	Bogbean
Meadow anemone	Pasque flower
Meadow cress	Bitter cress
Meadow saffron	Autumn crocus
Medicago sativa	Alfalfa
Melaleuca alternifolia	Tea tree
Melaleuca leucadendron	Cajuput
Melaleuca viridiflora	Niaouli
Melissa officinalis	Lemon balm
Mentha arvensis	Field mint
Mentha spicata	Spearmint
Mentha × piperita	Peppermint
Menyanthes trifoliata	Bogbean
Mercurialis perennis	Dog's mercury
Mexican sarsparilla	Sarsparilla
Mexican wild yam	Wild yam
Midsummer daisy	Feverfew
Milfoil	Yarrow
Milk vetch	Astragalus
Moneywort	Creeping Jenny
Monk's pepper	Chastetree
Mother's hearts	Shepherd's purse
Mountain box	Bearberry
Mountain grape	Oregon grape
Mountain tobacco	Arnica
Myrica cerifera	Bayberry
Myristica fragrans	Nutmeg
Myroxylon balsamum	Tolu
Myroxylon pereirae	Peruvian balsam
Myrtus communis	Myrtle
Naked ladies	Autumn crocus
Nasturtium officinale	Watercress
Neroli	Bitter orange
Night blooming cereus	Night blooming cactus
Nightcap	Californian poppy
Nosebleed	Yarrow
Oaklungs	Lungmoss
Ocimum basilicum	Basil
Oenothera biennis	Evening primrose
Oilnut	Butternut
Old man	Southernwood
Oleo europaea	Olive
Ononis spinosa	Restharrow
Ontario poplar	Balm of gilead
Orange root	Golden seal

Oregano	Marjoram
Origanum spp	Marjoram
Paeonia officinalis	Paeony
Panax ginseng	Ginseng
Panax quinquefolius	American ginseng
Paraguay tea	Maté
Parietaria judaica	Pellitory of the wall
Passiflora incarnata	Passion flower
Paullinia cupana	Guarana
Pawpaw	Papaya
Pelargonium graveolens	Rose geranium
Peruvian cat's claw	Cat's claw
Petasites hybridus	Butterbur
Petasites officinalis	Butterbur
Petroselinum crispum	Parsley
Peumus boldo	Boldo
Pfaffia paniculata	Paratudo
Phaseolus vulgaris	Beans
Phellodendron chinense	Phellodendron
Phytolacca americana	Poke root
Phytolacca decandra	Poke root
Picea abies	Norway spruce
Picrasma excelsa	Quassia
Pimenta racemosa	West Indian bay
Pimpinella anisum	Anise
Pimpinella saxifraga	Burnet
Pinus bark	Hemlock spruce
Pinus canadensis	Hemlock spruce
Pinus sylvestris	Pine
Piper methysticum	Kava kava
Piper nigrum	Pepper
Pipperidge bush	Barberry
Piscidia erythrina	Jamaica dogwood
Plantago lanceolata	Ribwort plantain
Plantago major	Common plantain
Plantago ovata	Isphaghula
Plantago psyllium	Isphaghula
Pogostemon patchouli	Patchouli
Polecat weed	Skunk cabbage
Poison oak	Poison ivy
Poke weed	Pokeroot
Polygala senega	Senega
Polygonum aviculare	Knotweed
Polypodium vulgare	Polypody
Populus alba	Poplar
Populus candicans	Balm of gilead

Populus tremula	Aspen
Poria cocos	Tuckahoe
Porter's lovage	Osha
Potentilla anserina	Silverweed
Potentilla erecta	Tormentil
Potentilla tormentilla	Tormentil
Potentwood	Muira-puama
Pot marigold	Marigold
Primula veris	Cowslip
Prunus avium	Cherry stalks
Prunus cerasus	Cherry stalks
Prunus persica	Persica
Prunus serotina	Wild cherry
Prunus spinosa	Blackthorn
Psyllium	Isphaghula
Pueraria lobata	Kudzu
Puerto Rica cherry	Acerola
Pukeweed	Indian tobacco
Pulmonaria officinalis	Lungwort
Pulsatilla vulgaris	Pasque flower
Pumilio pine	Pine
Purple cone flower	Echinacea
Purple medick	Alfalfa
Qing Hao	Sweet Annie
Qing Pi	Tangerine
Queen Anne's lace	Wild carrot
Queen of the meadow	Gravel root
Queen of the meadow	Meadowsweet
Queen of the night	Night blooming cactus
Quercus alba	White oak
Quercus robur	Oak
Quickset	Hawthorn
Quinsy berry	Blackcurrant
Ranunculus ficaria	Pilewort
Rat tail plantain	Common plantain
Rattlesnake root	Senega
Rattlewort	Black cohosh
Rehmannia glutinosa	Chinese foxglove
Red elm	Slippery elm
Red ink plant	Pokeroot
Red puccoon	Bloodroot
Rhamnus frangula	Alder buckthorn
Rhamnus purshianus	Cascara sagrada
Rhaphanus sativus	Black radish
Rheum palmatum	Rhubarb
Rhus aromatica	Sweet sumach

Rhus radicans	Poison ivy
Rhus toxicodendron	Poison ivy
Ribes nigrum	Blackcurrant
Rich weed	Stone root
Rio	Ipecacuanha
Roman chamomile	Chamomile
Rosa spp	Rose
Rosmarinus officinalis	Rosemary
Rubus idaeus	Raspberry
Rubus villosus	Blackberry
Rumex crispus	Yellow dock
Ruscus aculeatus	Butcher's broom
Ruta graveolens	Rue
Sabul serrulata	Saw palmetto
Saffron thistle	Safflower
Salix alba	White willow
Salix nigra	Black willow
Salvia officinalis	Sage
Salvia sclarea	Clary sage
Sambucus nigra	Elder
Sanguinaria canadensis	Bloodroot
Sanicula europaea	Sanicle
Santalum alba	Sandalwood
Sassafras albidum	Sassafras
Scabwort	Elecampane
Schisandra chinensis	Schisandra
Scolopendrium vulgare	Hart's tongue
Scot's pine	Pine
Scutellaria lateriflora	Skullcap
Sea onion	Squill
Seawrack	Bladderwrack
Selenicereus grandiflorus	Night blooming cactus
Senecio aureus	Life root
Senna alexandrina	Senna
Serenoa repens	Saw palmetto
Sesamum indicum	Sesame
Seven barks	Hydrangea
Seville orange	Bitter orange
Shave grass	Horsetail
Sheep's head	Maitake
Sheng Di Huang	Chinese foxglove
Shi Hu	Suk gok
Shu Di Huang	Chinese foxglove
Siamese ginger	Galangal
Silybum marianum	Milk thistle
Skunkweed	Skunk cabbage

Smallage	Celery
Small pimpernel	Burnet
Smilax aristolochiaefolia	Sarsparilla
Snake butter	Shiitake
Snowdrop tree	Fringe tree
Socotrine aloes	Aloes
Solanum dulcamara	Bittersweet
Solanum nigra	Black nightshade
Solanum tuberosum	Potato
Soldier's woundwort	Yarrow
Solidago vigaurea	Golden rod
Spilanthes oleracea	Paracress
Spindle tree	Wahoo
Spiny bamboo	Bamboo
Spiny rest harrow	Restharrow
Spotted cranesbill	American cranesbill
Squawroot	Black cohosh
Squaw weed	Life root
Stagbush	Black haw
Starflower	Borage
Starwort	Helonias
Stellaria media	Chickweed
Sticklewort	Agrimony
Sticky Willie	Clivers
Stillingia sylvatica	Queen's delight
Storkbill	American cranesbill
Styrax benzoin	Benzoin
Succory	Chicory
Suma	Paratudo
Swallow wort	Greater celandine
Sweet balm	Lemon balm
Sweet bay	Bay
Sweet wormwood	Sweet Annie
Symphytum officinalis	Comfrey
Symplocarpus foetidus	Skunk cabbage
Syzygium aromaticum	Cloves
Tabasco pepper	Cayenne
Tabebuia impetiginosa	Pau d'arco
Taheebo	Pau d'arco
Tamarindus indica	Tamarind
Tanacetum cinerariifolium	Pyrethrum
Tanacetum parthenium	Feverfew
Tao Ren	Persica
Taraxacum officinale	Dandelion
Tarweed	Gumplant
Teaberry	Wintergreen

Tetterwort	Greater celandine
Thoroughwort	Boneset
Thymus vulgaris	Thyme
Tian Hua Fen	Snakegourd
Tian Nan Xing	Arisaema
Tinnevally senna	Senna
Tilia cordata	Lime
Ti tree	Tea tree
Tolu balsam	Tolu
Tong kwai	*Dang Gui*
Toothache tree	Prickly ash
Tormentilla	Tormentil
Tremella fuciformis	Snow fungus
Trichosanthes kirilowii	Snakegourd
Trifolium pratense	Red clover
Trigonella foenum-graecum	Fenugreek
Tsuga canadensis	Hemlock spruce
Turkey rhubarb	Rhubarb
Turnera diffusa var. *aphrodisiaca*	Damiana
Tussilago farfara	Coltsfoot
Twitch	Couchgrass
Ulmus fulva	Slippery elm
Ulmus rubra	Slippery elm
Uncaria gambier	Pale catechu
Uncaria tomentosa	Cat's claw
Urtica dioica	Stinging nettles
Urtica urens	Annual nettle
Usnea spp	Usnea
Uva-ursi	Bearberry
Vaccinium myrtillus	Bilberry
Vaccinium oxycoccus	Cranberry
Valeriana officinalis	Valerian
Verbascum thapsus	Mullein
Verbena hastata	Blue vervain
Verbena officinalis	Vervain
Veronica officinalis	Speedwell
Veronicastrum virginicum	Black root
Viburnum opulus	Cramp bark
Viburnum prunifolium	Black haw
Viola tricolor	Heartsease
Viscum album	Mistletoe
Vitex agnus-castus	Chastetree
Vitis vinifera	Vine
Wax myrtle	Bayberry
Weeping tea tree	Cajuput
Weeping paperbark	Cajuput

West Indian cherry	Acerola
White birch	Silver birch
White bryony	Bryony
White man's foot	Common plantain
White pepper	Pepper
White poplar	Poplar
White walnut	Butternut
Whortleberry	Bilberry
Wild clove	West Indian bay
Wild garlic	Ramsons
Wild hydrangea	Hydrangea
Wild iris	Blue flag
Wild pansy	Heartsease
Wild rum cherry	Wild cherry
Winter squash	Pumpkin
Wolfiporia cocos	Tuckahoe
Woody nightshade	Bittersweet
Wu Wei Zi	Schisandra
Xiang Gu	Shiitake
Xi Yang Shen	American ginseng
Xue Jie	Dragon's blood
Yaw root	Queen's delight
Yerba maté	Maté
Yellow root	Golden seal
Yellow starwort	Elecampane
Yellow wood	Prickly ash
Yucca elata	Yucca
Zanthoxylum americanum	Prickly ash
Zanzibar aloes	Aloes
Zea mays	Cornsilk
Zhi Ke	Bitter orange
Zhi Shi	Bitter orange
Zi Cao	Lithospermum
Zingiber officinale	Ginger
Zizyphus jujuba	Chinese date
Zoom	Guarana

MEDICINAL TERMS

Abortifacient – causes abortion.

Adrenal cortex – part of the adrenal gland located above the kidneys, which produces several steroidal hormones.

Alkaloid – active plant constituent containing nitrogen and which usually has a significant effect on bodily function.

Allergen – any substance which triggers an allergic response.

Amino acids – the building blocks of proteins.

Amoebacidal – kills amoeba.

Analgesic – relieves pain.

Anaesthetic – causes local or general loss of sensation.

Anaphrodisiac – reduces sexual desire and excitement.

Anodyne – allays pain.

Anthroposophic – philosophy developed by Rudolf Steiner in the 1930s which teaches that health is related to internal vital force and energy.

Antibiotic – destroys or inhibits the growth of micro-organisms.

Anti-bacterial – destroys or inhibits the growth of bacteria.

Anti-fungal – destroys or inhibits the growth of fungi.

Anti-inflammatory – reduces inflammation.

Anti-microbial – destroys or inhibits the growth of micro-organisms.

Anti-oxidant – prevents or slows the natural deterioration of cells that occurs as they age due to oxidation.

Anti-rheumatic – relieves the symptoms of rheumatism.

Antiseptic – controls or prevents infection.

Antispasmodic – reduces muscle spasm and tension.

Anti-tussive – inhibits the cough reflex, helping to stop coughing.

Aphrodisiac – promotes sexual excitement.

Arteriosclerosis – build-up of fatty deposits in the blood vessels leading to narrowing and hardening of the arteries, and associated with heart disease and strokes.

Astringent – used to describe a herb which will precipitate proteins from the surface of cells or membranes thus producing a protective coating.

Bactericidal – kills bacteria.

Beta-carotene – an orange-yellow plant pigment which is converted in the body into vitamin A.

Bile – thick, bitter fluid secreted by the liver and stored in the gall bladder which aids the digestion of fats.

Bitter – stimulates secretion of digestive juices.

Blood clotting – the process by which the proteins in blood are changed from a liquid to a solid, by an enzyme, in order to check bleeding.

Blood sugar – levels of glucose in the blood.

Bronchial – relating to the air passages of the lungs.

Bulk laxative – increases the volume of faeces producing larger, softer stools.

Capillary permeability – the exchange of carbon dioxide, oxygen, salts and water between the blood in the capillaries and tissues.

Carcinogenic – causes cancer.

Carminative – relieves flatulence, digestive colic and gastric discomfort.

Cerebral circulation – blood supply to the brain.

Cholagogue – stimulates bile flow from the gall bladder and bile ducts into the duodenum.

Cholesterol – fat-like material present in the blood and most tissues which is an important constituent of cell membranes, steroidal hormones and bile salts. Excess cholesterol has been blamed for the build-up of fatty deposits in the blood vessels seen in arteriosclerosis.

Choleretic – increases the secretion of bile by the liver.

Circulatory stimulant – increases blood flow.

Citronellal – a volatile oil with a lemon aroma found in a number of herbs (including lemongrass) and used for flavourings and insect repellents.

Citronellol – a volatile oil with a rose-like aroma found in rose geranium and other species.

Cleansing herb – a herb that improves the excretion of waste products from the body.

Cooling – used to describe herbs that are often bitter or relaxing and will help to reduce internal heat and hyperactivity.

Coumarin – active plant constituent which affects blood clotting.

Decoction – herbal extract made by simmering usually roots, barks or berries in water for 20 minutes and collecting the liquid produced.

Decongestant – relieves congestion, usually nasal.

Demulcent – softens and soothes damaged or inflamed surfaces, such as the gastric mucous membranes.

Depressant – reduces nervous or functional activity.

Diaphoretic – increases sweating.

Diuretic – encourages urine flow.

Emetic – causes vomiting.

Emollient – softens and soothes the skin.

Essential fatty acid – a group of chemicals vital for maintaining health and needed for a number of bodily processes, including the production of prostaglandins.

Essential oil – volatile chemicals extracted from plants by such techniques as steam distillation; highly active and aromatic.

Expectorant – enhances the secretion or sputum from the respiratory tract so that it is easier to cough up.

Febrifuge – reduces fever.

Flavonoids – active plant constituents which improve the circulation and may also have diuretic, anti-inflammatory and antispasmodic effects.

***Gamma*-linolenic acid** – see Vitamins, Minerals and Dietary supplements, p. 434.

Haemostatic – stops bleeding.

Hormone – a chemical substance produced in the body which can effect the way tissues behave. Hormones can control sexual function as well as emotional and physical activity.

Hyperacidity – excessive digestive acid causing a burning sensation.

Hyperglycaemic – increases blood sugar levels.

Hypoglycaemic – reduces blood sugar levels.

Infusion – a herbal extract made by pouring boiling water on to a herb and leaving for 10 minutes before collecting the liquid: generally also called a herbal tea or tisane.

Laxative – encourages bowel motions.

Lipids – fat-like chemicals (such as cholesterol) which are present in most tissues and are important structural materials for the body.

Lubricant – reduces friction.

Menthol – a volatile oil with a peppermint aroma extracted from various mints (including peppermint), which is carminative, locally anaesthetic, decongestant and antiseptic. Used in a number of herbal products for colds and indigestion.

Mucilage – complex sugar molecules found in plants that are soft and slippery and provide protection for the mucous membranes and inflamed surfaces.

Nervine – herb that affects the nervous system and which may be stimulating or sedating.

Peripheral circulation – blood supply to the limbs, skin and muscles (including heart muscles).

Peristalsis – the waves of involuntary contractions in the digestive tract which move food and waste products through the system.

Phlegm – catarrhal-like secretion or sputum. In both Galenical and Oriental medicine phlegm is a more complex entity related to internal balance and sometimes associated with spleen deficiency.

Photosensitivity – sensitive to light.

Physiomedicalism – system of medicine developed in nineteenth century North America which focused on disease as a result of cold conditions.

Prostaglandins – hormone-like substances that have a wide range of functions in the body. They can act as chemical messengers and some also cause uterine contractions. Various series of prostaglandins are known usually designed PGE_1, PGE_2, etc.

Pungent – having an acrid smell and bitter flavour.

Purgative – drastic laxative.

Pyrrolizidine alkaloids – chemicals found in a number of plants (including comfrey, borage and coltsfoot) which, in excess, can be associated with liver damage although many regard the research evidence for this as inconclusive.

Qi (ch'i) – the body's vital energy as defined in Chinese medicine.

Relaxant – relaxes tense and overactive nerves and tissues.

Rubefacient – a substance which stimulates blood flow to the skin causing local reddening.

Saponins – active plant constituents similar to soap and producing a lather with water. They can irritate the mucous membranes of the digestive tract which, by reflex, has an expectorant action. Some saponins are chemically similar to steroidal hormones.

Sedative – reduces anxiety and tension.

Simple – a herb used as a remedy on its own.

Soporific – induces drowsiness and sleep.

Stimulant – increases activity.

Styptic – stops external bleeding.

Systemic – affecting the whole body.

Tannin – active plant constituents which are astringent and combine with proteins. The term is derived from plants used in tanning leather.

Thyroid – gland in the neck which controls metabolism and growth; it requires iodine for normal function.

Tincture – liquid herbal extract made by soaking plant material in a mixture of alcohol and water.

Tisane – see infusion.

Tonic – restoring, nourishing and supporting for the entire body.

Tonify – a tonic action: strengthening and restoring for the system.

Topical – local administration of a herbal remedy.

Venous return – the blood flow back to the lungs and heart from the body's extremities.

Volatile oils – complex, often aromatic, substances with a low boiling point which rapidly evaporate in the air. The smells associated with different herbs and extracts are often due to such oils.

Warming – a remedy which increases body temperature and encourages digestive function and circulation. Warming herbs are often spicy and pungent to taste.

Yang – aspect of being equated with male energy – dry, hot, light, ascending.

Yin – aspect of being equated with female energy – damp, cold, dark, descending.

VITAMINS, MINERALS AND SUPPLEMENTS

Amino acids – these building blocks for the body's various proteins are sometimes added to dietary supplements. The full complement is found in animal
products but plant proteins usually contain only a selection which is why
vegetarians should eat both pulses and grains together in order to balance
amino acid intake. The individual acids have a number of therapeutic uses
(including in rheumatoid arthritis, recurrent infections and fertility treatments). Amino acids which may be encountered in products are: arginine,
cysteine, cystine, histidine, isoleucine, leucine, lysine, methionine, phylalanine, taurine, tryptophan, tyrosine and valine.

Amylase – see Digestive enzymes.

Arginine – see Amino acids.

***Beta*-carotene** – a vitamin-A-type compound that is a very effective receptor of
free radical oxygen.

Biotin – a lesser known B-vitamin; deficiency is believed to contribute to severe
cradle cap in babies and dermatitis.

Calcium – essential to maintain healthy bones and teeth as well as involved in a
number of biochemical processes. Calcium is found in dairy products, leafy
vegetables, pulses, nuts and seeds (especially sesame). Absorption can be
affected by bran and a high-fat diet.

Choline – essential in human nutrition and fat metabolism, choline is related to
other B-vitamins and is a constituent of lecithin. It also forms acetyl-choline
which is important in the transmission of nerve impulses. Supplements have
been given for neurological disease, including Alzheimer's.

Chromium – this is included in a number of supplements aimed at the slimming
market. Deficiency is now believed to be associated with the development of
chronic degenerative diseases and it is also important in the production of
insulin which is needed to control blood sugar levels.

Co-enzyme Q10 – another popular ingredient of supplements, this occurs
naturally in heart, liver and muscles and is associated with the release of
energy. Production can be impaired by diet and ill-health and the co-enzyme
is thus promoted as a suitable energy-giving supplement, helpful for the
elderly, athletes or those in physically and mentally demanding work.

Copper – this is needed for the production of a number of enzymes involved in
brain metabolism and excess is believed to lead to mental disturbances. Taking
the contraceptive pill can raise blood copper levels with a consequent reduction in zinc absorption and post-natal depression has also been linked to high
copper levels in the body.

Cysteine – see Amino acids.

Cystine – see Amino acids.

Digestive enzymes – these are sometimes included in supplements to help with
the breakdown of food, although as a healthy digestive tract produces a well-
balanced cocktail of them it may not always be a good idea to add a few additional ones. The digestive enzymes most commonly encountered in
supplements are protease, which breaks down protein; amylase, which breaks

down starch; and lipase which breaks down fats.

Docosahexaenoic acid – see Essential fatty acids.

Eicosapentaenoic acid – see Essential fatty acids.

Essential fatty acids – these are classified by chemical structure and the two groups most commonly found in supplements are known as omega-six and omega-three acids. The omega-six group includes arachidonic acid and *gamma*-linolenic acid (GLA) while the omega-three category includes linoleic acid, *alpha*-linolenic acid and two commonly found in fish oil – eicosapentaenoic acid (EPA) and docosahexaenoic acid (DHA). In recent years these acids have been found to be of significant nutritional importance and lack of them is believed to contribute to a very wide range of common Western ills – including arthritis, skin diseases, menstrual and menopausal problems and heart disease. A number of acids can be metabolized in the body from linoleic acid but only when in its chemical *cis*-linoleic form. Commercially produced vegetable oils often convert this form into *trans*-linoleic acid in processing and this is less beneficial. *Gamma*-linolenic acid is found in evening primrose oil, borage oil and blackcurrant oil and these oils also contain substantial amounts of *cis*-linoleic acid. *Alpha*-linolenic acid is found in significant amounts in linseed, hemp seed and pumpkin seed oils with less in walnut and soy bean oils. Not all essential fatty acids are beneficial – erucic acid is believed to damage heart tissue, for example, and is found in high proportion in certain varieties of rape seed (and in trace amounts in some borage seed extracts). The essential fatty acids are important in the production of prostaglandins. More than 50 of these have been identified and they have wide-ranging and important functions in the body. The PGE_1 series is particularly beneficial and these are often at low-levels in people who are prone to allergies, depressives, alcoholics and diabetics. In the usual metabolic pathway *cis*-linoleic is converted to *gamma*-linolenic acid which in turn is made into *dihomogamma*-linolenic acid in the body which is then used to make PGE_1.

Folic acid – closely linked with B_{12}, folic acid is important for healthy function of the central nervous system and also in blood formation. Supplements in pregnancy are believed to reduce the risk of spina bifida.

Free radicals – these are combinations of molecules with highly reactive forms of oxygen which can react with other parts of the body to oxidise and destroy cells. They are believed to be responsible for a number of inflammatory conditions, drug-induced damage, degenerative arthritis, immunity changes and contribute towards ageing, cancer and cardiovascular disease. Substances which themselves react with and neutralize these free radicals are thus potentially extremely important. A number of herbs contain anti-oxidant chemicals and *beta*-carotene is one of the most effective freely occurring antidotes.

***Gamma*-linolenic acid** – see Essential fatty acids

Histidine – see Amino acids

Inositol – like choline, this is involved in fat metabolism and levels are often high in diabetics and those with kidney disease. It may be involved in nerve disorders found in diabetics.

Iron – this is essential for producing the haemoglobin of our red blood cells and is thus vital for oxygen transport around the body. Deficiency is common in menstruating women and can lead to iron-deficient anaemia. It is often included in multi-vitamin/multi-mineral supplements but excess can lead to constipation.

Isoleucine – see Amino acids.

Lactobacillus acidophilus – this is one of the beneficial bacteria found in the large bowel which help to process our food and remove toxins. It can become deficient due to dietary imbalance and over use of antibiotics so supplements can often be helpful. The bacteria also converts milk into yoghurt so eating live yoghurt can often be almost as effective. A number of other bacteria are also packaged in supplements notably the *Bifidobacterium* spp.

Lecithin – a dietary fat composed of choline, glycerol and certain fatty acids which is used to treat cholesterol problems and to help dissolve gall stones.

Leucine – see Amino acids.

Lipase – see Digestive enzymes.

Lysine – see Amino acids.

Magnesium – like potassium, magnesium is important in cell mechanism as well as needed for bone and teeth formation. Average daily requirement is around 400–800 mg and deficiency can be common if the diet is high in refined and heavily processed foods. As with calcium, bran can also reduce absorption. Magnesium supplements are often given for premenstrual problems.

Manganese – this element is found in bone, soft tissues, the liver, kidney and pituitary gland and deficiency can lead to birth defects and reduced fertility. It is found in leafy green vegetables, whole grains and tea. Since the body loses 4 mg of manganese a day supplements of this order would seem reasonable.

Methionine – see Amino acids.

Niacin – see Vitamin B$_3$.

Nicotinamide – also known as niacinamide, see Vitamin B$_3$.

Nicotinic acid – see Vitamin B$_3$.

Pantothenic acid – see Vitamin B$_5$.

Phosophorus – like calcium, this is important for bone and teeth formation. It is also needed to activate a number of the B vitamins. Deficiency is rare as it is found in many foods.

Phylalanine – see Amino acids

Potassium – this is present in every cell in our bodies and is important for healthy heart function, the nervous system and for maintaining normal blood glucose levels. Excessive use of diuretics can deplete the body's natural reserves of potassium and supplements are often then needed. Daily intake should be around 2–4 g and it is plentiful in fresh fruits, vegetables and whole grains. Potassium and sodium balance is important and meat eaters tend to have more sodium and could often benefit from additional potassium.

Propolis – a resinous substance collected by bees from buds, leafy stalks and twigs. It is reputedly an anti-infection compound.

Protease – see Digestive enzymes

Pyridoxine – see Vitamin B$_6$.

Riboflavin – see Vitamin B$_2$.

Royal jelly – a bee product used to feed the queen which allows her to become fertile. It is a rich source of vitamins and minerals and is used as a tonic supplement. Views on its efficacy vary and as a supplement it needs to be taken for several months before any real benefit can be seen. It should be avoided by those allergic to bee stings.

Selenium – a highly fashionable supplement in recent years, selenium deficiency has been associated with preventing heart disease and cancer so is frequently added to broad-spectrum supplements. It should be commonly found in vegetables and cereals as it is a naturally occurring trace element, however, over-cropping can deplete the soil so deficiency could be increasing.

Sodium – while potassium is found inside our cells, sodium tends to exist outside and this balance is important in the transmission of nerve impulses. Most dietary sodium comes from table salt as well as from use of monosodium glutamate (the "tasty powder" of Chinese cuisine). Excess can raise blood pressure and the average intake in the Western world is already well above minimum nutritional needs.

Taurine – see Amino acids.

Thiamin – see Vitamin B_1.

Tocopherol – see Vitamin E.

Tryptophan – see Amino acids.

Tyrosine – see Amino acids.

Valine – see Amino acids.

Vitamin A – a number of fat-soluble compounds, including retinol, retinal and retinoic acid only found in animal produce (liver, kidney, whole-fat milk, butter and egg yolk). A number of vitamin-A-type compounds are found in vegetables, generally as orange/yellow pigments – the most important is *beta*-carotene, and these are water soluble. Vitamin A is important for eye-function; it prevents drying of the eye and corneal changes as well as light-sensitive functions. Vitamin A is also important for maintaining the stability of cell membranes and is believed to be helpful in pregnancy to prevent birth defects. Vitamin A can be toxic in excess.

Vitamin B – a complex group of chemicals which are all water soluble and found in such foods as Brewer's yeast, meats, wholegrain cereals and vegetable proteins. They are chemically distinct but interact within the body in a number of metabolic processes. Deficiency of individual B vitamins is rare, but is sometimes found with vitamin B_{12} which is generally only found in animal products so can be missing from strictly vegetarian diets. The B vitamins are referred to both by number and name – which can be confusing.

Vitamin B_1 (thiamin) – important in energy production and carbohydrate mechanism.

Vitamin B_2 (riboflavin) – needed for production of enzymes mainly found in the liver and important in oxidising compounds to produce energy.

Vitamin B_3 (nicotinic acid – also known as niacin – and nicotinamide) – used in hydrogen transport and enzyme production. Nicotinic acid is important in cholesterol metabolism.

Vitamin B_5 (pantothenic acid) – regarded as a lesser B vitamin, B_5 is important in reactions involving carbohydrates, fats and amino acids.

Vitamin B$_6$ (pyridoxine, pyridoxal and *pyridoxamine)* – important in protein metabolism and needed by the body in direct proportion to the amount of protein consumed. B$_6$ is also involved in the metabolism of essential body chemicals including histamine, hydroxytryptamine and serotonin which is important in brain chemistry so deficiency of vitamin B$_6$ is can effect behaviour. Many women find vitamin B$_6$ supplements helpful for premenstrual problems.

Vitamin B$_{12}$ (cyanacobalamin) – important in cell formation and production of red blood corpuscles, a deficiency of B$_{12}$ can lead to pernicious anaemia. See also: Biotin, Choline, Folic acid, Inositol.

Vitamin C – helps to maintain healthy connective tissues and bones and is involved in the normal metabolism of cholesterol. Deficiency leads to scurvy – once common on long sea voyages – with bleeding and poor wound healing. Vitamin C is water soluble and also involved in the protection of cortisol by the adrenal glands. Vitamin C is a very widely used supplement and its supporters credit it with prevention from a range of ills from the common cold to cancer. It is an effective anti-oxidant and is also anti-viral and anti-bacterial. Dosages of up to 5 g a day can be safely taken, although in high doses it can contribute to diarrhoea. Vitamin C is found in fresh fruits and vegetables but is destroyed in cooking and breaks down rapidly after harvesting so is highest in the freshest vegetables.

Vitamin D – this is essential for normal calcium metabolism and deficiency can lead to rickets and other bone disorders. Regular exposure to sunlight has the same effect on calcium metabolism and nutritionists now believe there is little justification for vitamin D supplements since it can be synthesized naturally in the skin. Vitamin D is found in oily fish, dairy fats, egg yolk and liver.

Vitamin E – also known as tocopherol, vitamin E is sometimes called the "anti-old age" vitamin. The vitamin is fat soluble and found in many vegetable oils, nuts, lettuce and eggs. It is an anti-oxidant and is believed to act as nature's preservative, helping prevent fats from going rancid. It can help protect the lungs from pollutants and is often given as a supplement to those with high blood pressure or heart problems. A daily intake of 8–10 mg is believed essential for adults.

Vitamin K – a group of compounds involved in the production of blood clotting factors, especially prothrombin. It is found in many vegetables, liver, green tea and cereals and is routinely given in injection to new born babies who often have naturally low levels of vitamin K as the placenta cannot transmit fat soluble substances and Vitamin K, like a number of other vitamins, comes into this category.

Zinc – has become more important as a dietary supplement in recent years as its role in a number of metabolic processes has been recognized. Zinc is believed to help strengthen the immune system and is often combined with vitamin C as anti-infection supplements for the winter. It also affects prostate function and, again, is often included in products targeted at older men. It is also often recommended in inflammatory diseases (notably rheumatoid arthritis and bowel disorders). Hair loss and skin troubles can suggest zinc deficiency – as can white spots on the nails and an impaired sense of taste or smell.

FURTHER READING

Bartram, T. 1995 *Encyclopaedia of Herbal Medicine*, Grace Publishers, Christchurch

Bown, D. 1995 *Encyclopaedia of Herbs and their Uses*, Dorling Kindersley, London

Brooke, E. 1992 *A Woman's Book of Herbs*, The Women's Press, London

Chancellor, P. M. 1971 *Handbook of the Bach Flower Remedies*, C W Daniels, Saffron Walden

Chevallier, A. 1993 *Herbal First Aid*, Amberwood Publishing, Christchurch

Davis, P. 1995 *Aromatherapy: An A–Z*, 2nd Edition, C W Daniels, Saffron Walden

Erasmus, U. 1986 *Fats and Oils*, Alive Books, Canada

Foster, S., and Yue, C. *Herbal Emissaries*, Healing Arts Press, Rochester, VT

Frawley, D., and Lad, V. 1986 *The Yoga of Herbs*, Lotus Press, Santa Fe

Grieve, M. 1931 *A Modern Herbal*, Jonathan Cape, London

Griggs, B. 1981 *Green Pharmacy*, Jill Norman & Hobhouse, London

Gursche, S. 1993 *Healing with Herbal Juices*, Alive Books, Canada

Hobbs, C. 1995 *Medicinal Mushrooms*, Botanica Press, Santa Cruz

King, F. X. 1986 *Rudolf Steiner and Holistic Medicine*, Rider, London

Leung, A. Y. 1985 *Chinese Herbal Remedies*, Wildwood House, London

McIntyre, A. 1988 *Herbs for Pregnancy and Childbirth*, Sheldon Press, London

Mills, S. Y. 1991 *Out of the Earth*, Viking, London

Newell, C. A., Anderson, L. A., and Phillipson, J. D. 1996 *Herbal Medicines*, The Pharmaceutical Press, London

Ody, P. 1993 *The Herb Society's Complete Medicinal Herbal*, Dorling Kindersley, London

Ody, P. 1995 *The Herb Society's Home Herbal*, Dorling Kindersley, London

Schauenberg, P., and Paris, F. 1977 *Guide to Medicinal Plants*, Lutterworth Press, London

Strehlow, W., and Hertzja, G. 1988 *Hildegard of Bingen's Medicine*, Bear & Co, Santa Fe

Stuart, M. 1979 *The Encyclopaedia of Herbs and Herbalism*, Orbis, London

Tang, S. and Craze, R. 1995 *Chinese Herbal Medicine*, Piatkus, London

Tisserand, R. 1977 *The Art of Aromatherapy*, C W Daniels, Saffron Walden

Vogel, V. J. 1970 *American Indian Medicine*, University of Oklahoma Press

Weiss, R. F. 1988 *Herbal Medicine*, Beaconsfield Publishers, Beaconsfield

Wren, R. C. 1988 *Potter's New Cyclopaedia of Botanical Drugs and Preparations*, C. W. Daniels, Saffron Walden

Index

Herbs and ailments mentioned in the A to Z of Herbal Remedies and Supplements are already cross-referenced to relevant entries in the A to Z of Ailments and A to Z of Herbs so have been omitted from this Index to avoid duplication and unnecessary length. Refer to the main entry for each herb for a list of remedies in which it is contained and to the main ailment entry for a list of relevant remedies.